Psychocutaneous Medicine

BASIC AND CLINICAL DERMATOLOGY

Series Editors

Alan R. Shalita, M.D.

Distinguished Teaching Professor and Chairman
Department of Dermatology
State University of New York
Health Science Center at Brooklyn
Brooklyn, New York

David A. Norris, M.D.

Director of Research
Professor of Dermatology
The University of Colorado
Health Sciences Center
Denver, Colorado

Additional Volumes in Preparation

Psychocutaneous Medicine

edited by

John Y. M. Koo

University of California, San Francisco
San Francisco, California, U.S.A.

Chai Sue Lee

Henry Ford Hospital
Detroit, Michigan, U.S.A.

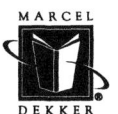

MARCEL DEKKER, INC.   NEW YORK · BASEL

Library of Congress Cataloging-in-Publication Data
A catalog record for this book is available from the Library of Congress.

ISBN: 0-8247-0979-9

This book is printed on acid-free paper.

Headquarters
Marcel Dekker, Inc.
270 Madison Avenue, New York, NY 10016
tel: 212-696-9000; fax: 212-685-4540

Eastern Hemisphere Distribution
Marcel Dekker AG
Hutgasse 4, Postfach 812, CH-4001 Basel, Switzerland
tel: 41-61-260-6300; fax: 41-61-260-6333

World Wide Web
http://www.dekker.com

The publisher offers discounts on this book when ordered in bulk quantities. For more information, write to Special Sales/Professional Marketing at the headquarters address above.

I would like to dedicate this book to Dr. Mark Lebwohl, Dr. Bruce Wintroub, Dr. Alan Menter, Dr. Tim Berger, Dr. Richard Fried, and all others who have supported my career steadily over the past many years and to my wife, Mrs. Nancy Koo, who took care of everything else outside of my career.

—JYMK

I would like to dedicate my efforts in this text to my loving grandmother, who passed away unexpectedly during the preparation of this text, to Dr. John Koo, who is the best mentor and friend in dermatology I can ever ask for, to Dr. Edward Krull, who continues to inspire me with examples to emulate, to Dr. Henry Lim, for supporting my career in dermatology, and, last but not least, to my mom and brother, Alex, for their love and sacrifice.

—CSL

Series Introduction

Over the past decade, there has been a vast explosion in new information relating to the art and science of dermatology as well as fundamental cutaneous biology. Furthermore, this information is no longer of interest only to the small but growing specialty of dermatology. Scientists from a wide variety of disciplines have come to recognize both the importance of skin in fundamental biological processes and the broad implications of understanding the pathogenesis of skin disease. As a result, there is now a multidisciplinary and worldwide interest in the progress of dermatology.

With these factors in mind, we have undertaken to develop this series of books specifically oriented to dermatology. The scope of the series is purposely broad, with books ranging from pure basic science to practical, applied clinical dermatology. Thus, while there is something for everyone, all volumes in the series will ultimately prove to be valuable additions to the dermatologist's library.

The latest addition to the series by Larry E. Millikan is both timely and pertinent. The authors are well known authorities in the fields of cutaneous microbiology and clinical skin infections. We trust that this volume will be of broad interest to scientists and clinicians alike.

Alan R. Shalita
SUNY Health Science Center
Brooklyn, New York

Preface

This publication is the first definitive textbook on psychodermatology and is an international, comprehensive, and practical book aimed at dermatologists, psychiatrists, and any other healthcare professionals with an interest in psychodermatology.

The aim of the book is to summarize the latest international scientific research in psychodermatology as well as the clinical aspects of psychodermatology with a psychopharmacology/theraupeutic direction. The editors are hopeful that the comprehensive yet practical and problem-focused approach to psychodermatology make this a reference that physicians can turn to again and again for guidance in taking care of patients with psychological aspects to their skin disease.

We are grateful to our contributing authors, who have taken time out from their busy schedules to prepare their chapters and share their clinical expertise. Finally, the completion of this project would not have been possible without the expertise and devotion of the editorial staff of Marcel Dekker, Inc.

John Y.M. Koo
Chai Sue Lee

Contents

Contributors

Matthias Augustin   University Clinics of Freiburg, Freiburg, Germany

Hilary Baldwin   State University of New York, Brooklyn, New York, U.S.A.

Burkhard Brosig   Justus-Liebig University, Giessen, Germany

Jane Choi   University of California, San Francisco, San Francisco, California, U.S.A.

J. A. Cotterill   Leeds, England

Raymond G. Dufresne, Jr.   Brown Medical School and Rhode Island Hospital, Providence, Rhode Island, U.S.A.

Richard D. Fried   Yardley, Pennsylvania, U.S.A.

Sylvia Garnis-Jones   McMaster University, Hamilton, Ontario, Canada

Uwe Gieler   Justus-Liebig University, Giessen, Germany

Iona H. Ginsburg   Columbia-Presbyterian Medical Center and New York Presbyterian Hospital, New York, New York, U.S.A.

William Gould Stanford University Palo Alto, California, U.S.A.

Francesc Grimalt University of Barcelona, Barcelona, Spain

Ramon Grimalt University of Barcelona, Barcelona, Spain

Aditya K. Gupta University of Toronto, Toronto, Ontario, Canada

Madhulika A. Gupta University of Western Ontario, London, Ontario, Canada

Brian H. Harvey Potchefstroom University for Christian Higher Education, Potchefstroom, South Africa

Giuseppe Hautmann University of Florence, Florence, Italy

Tom Hogarty Sheridan, Wyoming, U.S.A.

Sandy Duyen Hong UCLA Harbor Medical Center, Los Angeles, California, U.S.A.

Barry Douglas Jones McMaster University, Hamilton, Ontario, Canada

Thelda Kestenbaum University of Kansas Medical Center, Kansas City, Kansas, U.S.A.

Andrew W. Kneier University of California, San Francisco, San Francisco, California, U.S.A.

Caroline Koblenzer Moorestown, New Jersey, U.S.A.

Peter Koblenzer Philadelphia, Pennsylvania, U.S.A.

John Y. M. Koo University of California, San Francisco, San Francisco, California, U.S.A.

Jörg Kupfer Justus-Liebig University, Giessen, Germany

Don Kushon MCP Hahnemann University, Philadelphia, Pennsylvania, U.S.A.

Chai Sue Lee Henry Ford Hospital, Detroit, Michigan, U.S.A.

Ernest Lee University of California, San Francisco, San Francisco, California, U.S.A.

Paula S. Lin University of California, San Francisco, San Francisco, California, U.S.A.

Roger S. Lo* UCLA Medical Center, Los Angeles, California, U.S.A.

M. Musalek University of Vienna, Vienna, Austria

Volker Niemeier Justus-Liebig University, Giessen, Germany

Emiliano Panconesi University of Florence, Florence, Italy

Katharine A. Phillips Brown Medical School and Butler Hospital, Providence, Rhode Island, U.S.A.

Soraya Seedat University of Stellenbosch, Cape Town, South Africa

Mary E. Shepherd Dreyer Medical Clinic Aurora, Illinois, U.S.A.

Dan J. Stein University of Stellenbosch, Cape Town, South Africa and University of Florida, Gainesville, Florida, U.S.A.

Myriam Van Moffaert University Hospital, Ghent, Belgium

Bavanisha Vythilingum University of Stellenbosch, Cape Town, South Africa

Julia K. Warnock University of Oklahoma Health Sciences Center, Tulsa, Oklahoma, U.S.A.

Lee Thomas Zane University of California, San Francisco, San Francisco, California, U.S.A.

---

* Current affiliation: Weill Medical College of Cornell University, New York, New York, U.S.A.

1

General Approach to Evaluating Psychodermatological Disorders

John Y. M. Koo
University of California, San Francisco
San Francisco, California, U.S.A.

Chai Sue Lee
Henry Ford Hospital
Detroit, Michigan, U.S.A.

INTRODUCTION

Psychodermatology involves the many different types of conditions that lie between the fields of psychiatry and dermatology. Sometimes the underlying psychopathology plays an etiological role in the development of skin manifestations in patients who have no real skin disease, such as in delusions of parasitosis or neurotic excoriations. In other patients, psychological factors such as emotional stress can exacerbate bona fide skin disorders such as eczema or psoriasis. Also, many patients develop psychological or psychosocial problems as a result of the disfigurement caused by the skin disease.

It is well known among dermatologists that a significant proportion of patients have psychosocial issues associated with their chief complaint (1). To address the psychological component of the skin disorder, the easiest course of action would be to refer patients to a psychiatrist or some other mental health professional. However, this is not always feasible. Psychodermatological patients frequently refuse a referral to a psychiatrist. Some patients lack the insight to recognize the psychological aspects to their skin disease. Some fear the social stigma associated with coming under the care of a psychiatrist. Others may not be able to afford mental health visits.

Because so many different types of conditions lie between the fields of psychiatry and dermatology, it is helpful to have classification systems that will help the clinician understand what he or she is dealing with. In this chapter, two clinically useful ways to classify psychodermatological cases are discussed in detail: 1) by the category of psychodermatological condition and 2) by the nature of the underlying psychopathological condition. It is important to make a distinction between these categories and the underlying nature of the psychopathological condition because such distinctions help guide physicians to select the optimal approach to patients. In addition, it is helpful to become familiar with the various therapeutic options available, including nonpharmacological options. For patients who refuse to be referred to a psychiatrist, however, a pharmacological approach may be most feasible in a dermatological setting. The selection of appropriate psychotropic agents is generally dictated by the nature of the underlying psychopathologies that need to be treated. The pharmacological treatments for the major types of psychopathological conditions encountered in a dermatology practice are discussed in Chapter 28. Nonpharmacological treatments in psychodermatology are discussed in Chapter 27.

CATEGORIZING PSYCHODERMATOLOGICAL DISORDERS

Most psychodermatological conditions can be classified into five different categories (2): psychophysiological disorders, primary psychiatric disorders, secondary psychiatric disorders, cutaneous sensory disorders, and the use of psychotropic agents for purely dermatological (i.e., nonpsychiatric) indications (Fig. 1).

Psychophysiological Disorders

Psychophysiological disorders is a term used to describe psychodermatological cases with bona fide skin disorders in which the skin disorder is exacerbated by stress. This is the dermatological equivalent of conditions such as peptic ulcer disease or Crohn's disease, in which emotional factors are known to be an important variable that determines the onset and the natural course of the disease. Some examples of psychophysiological

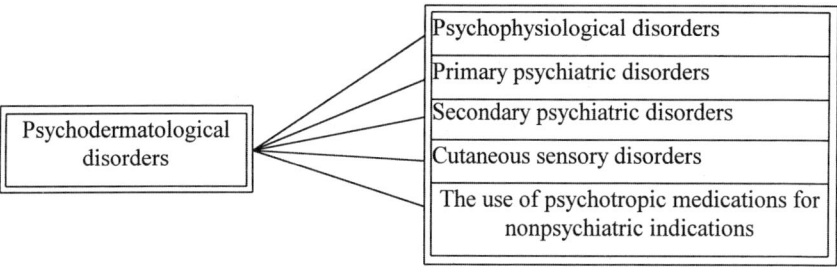

FIGURE 1 Classification of psychodermatological disorders. (Adapted from Ref. 11.)

conditions in dermatology are atopic dermatitis, psoriasis, acne vulgaris, seborrheic dermatitis, and dyshidrosis. For each of these psychophysiological conditions, there are patients who experience a close, chronological association between stress and exacerbation of their skin condition and patients whose emotional state have no effect on the natural course of their disease. In the medical literature, these two groups are often referred to as "stress responders" and "non–stress responders" (3). The relative proportion of stress responders versus non–stress responders appears to vary among different psychophysiological conditions, as determined by research involving 4576 subjects conducted by Griesemer (4) using patients in the Harvard health care system in Boston, Massachusetts (Table 1).

Primary Psychiatric Disorders

The term primary psychiatric disorders refers to cases in which the patient has no real skin disease but presents instead with serious psychopathology; all of the skin manifestations are self-induced. This category includes conditions such as neurotic excoriations, factitial dermatitis, delusions of parasitosis, and trichotillomania. These conditions are often seen as the stereotypes of psychodermatological disorders, even though there are fewer of these patients than psychophysiological cases because they are more blatantly psychogenic.

Secondary Psychiatric Disorders

The term secondary psychiatric disorders describes cases in which the patient develops psychological problems as a result of having skin disease, usually as a consequence of disfigurement. For certain conditions such as

TABLE 1   Incidence of Emotional Triggering of Common Dermatoses

Diagnosis	Proportion with emotional trigger (%)	Biological incubation between stress and clinical change
Hyperhidrosis	100	Seconds
Lichen simplex chronicus	98	Days
Rosacea	94	2 days
Dyshidrosis	76	2 days for vesicles
Atopic dermatitis	70	Seconds for itching
Urticaria	68	Minutes
Psoriasis	62	Days
Papular acne vulgaris	55	2 days
Seborrheic dermatitis	41	Days
Fungus infection	9	Days
Nevi	0	
Basal cell carcinoma	0	
Keratoses	0	

Total $N = 4576$.
Source: Ref. 4.

vitiligo or alopecia areata, the psychosocial impact of the skin disorder is the primary difficulty experienced by the patient because these conditions are generally not life-threatening or symptomatic.

Cutaneous Sensory Disorders

The term cutaneous sensory disorders refers to cases in which the patient has unpleasant sensations on the skin, such as itching, burning, stinging, crawling, or biting, with no apparent organic etiology; a psychiatric diagnosis may or may not be found. These cases are the dermatological equivalents of chronic pain syndrome. In approaching patients with cutaneous sensory disorders, cases can be divided into those with psychiatric findings and those without psychiatric disturbances. Among those with psychiatric findings, depression and anxiety are most frequently noted. In these cases, it is justified to try to treat the psychiatric condition whether or not there is a direct connection between the psychopathology and the abnormal cutaneous sensations, because patients who are depressed or anxious generally perceive discomfort of all types, including itch and pain, in an exaggerated manner. On the other hand, for patients who have no notable psychiatric disturbances, one can still use certain psychotropic medications for their nonspecific antipruritic or analgesic effect. This is very similar to the treatment of chronic pain syndrome in which the antidepressant amitriptyline is one of the treatments of choice, even if the patient is not depressed. If pruritus is the primary problem, doxepin (Sinequan) is the preferred agent. If various manifestations of pain, such as burning, stinging, biting, or chafing, are the primary sensations, amitriptyline is the preferred agent.

Use of Psychopharmacological Agents for the Treatment of Dermatological Conditions

In some clinical situations, psychotropic medications may be more efficacious in treating certain bona fide skin disorders than some of the traditional dermatological therapeutics. For example, the antidepressant doxepin is generally recognized as a more powerful antipruritic agent than most of the traditional antihistamines that dermatologists use for this purpose. Patients with chronic urticaria who do not respond to the usual antihistamines are often successfully treated with doxepin. Similarly, the antidepressant amitriptyline is one of the treatments of choice for postherpetic neuralgia, because its well-known analgesic effect can be helpful even for patients who are not depressed.

It is important to make the distinction between these different categories because it will help guide clinicians to select the optimal approach to patients. For example, patients with psychophysiological disorders or secondary psychiatric disorders usually welcome the opportunity to discuss their psychological status. In fact, sometimes they are frustrated if a dermatologist focuses only on their skin and not on what they perceive as important psychological variables that influence the natural course of their skin disorder. In addition, because in psychophysiological cases one is dealing with the skin and the mind simultaneously, the use of both somatic and psychological therapeutic modalities together may be more effective than either treatment alone. For example, in managing a recalcitrant case of psoriasis in which the patient's emotional stress appears to contribute to the flare of psoriasis, the simultaneous use of a more powerful psoriasis treatment in combination with counseling or an antianxiety agent to diminish stress may be more effective than either the somatic treatment or the psychological treatment alone. For secondary psychiatric cases, the approach may be somatic, such as resorting to a more powerful treatment because of the great emotional distress suffered by the patient, such as the use of oral antibiotics for mild acne. A psychological approach that takes the form of a referral to a support group such as the National Psoriasis

Foundation or the National Alopecia Areata Foundation may also be helpful.

In contrast, patients with primary psychiatric disorders, such as delusions of parasitosis, are usually extremely resistant to discussing their situation in psychological terms. In dealing with primary psychiatric cases, somatic modalities are at best supportive and are frequently no more than a temporizing measure.

For cutaneous sensory disorders in which no dermatological, medical, or psychiatric diagnosis can be made, it is important to be highly empirical in the approach to therapy. As in patients with chronic pain syndrome, successful treatment often involves therapeutic trials with various psychotropic medications with analgesic or antipruritic effect or both. Patients should be prepared for the possibility of long-term therapeutic trials with various psychotropic medications because improvements are generally seen slowly over months or even years.

COMMON PSYCHOPATHOLOGIES UNDERLYING PSYCHODERMATOLOGICAL DISORDERS

The second critical step in psychodermatology is to try to ascertain the nature of the underlying psychopathology, since selection of an appropriate psychotropic agent is generally based on the psychopathology involved. This is usually straightforward because the cases that dermatologists feel compelled to address are generally those that are so blatantly psychiatric that it is difficult to ignore. Among the dermatological cases that are "blatantly psychiatric," most fall into four underlying psychiatric diagnoses: anxiety, depression, delusion, and obsession-compulsion (2) (Fig. 2).

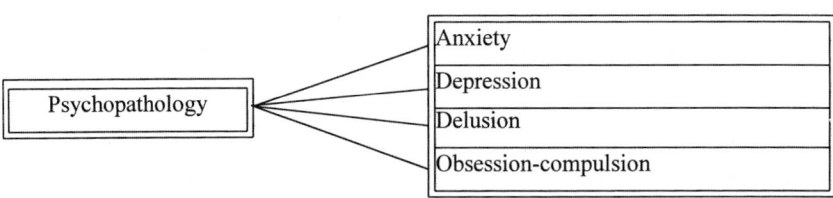

FIGURE 2 Common psychopathologies underlying psychodermatological disorders. (Adapted from Ref. 11.)

Anxiety

Patients with anxiety disorder report excessive anxiety and worry, which may revolve around valid concerns about money, jobs, marriage, health, etc. Patients may also report restlessness or feeling on edge, easy fatiguability, difficulty concentrating, irritability, muscle tension, and sleep disturbance. Other features often include palpations, dizziness, difficulty breathing, trembling, muscle aches and soreness, muscle twitches, clammy hands, dry mouth, urinary frequency, dysphagia, lightheadedness, abdominal pain, and diarrhea. The subjective anxiety or the associated physical symptoms are difficult to control and cause significant distress or impairment in functioning.

To help patients with excessive stress, the most obvious solution would be to find a real-life solution to the difficulties that the patients report. However, there are usually no easy solutions. In those situations, a nonspecific solution to the stress can still be beneficial. Nonspecific solutions to stress include nonpharmacological and pharmacological means. The nonpharmacological approach makes use of various modalities such as exercise, biofeedback, yoga, self-hypnosis, progressive relaxation, and other techniques taught in stress-management courses. For patients who do not have the time to take stress-management courses and relaxation exercises or those who are not psychologically minded, prudent use of antianxiety medications may be helpful to prevent a major flare of their skin condition.

Depression

Depression is frequently encountered in a dermatology practice. Patients report depressed mood or anhedonia. Feelings of worthlessness, hopelessness, and excessive guilt are common. Patients may also report somatic symptoms such as loss of appetite, weight loss, sleep disturbance, decreased energy, and difficulty concentrating. Preoccupation with physical health may occur. The symptoms may cause significant subjective distress and social or occupational dysfunction.

The easiest way to make a diagnosis of depression is to ask the patient questions such as "Are you depressed?" or "Have you been feeling very discouraged?" It is not unusual, however, for many patients to deny the fact that they are experiencing depression because they use denial as the primary method for coping with their depression. Frequently, this denial takes the form of somatization where they consciously or unconsciously focus on a physical complaint to diminish their awareness that they are feeling depressed.

When one encounters patients who deny their depression, it is frequently helpful to change the line of questioning to general medical inquiries. Patients are usually not defensive in responding to such questions. Consequently, one can obtain supporting evidence in making the diagnosis of depression by confirming the presence of physiological manifestations of depression such as insomnia and loss of appetite. Once the clinician is quite certain that the patient is suffering from depression, one should ask the patient open-ended questions regarding his or her personal, occupational, or financial situation in a sympathetic, nonjudgmental way. It is not unusual for depressed patients to come to realize the presence of depression as they talk about the difficulties in their lives. Once such an understanding is reached, it is much easier to obtain the patient's cooperation in treating underlying depression.

There are several nonpharmacological and pharmacological treatment options for depression. Nonpharmacological approaches include individual psychotherapies if there are definable psychological/interpersonal issues to be discussed and group therapies. It should be noted that pharmacological approaches and nonpharmacological approaches are not mutually exclusive.

Delusion

The type of psychotic patients most often seen by a dermatologist are patients with monosymptomatic hypochondriacal psychosis (MHP). Patients with MHP are psychologically "normal" in every way except for the presence of an "encapsulated" delusional ideation that revolves around one particular hypochondriac concern and, possibly, hallucinatory experiences that are compatible with the delusion (5–7). For example, the most common type of MHP seen by dermatologists is delusions of parasitosis. Many patients with delusions of parasitosis also experience formication, which is manifested as cutaneous sensations of crawling, biting, and stinging. MHP is very different from schizophrenia, in which in addition to the delusional ideation, patients have other psychological disturbances. The treatment of choice for delusions of parasitosis is the antipsychotic medication pimozide (Orap) (8–10).

Obsession-Compulsion

An obsession is a repugnant thought that repetitively intrudes into the thought process of the patient, whereas a compulsion refers to repetitious, stereotyped behavior that is very difficult for the patient to suppress. The diagnosis of obsessive-compulsive disorder (OCD) may be justified when either the obsession or the compulsion is of sufficient intensity to interfere with the patient's lifestyle or cause significant subjective distress. It should be emphasized that the diagnosis of OCD can be made without the presence of both obsession and compulsion because some patients present only with obsessions, whereas others present only with compulsive behaviors. For example, one patient may obsess about the "unsightly greasiness" of his or her face without engaging in any special activity to try to correct this "greasy complexion," whereas another patient may present with an irresistible compulsion to excoriate his or her acne without having any special thought process associated with the compulsion.

An obsession can be mistaken for a delusion because in both cases the patient presents with a mental preoccupation involving an overvalued idea. However, the key distinction between obsession and delusion is the presence or absence of insight on the part of the patient. Obsessive patients can usually acknowledge the bizarre, meaningless, or destructive nature of their obsessions and compulsions and yet be unable to stop the obsessive thought or the compulsive behavior. In contrast, delusional patients truly believe in the validity of their delusional thoughts. Frequently, patients with obsessive-compulsive behavior are even apologetic for their obsession or compulsion. For example, a patient with acne excoriée may say "I know I am not supposed to be doing this, and I know that if I keep picking on my acne I might really scar myself, but I can't stop picking on it because when I try to stop, I feel this tremendous urge to pick on my acne." The presence of such a compulsive urge intensifies until the patient finally gives in and engages in the compulsive activity, despite the presence of good insight, which helps differentiate OCD from a delusional disorder. There are many different manifestations of OCD or tendencies in dermatological practice. These include trichotillomania, onychotillomania, onychophagia, acne excoriée, and some cases of factitial dermatitis and neurodermatitis.

Like anxiety and depression, there are nonpharmacological (e.g., behavioral therapy) as well as pharmacological approaches to obsessive-compulsive disorders. Although the anti–obsessive-compulsive medications can be very helpful in overcoming one's obsessive tendencies or compulsive behaviors, it is still critical that patients keep up their own efforts and vigilance in controlling their compulsive behavior. If patients have no motivation to stop the destructive behavior, simply putting them on medications is not likely to be helpful.

The choice of a psychotropic medication is based on the nature of the underlying psychopathology involved. For example, if the underlying psychopathology involves depression, the treatment would be an antidepressant. It does not matter whether the patient presents with a primary psychiatric disorder such as neurotic excoriation resulting from depression, a psychophysiological disorder such as psoriasis exacerbated by depression, or secondary depression resulting from disfigurement. As long as the underlying psychopathology is depression, an antidepressant would be the most appropriate choice. The same holds for anxiety, delusion, and obsession-compulsion, where the use of antianxiety agents, antipsychotic agents, and antiobsessive-compulsive agents, respectively, may be indicated. Simply knowing the category of psychodermatological condition does not help one choose the appropriate psychotropic medication.

The determination of the exact category of psychodermatological condition and the decision about the underlying psychiatric diagnosis are made independently of each other. Any one of the psychopathologies, such as anxiety, depression, delusion, and obsession-compulsion, can be found in any one of the different categories of psychodermatological disorders. Moreover, it is important to recognize that the dermatological labels used to diagnose psychodermatological patients may not give any information as to the true nature of the underlying psychopathology involved. For example, when a patient presents with self-induced skin lesions, the diagnosis of neurotic excoriations may be given. Even though this term contains the word "neurotic," the nature of the underlying psychopathology may not involve neurosis; patients may excoriate their skin in response to a variety of other psychopathologies such as anxiety, depression, or obsession-compulsion. Similarly, the term trichotillomania conveys only that the patient is pulling out his or her own hair. It does not give any clue as to the reason for the behavior. Even though the majority of patients with trichotillomania complain of obsessive-compulsive types of symptoms, some patients will pull out their hair when they are extremely depressed or anxious. Some rare patients suffer from a psychodermatological condition called trichophobia, in which they hold a peculiar delusion that they have to pull out something from their hair root "for the hair to grow normally." If such ideation exists, even though the patient has trichotillomania, the underlying psychiatric diagnosis is that of delusional disorder, and the patient is most appropriately treated with an antipsychotic agent. Therefore, for each individual case, it is important for dermatologists to learn to go beyond the dermatological label and to try to assess the nature of the underlying psychopathology in order to guide the psychopharmacological therapy. In most cases, this can be accomplished simply by asking the patient direct questions, such as "Have you been feeling depressed?" or "Have you been feeling nervous and edgy?" Even though one cannot directly ask patients whether or not they are psychotic, usually truly psychotic patients are so blatantly psychotic that questions are not needed to make the diagnosis.

CONCLUSION

In approaching psychodermatological patients, it is important to have strategies that will help the clinician understand what types of psychodermatological cases one is dealing with. Two strategies that will help guide physicians to select the optimal approach to patients are outlined in this chapter: 1) by the category of psychodermatological condition and 2) by the nature of the underlying psychopathological condition. The idea of diagnosing and treating psychiatric problems may seem intimidating to an average practicing dermatologist. However, the cases that dermatologists feel compelled to address are generally those that are so blatantly psychiatric that it is difficult to ignore, and most of those fall into four underlying psychiatric diagnoses as discussed here. The selection of appropriate psychotropic medications is dictated by the nature of the underlying psychopathologies that need to be treated. Moreover, it is not at all unusual for a nonpsychiatrist to be prescribing psychotropic agents. For the past several decades, a significant proportion of patients with conditions such as anxiety and depression have been treated with psychotropic agents prescribed by primary care physicians. Even though these patients can be very challenging, the dermatologist who has an open mind, a thorough knowledge of the differential diagnosis, and good interpersonal skills can be effective in helping significant proportion of these patients who might otherwise be lost between the two specialties of dermatology and psychiatry.

REFERENCES

1. Klauder JV. Emotions and bodily changes. In: Dunbar HF, ed. Emotions and Bodily Changes: A Survey of Literature on Psychosomatic Interrelationships, 1910–1953. New York: Columbia University Press, 1954:598–648.
2. Koo JYM. Psychotropic agents in dermatology. Dermatol Clin 1993; 11(1):215–224.
3. Gupta MA, Gupta AK, Ellis LN, et al. Some Psychosomatic aspects of Psoriasis. Adv Dermatol 1990; 5:21–30.
4. Griesemer RD. Emotionally triggered disease in a dermatology practice. Psychiatr Ann 1978; 8:49–56.
5. Munro A. Monosymptomatic hypochondriacal psychosis. Br J Psychiatry 1988; 153(suppl):37–40.
6. Munro A, Chmars J. Monosymptomatic hypochondriacal psychosis: a diagnostic checklist based on 50 cases of the disorder. Can J Psychol 1982; 27:374–376.
7. Bishop ER Jr. Monosymptomatic hypochondriacal syndromes in dermatology. J Am Acad Dermatol 1983; 9:152–158.

8. Damiani JT, Flowers FP, Pierce DK. Pimozide in delusions of parasitosis. J Am Acad Dermatol 1990; 22(pt 1):312–313.

9. Hamann K, Avnstorp L. Delusions of infestation treated by pimozide: a double-blind crossover clinical study. Acta Derm Venereol (Stockh) 1982; 62:55–58.

10. Holmes VF. Treatment of monosymptomatic hypochondriacal psychosis with pimozide in an AIDS patient [letter]. Am J Psychiatry 1989; 146(4):554–555.

11. Koo J. Psychodermatology: a practical manual for clinicians. Curr Prob Dermatol 1995; 7:203–225.

2

The "Third Ear" of the Dermatologist
How a Dermatologist Can Improve the Psychological
Quality of Life of Patients Who Consult for a
Dermatosis Not Considered Psychocutaneous

Francesc Grimalt
University of Barcelona
Barcelona, Spain

INTRODUCTION

Dermatological patients whose psychological life would improve with a psychiatric-psychological treatment can be divided into two groups. The more familiar group, with fewer members, is formed by the greater part of psychocutaneous dermatosis, that is: 1) dermatoses that are primarily psychiatric (delusions of parasitosis, dysmorphophobias, glossodynias), 2) dermatoses primarily emotional in origin (dermatitis artefacta, neurotic excoriations, tricho- and onychotillomania, psychogenic purpura, and pathomimicry), and 3) dermatoses due to accentuated psychological responses (hyperhidrosis, flushing). In these dermatoses, the clinical diagnosis already includes the certainty of a psychiatric participation. It is not the patient with all his or her personal characteristics that makes one suspect the existence of psychiatric participation, but the illness itself. If the psychiatric pathology is not taken care of, these patients cannot be helped.

The other, much bigger group includes all the consultations in which the personal characteristics of the patient give rise to the suspicion of an important psychological factor—that is, what determines the psychological participation is not the illness but the patient. In this second group we include a subgroup of variations (e.g., vesicular eczema of the palms and soles, atopic dermatitis in the adult, lichen planus) that, depending on the psychological characteristics of patients who present them, should or should not be considered psychocutaneous disorders. They are to be considered psychocutaneous if emotional precipitating or perpetrating factors of the patient are suspected, diagnosed, and are important. (This consideration is not established by the name of the disorder but for the way in which the patients refer to it.) An excoriated acne could be a psychocutaneous dermatosis, but not all excoriated acnes have a psychiatric alteration. In an intensely excoriated acne the psychiatric participation is evident. On the other hand, in an acne with discrete excoriations, it is not these but the characteristics of the patient that could make one suspect of coexisting psychiatric alterations. Clinical experience makes one accept that if it were possible to produce multiple duplicates of the clinical image of some discrete hyperchromias of the face and compare several patients of the same sex, age, and social condition, these spots would affect each one differently psychologically.

The last group of psychocutaneous illnesses is a subset of the second group, made up of patients capable of consulting dermatologists. The second group is not constituted by illness, but by people looking for help. A frequent characteristic case is the patient referring worriedly to a discrete middle facial seborrhoeic eczema, which makes the dermatologist suspect of psychological alterations. If these were demonstrated and treated, it would improve the patient's quality of life. Many other examples could be added: patients consulting for minimum pruritous, psoriatic scaling of the scalp, itchy nummular-like eczema of the ankles in winter, men with so-called candidal balanitis, patients with plantar corns that provoke excessive pain, psoriatic plaques in a patient at an age when psoriatic patients generally accept their skin problem, older patients who consult for long-lasting seborrhoeic keratosis, photoaging wrinkles in a 60- to 70-year-old woman, "falling hair," cherry angiomas of the trunk, etc.

The psychiatric alterations of these patients may be slight states of anxiety, with or without masked depressive alterations. In some patients obsessive tendencies may be observed and, in a few, slight phobias. Most cases are only a transitory distress (1). None of them has important psychiatric alterations. If they had, they would have previously consulted a psychiatrist.

Masked depression (which is frequently hidden in dermatological consultations) is characterized by the lack of a specific symptom of depression, sadness. Patients with masked depression frequently somatize their problem. Those who do so in the skin consult the dermatologist. During the visit of some of these patients, it is evident that if they had not been anxious or depressed they would not have felt it necessary to consult.

Perceptive dermatologists open to the psychological aspects of their patients have a "third ear," which allows them to "hear" beyond the patient's explanation and makes them automatically suspect an alteration in the psychological state of their daily patients. This suspicion is established by the general attitude of some patients, what they say, but, above all, the way in which they explain. A systematic and specific questionnaire helps to accept or reject a suspected psychological alteration.

Psychiatrists are the only experts in psychiatric diagnostic and treatment. Patients seen in hospitals can easily accept the transferral to a liaison center. On the other hand, the patients we are referring to are visited in private offices and they should receive psychiatrical treatment from the dermatologist as, due to the stigma of mental illness in our society, these patients would be upset to be referred to a psychiatrist, they would not go, and would be lost, without psychiatrist, dermatologist, without being cured of either their dermatosis or improvement of the psychological alteration.

The necessary therapeutic management can be made with or without psychotropic drugs. In some of these patients psychiatric treatment is the only way to cure their dermatosis. In all of them this treatment improves the patient's psychological quality of life. The only person who could give them this improvement is the consulted dermatologist.

SUSPICION OF HIDDEN PSYCHIATRIC ALTERATIONS IN PATIENTS CONSULTING DERMATOLOGISTS FOR A SKIN DISORDER NOT CONSIDERED PSYCHOCUTANEOUS IN ORIGIN

Sensitive dermatologists have acquired enough experience to automatically suspect that a psychological alteration may exist in a patient who does not consult for a psychocutaneous dermatosis. The reasons for suspicion are multiple:

1. General behavior of patient.
2. Content of explanation.
3. Manner of explaining.

A determined patient may present one or several reasons for suspicion.

Patient's General Aspect and Behavior

The following behaviors may give rise to the suspicion that a patient suffers from a psychological disorder:

> Avoidance of the doctor's eyes. Doctor's greeting may hardly be answered.
>
> General attitude producing a rather disagreeable or surprising impression.
>
> Patient with tense aspect and sitting on the edge of the chair.
>
> Patient sitting with dejected aspect, fallen shoulders, tilted head and trunk, or leaning excessively on one or both arms of the chair.
>
> Patients with an aspect of being in a hurry to speak, to free themselves from the burden of the series of prepared explanations and complaints. In this hurry they may avoid replying to our usual, initial greeting.
>
> Mother accompanied by one or two daughters, all in mourning and with afflicted aspect (probably recent loss of a husband-father).
>
> An older woman, alone, with a sad aspect.
>
> Any patient with an aspect or behavior that calls doctor's attention.

Patient's Explanation of Problems

The following behaviors may also indicate psychological disorders:

> When the explanation of the symptoms becomes a series of complaints.
>
> When cutaneous problems are explained as in other patients, but with a sight accent of complaint.
>
> When a patient consults for a variety of unrelated cutaneous disorders (polyconsultation), especially when some extracutaneous troubles are included.
>
> When the explanation is made with a vehemence not usually found in other patients. For example, when referring to a pruritus, expressions like "terrible," or "enormous" are used, increasing the tone of some syllables or letters ("teeerrible!"). The patient may comment with exaggerated facial expressions upon the great pleasure provoked by scratching. Some patients lower their voices and smile slightly, requesting the physician's complicity in what, in a way, is considered as excess.
>
> When the patient describes a pain as the action of "gnawing, dragging, plowing" or refers to sensations of "burning, or hot" or being

"trapped." Patients with real physical pain habitually use terms like "intense," "dull," or "pulsating."

When patients explain slowly and in a low voice, with an aspect of tiredness.

When a patient refers to "strange things," that is to say, concerning real, objective lesions, they explain symptoms not shown by other patients with the same skin condition.

When the dermatologist cannot see a lesion in any area that the patient tries to point out, especially in the mouth or on the face (always when there is a disproportion between what the patient explains and what the doctor may observe).

When the patient explains his or her disorders with a previously noted list.

When consulting for alopecia, the patient shows the well-known plastic bag with the fallen hairs from the last hair wash.

When we are asked to excise, electrofulgurate, or to treat in any way a minimal or banal lesion that other patients with similar lesions do not request treatment for. If the request is exaggerated, suspicion may arise at once. When it is reasonable, later visits with reiterative, strange requests may follow.

Always when a patient referring to a skin condition uses the expression "I am fed up with it."

When a patient answers "Fatal!" to the question "How do you feel?"

A SHORT SYSTEMATIC PSYCHIATRIC QUESTIONNAIRE

We may suspect in any patient consulting us a concomitant psychological psychiatric alteration. To reject or to accept a suspected disorder, a specific questionnaire is needed. In this chapter the author offers the questionnaire he uses to dermatologists uninitiated in this subject.

In the practice of psychiatry and in the aim of investigation, detection questionnaires may be necessary for psychiatrists or any doctor wanting to compare results with those of other colleagues. Questionnaires specific for psychiatrists are too complete for use in daily dermatological consultation.

The questionnaire I use with my patients begins by asking about the quality and duration of sleep. A psychiatrist may ask direct, specific questions about mental welfare, but in our case patients have come to be asked about the skin. A patient who has come to tell us how much hair he is losing or another patient who applies too much emphasis on explaining the sting in her soles where no objective lesions can be seen may be surprised but will accept being asked about his sleep conditions.

In some cases I ask first about the home environment, the relationship among family members, and the patient's job (e.g., if their work allows them to get as much sleep as they need), that is, I try to initiate some kind of empathy. If these questions about domestic and work environment are not asked at the beginning, they will usually come up later because patients tend to explain why they sleep so little and are irritable or tired. Once the questionnaire has been initiated, some patients may show clear reluctance to answer the questions, but most of them seem pleased with the opportunity to talk about aspects not usually addressed in doctors' offices. Even with collaborative patients, the difference between the great narrators and the ones who need to be continuously asked is surprising.

The questionnaire presented here is used routinely in patients in whom some psychological alteration is suspected. It is no better than any other.

Systematic Questionnaire

In the last 3 months:

1. How many hours do you sleep? Do you sleep less on account of not having enough time or not being sleepy?
2. Do you sleep satisfactorily? Of the 30 days in the month, how many do you sleep badly: 2 or 3, 5 or 6, 15, more than 15, most days? Do you take tablets to get to sleep? (In older patients it is necessary to ask the relative about naps. What time do they go to bed; some old people go to bed rather early.)
3. Do you have difficulty in getting to sleep? (Primary insomnia.) How long does it take? Once asleep, do you sleep well for the rest of the night?
4. Do you wake a few hours after getting to sleep? (Secondary insomnia.) Do you wake many times during the night but get back to sleep easily?
5. Do you wake up some hours before the time to get up, and are you unable to get to sleep again for several hours in spite of wanting to? (Tertiary insomnia.)
6. Do you wake well? Do you wake up feeling tired? How long do you need to be properly awake? After drinking a cup of coffee, some tea, after a shower, in the middle of the morning, at noon? Not at all?
7. When do you feel at your best? In the morning, at noon, in the evening, at night?
8. Are there some days that you make a big thing of something? How many days a month?

9. Are there some days that you feel rather tired, regardless of what you have done? How many days a month?
10. Are there some days that this tiredness is accompanied by a sensation of sadness? Do you have a reason to feel sad? (To women: Are there some days that you feel like crying, even for no reason? Do these days coincide with the days previous to menstruation?)
11. If several things go wrong at home or at work, does it make you angry (even if you are able to contain it) or does it make you feel rather sad?
12. Do things like a loud TV set, children shouting and playing, a noisy motorbike, get on your nerves?
13. Are you more irritable than usual? Do you get angry easily?
14. Do you agree with what your spouse has said? Do you consider something should be added to what has been mentioned here? Do you know something he or she may be worried about and has not mentioned?
15. If at that point of the questionnaire it is has been discovered that the patient feels both anxious and depressed, to know if a sedative antidepressant or a stimulant one is preferable, or if an anxiolytic drug should be added, the following question may be helpful: consider that on that table, in front of you, there are some scales. On one dish we would put your irritability, your contained rage; on the other your sadness, tiredness, your desire to do little. In your case, in the last 3 months, which dish would be the heaviest?

Addenda to the Questionnaire

When beginning the questionnaire, a patient, especially if he is young, may try to avoid answering directly, saying "it depends ... " That answer may hide several attitudes to the questionnaire. One could be the lack of desire to collaborate because the patient considers the questions unrelated to the consultation. But, when the patient is pressed—"All right, it depends, but even so, of the 30 days in a month, how many days ... ?"—he will soon realize that there is a firm decision to conduct the questionnaire in a precise way. Some patients may have thought that they came to show only their skin and may show some reluctance to answer questions. It is necessary to know how to recognize patients who find the questionnaire too disagreeable. In such cases you should not continue.

Comments on Answers to Questions

Difficulties in getting to sleep (initial insomnia) as well as waking up several times during the night (secondary insomnia) suggest anxiety. To wake at 3 or 4 A.M. and not be able to get to sleep again, even though wanting to, is characteristic of depressive disorder (tertiary insomnia).

Referring to circadian rhythm (*circum die*, "around the day"), subjects are divided in two groups: those who are "lark-like" are more euphoric in the morning, and those who are "owl-like" feel best at night. Depressed patients tend to feel better at night or in the afternoon than in the morning. It is frequent that both anxious and depressed patients wake up feeling rather tired, but the anxious are wide awake sooner.

Excessive tiredness, "feeling bad on the whole," apathy, loss of pleasure in going out, traveling, shopping, chronic leg and back pain, the fact that domestic tasks or work are done without enthusiasm point to a depressive disorder. Sadness, a desire to cry, feeling bad among people, preferring to be alone also suggest depression.

The person who reacts angrily to an adverse situation is usually an anxious person. The one who is devastated is usually depressive.

"I am rather stressed" constitutes a frequent expression of some patients who with that euphemism refer to the degree of psychological participation they accept to play a role in their condition. The paradigm of such acceptance lies in the expression "it is the stress provoked by work, you know?"

Anxious people do not tolerate unexpected noises that make them start. Depressive people tolerate neither excessive noises nor children shouting. This should not be confused with the tendency of obsessive people to refuse contact with others ("miscommunication").

Persons lacking preparation for their normal work tend to be depressed. Subjects with a tendency to depression do not plan their work. It is done by force when it appears. When a depressed person improves, he or she plans what is to be done during the following days.

On an intellectual and cultural level, women are usually better psychologists than men. They answer more precisely than men do. Sometimes it is helpful to ask the opinion of the spouse present, especially when the person being questioned is a man. In our environment, men usually accept the problems referred to by their wives as real. Men tend to answer with set phrases, without real value, with established concepts.

A man will sometimes feel a compulsion to explain conflictive domestic or work situations. But, possibly due to unconscious shame or pride, he does not do so. In contrast, the wife, on hearing the questions put to her husband, soon grasps what the dermatologist is looking for. (It could be, for example, the problem of a drug abuser son or a daughter-in-law who is living with them who has values different from their own.) The woman may, out of respect, abstain from interfering in the questionnaire process. She might have been able to answer the questions correctly, but she needs to be directly questioned to answer.

Conflicts at work usually affect men more than women, whereas domestic and family problems are more likely to affect women. Previous treatment for a depressive disorder by a primary physician or by a psychiatrist has been called "psychiatric level," which is a useful indicator. Parents who have lost a child, especially mothers, have a high likelihood of suffering psychiatric disorders, no matter how many years have passed since the event. Elderly, widowed women living alone, without children or with children living far away, may feel alone, more depressed than anxious.

It is important to carefully consider couples without children at home or one spouse taking care of the other in a situation that permits him or her to go out only for pressing matters. Such patients' horizons may be rather limited and gloomy. Some of these patients may consult a dermatologist for gloso- and orodynia. Even if they are in an economic position to hire caregiving assistance, they may not consider doing so if they are not pressed by us. Children who are consulted can usually confirm such financial possibilities and may comment that, for example, their mother prefers to take personal care of their father. Employing a person to do this would permit the spouse to engage in outside activities such as yoga classes, swimming, gymnastics, or shopping, which might help them more than an antidepressant drug.

The presented questionnaire permits acceptance or rejection of the suspicion of a psychological trouble.

Ratio of Anxious to Depressive Symptoms

When writing a prescription, it is necessary to have established the ratio between the two main aspects of depressive disorders in each patient: irritability and sadness. For this purpose I use an example. As the final question of my questionnaire I tell the patient to imagine a set of scales on my desk. (Anxious, not depressed, patients do not need the scales' example: they are only irritable.) On one plate he should put his irritability, or his rage, on the other plate, his tiredness, his sadness. For the previous 3 months does one plate weigh more than the other? Or do they weigh the same? (It is better not to use the expressions "anxiety" and "depression" with patients.) When you put the question in this way, patients answer quite well. Four possible outcomes include:

1. More irritability than tiredness.
2. Similar degree of tiredness and irritability.
3. More tiredness than irritability.
4. Only tiredness.

When there is more irritability than tiredness, psychiatrists use paroxetine 20 mg as an excellent sedative antidepressant. It is rather unusual for a depressed patient consulting us to present with such a degree of irritability. An anxiolytic may be added. When the scales show that there is more tiredness than irritability, and when only tiredness is found, a stimulant antidepressant is preferable. When the ratio of irritability to tiredness found in the scales shows a similar degree of irritability and tiredness, sertraline may be prescribed. An anxiolytic may be added.

REFERENCES

1. Goldberg D. A classification of psychological distress for use in primary care. Settings Soc Sci Med 1992; 35:189–193.
2. Grimalt F. Sospecha de alteraciones psiquiátricas ocultas en pacientes dermatológicos que consultan por dermatosis no consideradas como psicocutáneas. In: Grimalt F, Cotterill JA, eds. Dermatología y Psiquiatría: Historias Clínicas Comentadas. Madrid: Editorial Aula Médica, 2002.
3. Grimalt F. Interrogatorio psiquiátrico sistemático. In: Grimalt F, Cotterill JA, eds. Dermatología y Psiquiatría: Historias Clínicas Comentadas. Madrid: Editorial Aula Médica, 2002.

3

Liaison Dermatology

Iona H. Ginsburg
Columbia Presbyterian Medical Center and New York Presbyterian Hospital
New York, New York, U.S.A.

Liaison dermatology may be defined as a branch of liaison psychiatry, the subspecialty of psychiatry that focuses on clinical service, teaching, and research at the borderland of psychiatry and medicine. In 1811 Benjamin Rush, a clinician and professor of medicine in Philadelphia, noted that the human being is, "in the eye of the physician, a single and indivisible being, for so intimately united are [the] soul and body, that one cannot be moved without the other. The actions of the former upon the latter are numerous and important." However, development of liaison psychiatry in the United States has taken place only since the 1930s. The complex interplay of biological and psychosocial factors in the development, course, and outcome of all diseases is central to the concept of psychosomatic disorders (1).

During this period, a number of psychiatrists, such as Menninger and Wittkower, and dermatologists, such as Obermayer and Stokes, worked at the interface between psychiatry and dermatology. But as the sophistication of scientific techniques increased enormously and as a result a burgeoning of knowledge about the pathophysiology of skin disorders and wider spectrum of available treatments, attempts at an integrated understanding tended to recede (2).

In recent years especially, there has been a renaissance of interest and a more vivid awareness of the importance of psychological factors in skin disease. A British study of 196 dermatology outpatients and 40 inpatients disclosed that 30% of the outpatients and 60% of the inpatients had high scores on the General Health Questionnaire, a screening instrument to detect such symptoms as anxiety and depression in medical patients. In addition, half the high scorers in each group were found to have clinically significant depression on a depression measure. Thus the groups in the study had a significantly higher prevalence of psychiatric disorder than the general population and general medical inpatients, respectively (3).

When 149 dermatology patients were referred to a psychiatry liaison clinic located physically within a dermatology department, a very high proportion was found to have psychiatric pathology, with only 5% of the group judged to have no psychiatric problem. The most common diagnoses were depression and generalized anxiety, with an additional 14% diagnosed with severe depression. Body dysmorphic disorder (or dermatological nondisease) accounted for 34% of the dermatology categories, with exacerbation of chronic skin diseases in 32%, symptoms out of proportion to the skin disease in 19%, and scratching without physical signs of illness in 11% (4).

An Italian study of a large number of patients involved the analysis of 2579 usable questionnaires, using a brief general health questionnaire (GHQ12), finding a psychiatric morbidity of 25.2%. The questions were general, eliciting chiefly symptoms of anxiety and depression, distress rather than specific psychiatric disorders. Women were more vulnerable than men (30.6% vs. 17.6%), with widowed people displaying more distress (40.1%) than married (24.5%) as well as those who were unmarried (25.4%) and separated/divorced (22.9%). Health-related quality of life was found to be a stronger predictor of psychiatric problems than clinical severity rated by physicians. The dermatological conditions with prevalence of over 30% included acne, pruritus, urticaria, alopecia, and herpesvirus infections, as well as patients without objective indication of dermatological disease (5).

Insofar as specific psychiatric syndromes, body dysmorphic disorder is of particular importance (see Chapter 11). In a study focused on the rate of body dysmorphic disorder, 268 patients in outpatient settings filled out two questionnaires, with the results showing a 12% rate (6). Since these patients are preoccupied to an intense degree, sometimes impairing their capacity to relate to others and their daily functioning, with a nonexistent or minimal physical defect, they are likely to be dissatisfied with their treatment results. It would clearly be advantageous to the patient, as well as the physician, if these patients were to be readily identified so that appropriate treatment could be instituted.

Perhaps the most distressing and weighty issue is the question of suicide in dermatological patients. Cotterill and Cunliffe report on 16 patients, most with body dysmorphic disorder (dysmorphophobia) or acne, which are special areas of interest for each, respectively (7). In their patients, facial scarring, especially in men, and body image problems, especially in women with facial complaints, were related to severe depression and suicide. They also point out that patients with disabling chronic skin disorders, as well as those with marked psychiatric problems who happen to also suffer from a skin disease, may also be in danger of killing themselves. A study of 217 psoriasis patients found that 9.7% wished to be dead and 5.5% indicated active suicidal ideation at the time of the study, a higher rate than in epidemiological surveys of the general population (8).

It is important for dermatologists to develop a higher level of awareness about this problem and to screen patients for depression, especially patients with chronic skin disorders and body dysmorphic disorder. Patients who do not improve with the usual spectrum of dermatological treatments for their condition may be noncompliant with treatment or may be experiencing intense stress in their lives, which then, through various psychophysiological pathways (see Chapter 5), may perpetuate the skin disorder. Some of these patients may also be vulnerable.

If the clinician suspects that a patient may be depressed or if he falls into one of the groups just mentioned, questioning can be folded into the general medical inquiry. How is your sleep? Appetite? Energy level? Concentration? Do you ever feel sad? Do you ever feel that life is not worth living? If the patient is depressed, she can be referred to a psychiatrist for consultation, or if a medical center in the area has a liaison dermatology clinic, the patient may be referred there.

A considerable number of patients present to dermatologists who would be more accurately addressing their difficulties if they saw a psychiatrist. These include patients fully discussed in other chapters, such as those with body dysmorphic disorder, delusional disorders focused on the skin (parasitosis, bromosis, etc.), and self-mutilating syndromes (trichotillomania, acne excoriée, neurotic excoriations, dermatitis artefacta, etc.). Of course, many such patients should see a dermatologist as well to treat self-induced skin lesions as well as to ascertain that no skin disorder is causative or coexists with what is primarily a psychiatric disorder.

However, these patients have chosen to consult a dermatologist, not a psychiatrist. And on a very concrete level, there is a degree of logic to it. After all, these lesions or sensations or abnormalities do appear on the skin. And not infrequently dermatological patients who have decided that their difficulties lie in their skin may be resistant to referral to a psychiatrist.

However, if referral is approached in a manner that is appreciative of the patient's sensitivities, it may well be successful. First, in order for a patient to even consider a suggestion so counterintuitive as consulting a psychiatrist when it is clear to the patient that the problem lies in her skin, she must come to trust the dermatologist. This rapport would be expected to develop during the course of several visits to the office in which the patient feels, with good reason, that the dermatologist is an ally in the struggle to understand and control or cure the disease.

In introducing the idea of a consultation, the dermatologist might frame the suggestion by referring to what the patient may have told him about his feelings of tension or depression or about the stresses he is undergoing in his life, including the stress of the illness. If a patient's complaint is of a sensory dysesthesia, including pruritus and delusions of parasitosis, often speculating about the role of neurotransmitters may influence him to consult with a psychiatrist as a person skilled in prescribing medications that can alter the "chemical imbalance."

It is important that the dermatologist make clear that this would be a consultation, not a transfer of care. If the patient feels she is being abandoned, resistance would be heightened and the patient might well feel hurt and angry. It is vital to have phone contact, at least, with the psychiatrist after the consultation, which may result in treatment with medication, psychotherapy, behavioral therapy, group therapy, etc. Many patients tend to be far more amenable to a consultation if this occurs on dermatological turf, in the dermatology clinic.

In their classic paper, Gould and Gragg describe the work they had been doing since 1972, when they started a dermatology-psychiatry liaison clinic at Stanford University (9). To summarize various aspects of their clinic, since many which have sprung up since follow a very similar format, they held the clinic once a week in the outpatient dermatology department while the regular clinics were going on. Patients were referred by residents, attendings, and sometimes by private practitioners. The patients were specifically informed that a dermatologist and psychiatrist would see them simultaneously and that a resident might be present. At the session the reason for referral is discussed, a dermatological examination is performed, and a complete history, including physical and psychiatric issues, is elicited. There is not a rigid structure to the meetings, with all physicians present participating, although Dr. Gragg most often dealt with psychiatric issues and Dr. Gould and the resident with dermatological ones. At Stanford a resident is assigned to the clinic for 3–6 months, thus being able to appreciate, by evaluating a number of patients, how intertwined the physical is with the mental. In their review of 60 consecutive patients, 40% were seen once or twice, 40% three to six times, and the rest for longer.

The most frequent diagnoses in this group were eczema, pruritus, acne, psoriasis, and prurigo nodularis. A major problem was a high rate of missed appointments, patients presumably displaying their resistance in this way. They point out that "the liaison clinic is a way for dermatology residents to observe at first hand techniques of interviewing, strategic questioning and listening which can be applied to the types of patients they will soon be seeing in their practices."

In my opinion, the model set forth by Gould and Gragg is highly effective as a clinical contribution to the care of dermatology patients as well as an effective teaching technique. Since it is the rare clinician who has training in both disciplines, having both a dermatologist and psychiatrist evaluating their complaints is a great advantage to patients who require this attention. It is usually immensely reassuring to patients that their skin as well as their psyche is being evaluated.

Liaison clinics at other centers may meet twice a month rather than weekly; some are more focused on clinical services to patients rather than teaching; some may not be staffed by practitioners of both disciplines, although most appear to be. But the patients and their diagnoses, which comprise the body of this book, are very similar. Psychopharmacological treatment will often be initiated in the liaison clinic, as will a tactful referral for ongoing psychiatric treatment.

Does psychological intervention actually help people afflicted by chronic skin conditions? A British study found that of 64 patients with chronic or intractable conditions, 12 remitted and 28 showed some improvement up to 5 years after undergoing assessment (10). They concluded that liaison between dermatology and psychiatry proved a valuable adjunct to the standard dermatological treatments. Other studies also suggest a need for psychiatric and psychological services for some dermatological patients (11–14).

However, the actual existence of a liaison dermatology presence is highly variable, not only in the United States but in other parts of the world as well. In a survey of dermatology clinics in Germany, Gieler et al. found that of 69 questionnaires, 85% of the clinics indicated that they take psychosomatic aspects into consideration in their work, with 5% of the clinic dermatologists having additional psychotherapeutic certification (15).

It is striking that in a 2-year study of 889 referrals to liaison psychiatry at the medical center of Istanbul University, referrals from dermatology were the third most frequent, after internal medicine and surgery (16). The development of a "bifocal strategy" in Belgium defines its goal of defusing the somatization process through close collaboration between the physician treating the somatic disorder and the liaison psychiatrist, giving as an example improvement in varying degrees in 68% of 50 psoriasis patients.

Liaison dermatology is based on the biopsychosocial model so eloquently described by Engel: "to provide the basis for understanding the determinants of disease and arriving at rational treatments and patterns of health care, a medical model must also take in to account the patient, the social context in which he lives, and the complementary systems devised by society to deal with the disruptive effects of illness" (18). That the awareness of this reality is increasing in so many countries is an exciting development, which can only lead to vastly improved medical services for our patients and to approaching still closer to physicians' determination to provide the best care possible.

REFERENCES

1. Lipowski ZJ. History of consultation–liaison psychiatry. In: Textbook of Consultation–Liaison Psychiatry. Rundell JR, Wise MG, eds. Washington, DC: American Psychiatric Publishing, 1996:3–4.
2. Koblenzer CS. Psychocutaneous Disease. Orlando, FL: Grune & Stratton, 1987:12.
3. Hughes JE, Barrachlough BM, Hamilton LG, White JE. Psychiatric symptoms in dermatology patients. Br J Psychiatry 1983; 143:51–54.
4. Woodruff PWR, Higgins EM, du Vivier AWP, Wessely S. Psychiatric illness in patients referred to a dermatology-psychiatry clinic. Gen Hosp Psychiatry 1997; 19:29–35.
5. Picardi A, Abeni D, Melchi C, Puddu P, Pasquini P. Psychiatric morbidity in dermatologic outpatients: an issue to be recognized. Br J Dermatol 2000; 143:983–991.
6. Phillips KA, Dufresne RG Jr, Wilkel CS, Vittoio CC. Rate of body dysmorphic disorder in dermatology patients. J Am Acad Dermatol 2000; 42:436–441.
7. Cotterill JA, Cunliffe WJ. Suicide in dermatological patients. Br J Dermatol 1997; 137:246–250.
8. Gupta MA, Schork NJ, Gupta AK, et al. Suicidal ideation in psoriasis. Int J Dermatol 1993; 32:188.
9. Gould WM, Gragg TM. A dermatology-psychiatry liaison clinic. J Am Acad Dermatol 1998; 9:73–77.
10. Capoore HS, Rowland Payne CM, Goldin D. Does psychological intervention help chronic skin conditions? Postgard Med J 1998; 74:662–664.
11. Humphreys F, Humphreys MS. Psychiatric morbidity and skin disease: what dermatologists think they see. Br J Dermatol 1998; 139:679–681.
12. Driscoll MS, Rothe MJ, Grant-Kels JM, Hale MS. Delusional parasitosis: a dermatologic, psychiatric and pharmacologic approach. J Am Acad Derm 1993; 29:1023–1033.
13. Millard L. Dermatological practice and psychiatry. J Dermatol 2000; 143:919–922.

14. Stoberl C, Gusale M, Partsch H. Artificial edema of the extremity. Hautarzt 1994; 45:149–153.

15. Gieler U, Niemeier V, Kupfer J, Brosig B, Schill WB. Psychosomatic dermatology in Germany: a survey of 69 dermatological clinics. Hautarzt 2001; 52:104–110.

16. Ozkan S, Yucel B, Turgay M, Gurel Y. The development of psychiatric medicine at Istanbul Faculty of Medicine and evaluation of 889 psychiatric referrals. Gen Hosp Psychiatry 1995; 17:216–223.

17. Jonckheere P, Stockebrand B. The bifocal strategy: a new model for flexible liaison between departments of somatic medicine and psychiatrists and psychologists. Acta Clin Belg 1999; 54:72–79.

18. Engel GL. The need for a new medical model: a challenge for biomedicine. Science 1977; 196:129–135.

4

International Consensus on Care of Psychodermatological Patients

John Y. M. Koo
University of California, San Francisco
San Francisco, California, U.S.A.

Chai Sue Lee
Henry Ford Hospital
Detroit, Michigan, U.S.A.

Thelda Kestenbaum
University of Kansas Medical Center
Kansas City, Kansas, U.S.A.

Iona H. Ginsburg
Columbia-Presbyterian Medical Center and New York Presbyterian Hospital
New York, New York, U.S.A.

Hilary Baldwin
State University of New York
Brooklyn, New York, U.S.A.

Tom Hogarty
Sheridan, Wyoming, U.S.A.

Don Kushon
MCP Hahnemann University
Philadelphia, Pennsylvania, U.S.A.

Richard D. Fried
Yardley, Pennsylvania, U.S.A.

Peter Koblenzer
Philadelphia, Pennsylvania, U.S.A.

Caroline Koblenzer
Moorestown, New Jersey, U.S.A.

William Gould
Stanford University
Palo Alto, California, U.S.A.

Mary E. Shepherd
Dreyer Medical Clinic
Aurora, Illinois, U.S.A.

J. A. Cotterill
Leeds, England

Matthias Augustin
University Clinics of Freiburg
Freiburg, Germany

Emiliano Panconesi
University of Florence
Florence, Italy

SUMMARY

Psychodermatology involves the many different types of conditions that lie between the fields of psychiatry and dermatology. These conditions range from patients who experience exacerbation of a real skin disease with emotional stress to those who are devastated emotionally by the disfigurement of their skin disease and those with serious underlying psychopathologies who self-inflict skin lesions. Psychodermatology is a discipline that strives to encourage a more comprehensive and humanistic approach to the management of dermatology patients with psychological overlays to their chief complaint. An international group of dermatologists and psychiatrists who have an interest in the field of psychodermatology has developed a concensus statement on the care and management of psychodermatological disorders. The hope is that this consensus statement will promote the delivery of quality care for these patients and assist those outside our profession in understanding the complexities and scope of care provided by dermatologists.

INTRODUCTION

An international group of dermatologists and psychiatrists who have an interest in the field of psychodermatology has convened to develop a concensus statement on the care and management of psychodermatological disorders. The development of a consensus statement will promote the delivery of quality care and assist those outside our profession in understanding the complexities and scope of care provided by dermatologists.

DEFINITION

Psychodermatology involves the many different types of conditions that lie between the fields of psychiatry and dermatology. These conditions range from patients who experience exacerbation of a real skin disease with emotional stress, to those who are devastated emotionally by the disfigurement of their skin disease and those with serious underlying psychopathologies who self-inflict skin lesions. The field of psychoneuroimmunology has emerged to explain the mechanisms underlying the complex interactions between stress, including psychological stress, and the body in terms of the alterations in the nervous, endocrine, and immune systems. In addition, psychodermatology covers other topics such as the use of psychotropic medications to treat certain bona fide skin diseases and the management of cutaneous sensory disorder. The psychodermatological model strives to provide a more comprehensive biopsychosocial approach to the management of dermatology patients. The concerns of psychodermatology go beyond just treating pathologies; they also cover the psychosocial implications of normal physiological events such as aging and the need for a sense of cutaneous well-being. In short, psychodermatology is a discipline that strives to encourage a more comprehensive and humanistic approach to the management of dermatology patients with psychological overlays to their chief complaint.

RATIONALE

Scope

Many patients with skin disease have psychological aspects to their disease. It has been estimated that at least one third of dermatology patients have psychological or psychosocial issues associated with their chief complaint. The exact percentage in any particular dermatological practice depends on the diagnosis, on individual factors, and on the interest of the dermatologist. However, some patients have such blatant psychopathological conditions, such as delusions of parasitosis, neurotic excoriation, or trichotillomania, that even the least psychologically minded dermatologist feels compelled to address the psychological issues.

Issues

Morbidity

In terms of morbidity, it is frequently the case that the psychosocial impact of skin disease may figure more prominently in the patient's experience than does the strictly physical pathology. For example, patients with acne frequently suffer more from the psychosocial consequences of acne, such as self-conciousness, embarrassment, and low self-esteem, than from the purely physical symptoms such as pain and bleeding. Suicidal ideation appears to be more prevalent among psoriasis and acne patients than among general medical patients. For certain conditions such as vitiligo or alopecia areata, the psychosocial impact of the skin disease is the primary difficulty experienced by the patient because these conditions are generally not life-threatening or symptomatic. In fact, the true value of dermatological intervention cannot be fully appreciated if one disregards the psychosocial benefits. In other words, dermatology as a specialty can easily be trivialized if one assesses it strictly from a physical point of view.

Mortality

In terms of mortality, it is well known that certain subsets of psychodermatological patients, such as those with delusional disorders or dysmorphophobia (body dysmorphic disorder), are at a high risk for committing suicide. Patients with delusional disorders or dysmorphophobia have real psychiatric disorders that need psychiatric referral. However, those patients who most need psychiatric help are often the least likely to accept it. This is particularly true of patients with dermatological delusional disorders who see their problems entirely in dermatological terms, while the dermatologists see these problems in psychological or psychiatric terms.

Bridging this gap in communication is often difficult, and the clinician needs to be much more cautious and diplomatic when interacting with those patients.

APPROACH TO PATIENTS

A proper approach to psychodermatological patients is the critical first step in trying to optimize the outcome of the interaction. Without the proper approach to these patients, it may be impossible to establish an adequate rapport and functional working relationship. Without these prerequisites, it is very difficult to proceed to the next step, namely diagnosis and treatment.

1. It is critical to minimize the chances of the patient feeling rejected (implicit or explicit), trivialized, or abandoned by the dermatologist, the nurse or assistant, and the office staff. The dermatologist may feel that the patient has chosen the wrong physician. However, it is important to recognize the fact that the patient, using his or her best judgment, has chosen the dermatologist to be the designated caregiver. In view of this, it is important to respect their decision if it is in the patient's best interest and to try one's best to deliver optimal care with a nonjudgmental, accepting, and helpful demeanor.

2. The dermatologist is encouraged to take an empathic stance, whereby he or she, without agreeing with the patient's pathological ideation, communicates to the patient that they know what the patient is going through.

3. The dermatologist is encouraged to convey as much hope to patients as possible. Some of the sicker psychodermatological patients, such as those who are depressed or psychotic, are frequently in a state of despair. Once again, without agreeing with their ideation, the dermatologist should demonstrate a willingness to help and to encourage the patient to not give up.

DIAGNOSIS

Other than psychophysiological disorders, where a bona fide skin disease such as psoriasis is made worse by stress, in most other cases of psychodermatological conditions the skin manifestations are likely to be nonspecific. Therefore, the determination of a specific diagnosis within psychodermatology usually relies on the history, the appearance and distribution of skin lesions, and the psychological evaluation of the patient.

It is important to rule out a primary dermatological or other real organic disorder masquerading as a psychodermatological condition. Real skin conditions do not necessarily follow the descriptions in the textbooks. Sometimes a typical fungal infection, blistering disease, etc., can mimic the bizarre, unnatural appearance of self-induced lesions.

It is important not to make a psychiatric diagnosis based only on skin findings. One must remember that psychopathology is not a "diagnosis of exclusion." In order to make a psychiatric diagnosis, there must be positive psychiatric findings. A lack of a ready organic explanation for the skin manifestation is not sufficient to assume that the patient has an underlying psychiatric condition. Similarly, it is important to recognize that the terms used by dermatologists, such as neurotic excoriations and trichotillomania, are dermatological terms and have no implication about the true nature of the underlying psychopathology. For instance, the term trichotillomania conveys only that the patient is pulling out his or her own hair; it does not give any clue as to the reason for the behavior. Even though the majority of patients with trichotillomania complain of obsessive-compulsive types of symptoms, some patients pull out their hair when they are extremely depressed or anxious.

It is important for the dermatologist to try to ascertain, to the best of his or her ability, the nature of the underlying psychopathology, such as anxiety, depression, psychosis, obsessive-compulsive disorder, personality disorder, etc. This is because the approach to the patient may differ depending on the nature of the underlying psychopathology. Moreover, if the clinician wishes to use psychotropic medications in cases where no other help is available, the exact category of psychopharmacological agent to be used is frequently determined by the nature of the underlying psychopathology.

It is important to recognize different categories of psychodermatological conditions: psychophysiological disorders (bona fide skin disorders such as psoriasis or eczema in which the skin disorder is exacerbated by emotional factors such as psychological stress), primary psychiatric disorders (self-induced skin conditions such as neurotic excoriation or trichotillomania), secondary psychiatric disorders (patients develop emotional problems as a result of having skin disease, usually as a consequence of disfigurement), and cutaneous sensory disorders (dysesthesia).

It is important to ascertain whether substance abuse may be complicating both the diagnosis and the management of the case.

Even though diagnostic procedures such as skin biopsies are usually nonspecific in self-induced types of psychodermatological cases (trichomalacia in trichotillomania is a notable exception), it may be justified to do skin biopsies, stool samples for ova and parasites, etc., in self-induced cases if, in the judgment of the dermatologist, it is worthwhile to do them to avoid "power struggles" and to facilitate the building of rapport by convincing the patient that his or her complaints are being taken seriously. However, in this instance it is important for the dermatologist to make sure that the patient does not mistakenly take the willingness of the dermatologist to conduct diagnostic procedures as a sign that the dermatologist agrees with the ideation. It is also recommended that the dermatologist make a verbal contract with the patient prior to conducting these procedures so that the patient will be more open-minded if the result is negative.

WORKING WITH A PSYCHIATRIST

Prior to discussing therapeutic options, it should be recognized that, if at all possible, psychodermatological cases should be referred to a psychiatrist. However, this referral process may be most optimally conducted if the dermatologist has also expressed his or her willingness to follow the patient with the psychiatrist so that the patient does not feel "abandoned." The provision of a multidisciplinary liaison clinic within a dermatology department in a university setting may be a particularly useful way of obtaining skilled psychiatric help for the patient. In some instances it may be the judgment of the dermatologist that even broaching the subject of a psychiatric referral could be detrimental to the doctor-patient relationship; in such cases, a suggestion for a psychiatric referral may never be brought up.

1. Psychiatric referral should be made with care and empathy and not "discussed out of hand."
2. It is important for the dermatologist to establish a working relationship with a psychiatrist so that the care of the patient may be properly coordinated.
3. For those cases where the patient is resistant to being followed by a psychiatrist but is still willing to be seen on an infrequent basis, the psychiatrist may act as a consultant helping the dermatologist to manage the psychological aspects of the case.
4. Psychodermatological cases, just like anything else in medicine, encompass a whole spectrum of severity. For those cases involving anxiety, depression, etc., where the intensity of the psychopathology is mild and manageable and where the patient is reluctant to be referred to a mental health professional, the dermatologist is encouraged to expand his or her knowledge and expertise in psychodermatology and handle these cases.

5. Even if the patient is resistant to being referred to a psychiatrist or other mental health professional, there are some situations where extra urging by the dermatologist may be needed. Some examples of this are as follows: (a) if the dermatologist decides that the psychopathology involved is clearly beyond his or her capacity to analyze or treat; (b) if the psychopathology is escalating, despite the dermatologist's best efforts; (c) if the patient shows no improvement despite the dermatologist's best efforts to address the psychosocial aspects of the case; (d) in homicidal/suicidal cases.

MANAGEMENT

In situations where referral to a mental health professional is not feasible, it is within the scope of acceptable dermatological practice to try to address the psychosocial aspects of the patient's care as long as the dermatologist is knowledgeable and competent in the care given the patient.

Ideally, one should recognize the possible added benefit of a multidisciplinary treatment approach rather than a single therapeutic approach used alone. However, it is also recognized that, within the limited setting of a dermatology practice, judicious, knowledgeable, and responsible use of psychopharmacology may be more helpful to the patient than to ignore the psychodermatological problem.

The therapeutic plan, such as the choice of psychotropic medication to be used, is, in large measure, contingent upon the nature of the underlying psychopathology. The following therapeutic options are available to the dermatologist or, better, can be made available through a referral.

1. Psychopharmacology

    (a) Antianxiety medications for anxiety [e.g., alprazolam (Xanax), buspirone (BuSpar), lorazepam (Ativan)] (some antihistamines may have antianxiety effects).
    (b) Antidepressants for depression [e.g., doxepin (Sinequan), fluoxetine (Prozac), sertraline (Zoloft)].
    (c) Antipsychotic medications for delusion [e.g., pimozide (Orap), olanzapine (Zyprexa), risperidone (Risperdal)].
    (d) Anti–obsessive-compulsive medications for obsessive-compulsive disorder [e.g., fluoxetine (Prozac), paroxetine (Paxil)].
    (e) If one psychotropic medication does not work adequately, it is recommended that a different agent be tried or that the dose be optimized.

(f) The use of psychotropic medications requires ongoing monitoring for efficacy and side effects.

(g) Sometimes, a creative combination of medications or an empirical trial of an alternative category of medications may be needed. For example, a delusional patient who does not respond adequately to antipsychotic agents may, in fact, respond to serotonin reuptake inhibitors.

(h) It is important to inform the pharmacist that many medications have usages other than their primary, indicated usage. For example, it is important for the pharmacist to know that doxepin can be used as an antipruritic or antianxiety agent as well as an antidepressant.

2. Behavioral Therapy

   For psychodermatological patients with recalcitrant behavioral disorders, such as itch-scratch cycle or chronic picking, a referral to a behaviorist may be indicated in addition to other treatment modalities.

3. Psychotherapy

   Psychotherapy is usually not feasible for a dermatologist to conduct due to a general lack of training and time. However, referral to a therapist for different types of therapeutic options such as brief crisis therapy, psychoanalysis, counseling, problem-oriented psychotherapy, etc., could be helpful.

4. Supportive Group Treatment

   The dermatologist should never minimize the importance of patient education and supportive group treatment for psychoder-matological patients. This is true even if a mental health professional is involved simultaneously in the care.

5. Stress Reduction

   Various methods of stress reduction, such as exercise, hypnosis, biofeedback, meditation, etc., can be helpful, especially in primary psychiatric cases or psychophysiological cases, where anxiety and stress are prominent elements in the patient's overall clinical picture.

Apart from and in addition to the above therapeutic options, it is also important to recognize that how the dermatologist interacts with the patient has important positive (or negative) management implications.

DISCLAIMER

Adherence to the consensus statement will not ensure successful treatment in every situation. Further, the consensus statement should not be deemed inclusive of all proper methods of care or exclusive of other methods of care reasonably directed to obtaining the same results. The ultimate judgment regarding the propriety of any specific procedure must be made by the physician in light of all the circumstances presented by the individual patient.

5

Stress and Emotions in Skin Diseases
Physiology, Pathology, and Clinical Aspects

Emiliano Panconesi and Giuseppe Hautmann
University of Florence
Florence, Italy

INTRODUCTION

Behavioral and psychological experiences involving stress are proposed to us by our patients every day, but the more simple aspects have been studied more in animals than in humans, and it is well documented that reactions to weaning, overcrowding, hierarchic challenge, exposure to unfamiliar surroundings, isolation, anger, frustration, and helplessness provoke a precise flight-fright response in animals. The same and other similar situations are everyday experiences for modern humans (1), whose various responses may be psychological and/or physical. Since stress can be caused by environmental as well as psychological factors, it is easy to perceive that there is a relationship between everyday stress and defense mechanisms and disease susceptibility and that the physical and psychological spheres are often both involved in the process. The result is a unitary concept of human pathology, and the problem is to determine the entity of the emotional component in any disease. The body (soma) and the mind (psyche) constitute a single unit, and physicians should do the utmost to consider and treat them as such.

The term psychosomatic is an accepted part of current medical terminology that has been incorporated into everyday language. Psychosomatic medicine (2) proposes the examination of psyche and soma as a unit "in sickness and in health," and it is often imperative to intervene in both areas to reestablish the altered equilibriums evidenced in diseased (dis-eased) subjects. It was inevitable that any organ (including the skin) and its diseases become the object of medical observation and interpretation from a psychosomatic point of view because the effects of emotional stress on human physiology are enormous.

The skin is the largest organ of the body, and it can respond in various ways during periods of emotional stress. The most typical and evident cutaneous responses to stressful situations include, in particular, blushing, pallor, increased perspiration, and increased activity of the sebaceous glands. In addition, we are familiar with the deleterious effects of stress on the course of various inflammatory diseases in general medicine, such as asthma, rheumatoid arthritis, multiple sclerosis, and ulcerative colitis. Similarly, a number of skin disorders are triggered or exacerbated by stress, e.g., psoriasis, atopic dermatitis, acne, and urticaria.

Furthermore, the cutaneous sensory nervous system both conducts sensory impulses and induces local inflammatory responses. Thomas Lewis (3) clarified the concept of the "triple response that is observed in human skin in response to an injury." This triple response refers to the morphological manifestations of wheals, local erythema, and flare reactions in response to external stimuli. Lewis (3) proposed that injury to the skin provokes stimulation of sensory nerves, with consequent transmission of impulses to the spinal cord and antidromic stimulation of connecting fibers which innervate the adjacent skin. Over 30 years later in the late 1960s, Jancso et al. showed that denervation of sensory nerves could block inflammatory responses in the skin, and they postulated that such inflammatory responses were due to release of neurohormones (4).

Extensive research has been done during the last 30 years to identify the neurohormones hypothesized by Lewis and Jancso. Now we know that neurogenic inflammation (with vasodilatation, exudation of plasma, and migration of leukocytes caused by antidromic stimulation of dorsal roots) is due to release of neuropeptides (NPs) from unmyelinated sensory nerve endings, a process involving various immune cells through specific neuropeptide receptors (5–8). Numerous neuropeptides have been identified in the skin by immunohistochemical staining and/or radioimmunoassay, and some of these neuropeptides, in particular substance P (SP), vasoactive intestinal peptide (VIP), calcitonin gene–related peptide

(CGRP), and neuropeptide Y (NPY), have been extensively studied in relation to their role in cutaneous inflammatory reactions (see Tables 1–3 for the biological effects of these neuropeptides on various components of cutaneous tissue).

Substance P–positive nerve fibers are present in the dermis, epidermis, Meissner's corpuscles, and around the sweat glands in normal human skin. Substance P increases vessel permeability by activating the NK-1 receptors on postcapillary venules and causing release of histamine from the mast cells (5–7). The fact that the flare component of the triple response can be inhibited by the H-1 receptor antagonist (5–7) suggests that the flare response is a reaction to histamine released by mast cells.

CGRP, one of the most abundant neuropeptides, is distributed widely throughout the skin. It is commonly found together with substance P (5–7), and CGRP-positive and substance P–positive nerve fibers are similarly distributed in the skin. Intradermal injection of CGRP induces localized erythema that can last for several hours.

Vasoactive intestinal peptide is found mainly in nerve fibers near the arteriolar walls and acini of sweat glands (5–7). Intradermal injection of VIP causes a wheal-and-flare response, and as the axon-reflex flare response fades the increase in blood flow produces an area of localized erythema (5–7).

Finally, neuropeptide Y, a potent vasoconstrictor agent often found in adrenergic neurons, produces vasoconstriction, thus increasing blood pressure, and it can modulate the release of CGRP (5–7).

TABLE 1 Biological Actions of Substance P

Target	Action
Endothelial cells	Stimulates proliferation, increases permeability, upregulation of ELAM-1
Fibroblasts	Stimulates proliferation
Keratinocytes	Stimulation of IL-1, GM-CSF synthesis and secretion, comitogen with CGRP, LTB4
Lymphocytes	Stimulates proliferation and IL-2 synthesis, increases IgA, IgM mRNA production
Macrophages	Stimulates IL-1, IL-6 secretion
Mast cells	Degranulation, stimulates proliferation, and survival in culture
Monocytes	Increases chemotaxis, phagocytosis, and arachidonic acid synthesis
Neutrophils	Stimulates chemotaxis, phagocytosis

TABLE 2   Biological Actions of Calcitonin Gene–Related Peptide

Target	Action
Endothelial cells	Proliferation upregulation of ELAM-1
Keratinocytes	Proliferation in association with SP
Langerhans cells	Inhibits antigen presentation
T lymphocytes	Chemotactic T-cell proliferation
Mast cells	Degranulation

The skin is a fundamental organ of communication that plays an important role in socialization throughout one's life cycle. It has long been recognized that psychosomatic factors play a role in dermatological disease, and we believe, like Ironside (9), that an organ system is particularly vulnerable to psychosomatic influence when: 1) several etiological factors, including genetic and constitutional predisposition, are operant, 2) emotional factors mediated by the central nervous system (CNS) are in play, 3) intrapsychic processes involving self-concept, identity, or eroticism are involved, 4) the organ system is prone to "conversion" and conditioning due to emotions stimulated by psychological problems, and 5) social values and standards are related to the organ system. In their well-known *Textbook of Dermatology*, Rook and Wilkinson (10) open the chapter on "Psychocutaneous Disorders" by stating that "the role of emotional factors on diseases of the skin is of such significance that if they are ignored the effective management of at least 40% of the patients attending departments of dermatology is impossible." These percentages are even higher for the psycho-influenced dermatoses; Obermayer (11) reported psychological influences in 66% of patients, and Medansky and Handler wrote that for them, "almost 80% of dermatologic patients had a psychogenic overlay" (12). Many individuals communicate emotional distress via their skin, and a wide variety of personal and family problems may underlie the presenting dermatological problem. For example, many women who present with complaints of hair loss that are objectively

TABLE 3   Biological Actions of Vasoactive Intestinal Polypeptide

Target	Action
Endothelial cells	Proliferation
Lymphocytes	Inhibits NK cell activity
Mast cells	Degranulation
Neutrophils	Chemotaxis; inhibits proliferation

disproportionate to the actual severity of the alopecia have been found to have marital difficulties and/or to be suffering from depression (13). Individuals with immature psychological coping mechanisms who otherwise receive inadequate nurturing or insufficient attention from others may derive secondary gain from a visible skin conditon. Alternatively, an unaesthetic condition can increase an individual's self-consciousness and lead to social stigmatization, resulting in social withdrawal, underachievement at school or work, and even serious psychological problems, especially in adolescents or subjects under stress. For example, psoriatic lesions can be particularly unsightly, and the real or imagined social stigma can have a profoundly adverse effect on the affected individual's quality of life, sometimes with significant disease-related stress that can, in turn, have an adverse effect on the course of the disease. Many clinical observations have indicated that psychoneuroimmunological factors can have important applications in dermatology. Psychological stress has been associated with increased CNS levels of opioid neuropeptides, and it has also been reported to exacerbate certain dermatological conditions that have both psychosomatic and immunological components, such as chronic idiopathic urticaria, atopic dermatitis, and psoriasis (1,5–7,14). However, we believe that some stressing factor(s) can be individuated in practically all subjects with a dermatosis.

PSORIASIS

Psoriasis is a common, chronic, erythematous dermatosis presenting squamous accumulations; the lesions may be circumscribed or disseminated and arise preferentially on the elbows, knees, and scalp. The disease is presumed to be genetically determined, and subjects present typical histological markers (capillary dilatation, sterile epidermal microabscesses, parakeratosis) and accelerated epidermal turnover (Fig. 1). The lesions and the markers are negatively influenced by acute and chronic emotional stress. Arnetz et al.'s study (15) of psychoendocrine and metabolic reactions of psoriatics and matched healthy subjects during standardized stressor exposure (color-word conflict test and forced mental arithmetics) showed similar psychological and biochemical variables for the two groups under resting conditions, but the psoriatic group experienced significantly higher strain levels during stressor exposure. Both groups showed increased blood pressure, pulse rate, plasma glucose, and urinary adrenaline excretion during exposure, but the psoriatics showed more pronounced increases in the latter two.

Decades of observations have made it evident to physicians and patients alike that stressing life events and various psychosocial factors can

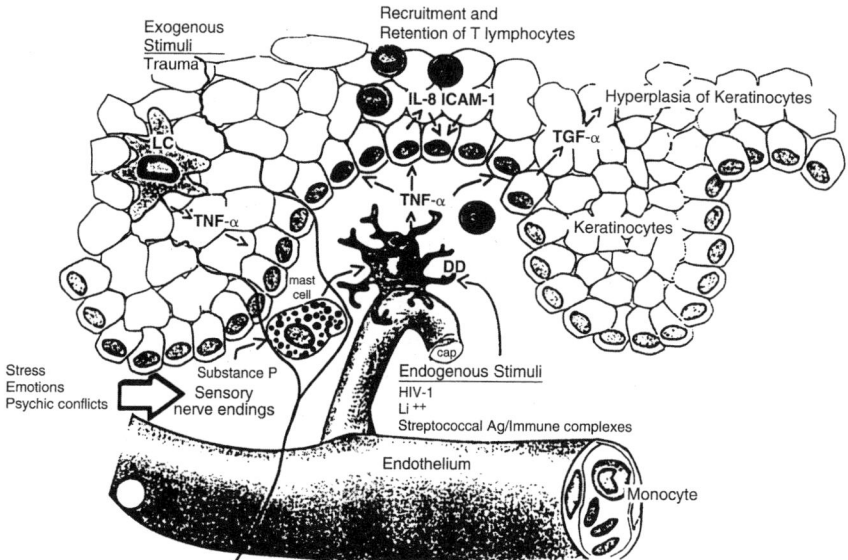

FIGURE 1 Exogenous and endogenous stimuli can trigger the onset of psoriasis. TNFα: tumor necrosis factor–alpha IL-8: interleukin-8; ICAM-1: intercellular adhesion molecule-1; DD: dendrocyte; Li++: lithium salts; TGF-α: transforming growth factor-alpha; Ag: antigen; LC: Langerhans cell. (From Ref. 14.)

be important in triggering the onset or exacerbation of psoriasis, and this has been confirmed by several studies of large case series. Farber and Nall reported that 33% of 5600 patients noticed the appearance of new lesions at a time of worry (16). Braun-Falco et al. reported that in 42% of 536 patients, worry precipitated an exacerbation of psoriasis (17). Fava et al. (18) correlated the appearance or exacerbation of psoriasis with stressful events in 80% of patients. Seville (19) did a 3-year follow-up study of 132 subjects with psoriasis and reported that a specific stress had occurred within 1 month before the appearance of psoriasis in 39% of subjects (19). Farber et al. also reported larger areas of lesions in psoriatics with higher levels of distress than in those who were relatively emotionally stable and that remissions were less frequent in distressed subjects (21).

The characteristic features of psoriasis include symmetry of lesions, exacerbations, and remissions, exogenous and endogenous Koebner phenomena, and the triggering role of stress. However, it is still not clear how stress influences the inflammatory and proliferative processes of psoriasis. Farber's proposal that neuropeptides play a role in the pathogenesis of psoriasis was based on the correlation that stress exacerbates psoriasis and symmetrical distribution (21). The theory is that the release of substance P and other neuropeptides from unmyelinated terminations of sensory nerve fibers in the skin causes local neurogenic inflammatory responses that trigger psoriasis in genetically predisposed individuals.

Stressful events can alter levels of substance P in the central and peripheral nervous systems. Stress was reported to increase levels of substance P in the adrenal glands by activating the descending autonomic fibers in an animal model (22). It is possible that descending autonomic paths can cause release of cutaneous neuropeptides because there are interneurons in the spinal cord for substance P–containing nerves and some of the descending autonomic fibers innervate opoid interneurons in the dorsal horn (23). However, local release of neuropeptides from sensory nerves in the skin has not been measured after stressful stimuli in either animals or humans.

Stressful conditions stimulate the hypothalamic-pituitary-adrenal axis, resulting in increased blood levels of adrenocorticotropic hormone (ACTH), corticosteroids, and adrenalin. In addition to these known conventional endocrine changes, there are reports indicating that the levels of nerve growth factor (NGF) rise significantly under various stressing conditions (24,25). NGF can influence an inflammatory reaction in a number of ways, and it is involved with the mechanisms of T-lymphocyte proliferation and activation and mast cell degranulation (26,27). Thus, in psoriatics stress-induced neurohormonal agents like SP and NGF could contribute significantly to the inflammatory processes of psoriasis.

Increasing numbers of biochemical and clinical studies support the idea of a functional role for cutaneous nerves and neuropeptides in the pathogenesis of psoriasis. Weddell et al. found increased numbers of neural filaments in both lesional and symptomless psoriatic skin (28). The development of immunohistochemical staining made it much easier to stain cutaneous nerves and neuropeptides, resulting in reports of an increased number of substance P–containing nerves in psoriatic epidermis (29). Other investigators have published similar findings and also demonstrated VIP containing nerves in psoriatic plaques (30,31). The results of a double-labeled immunofluorescence study to identify the nerves and neuropeptides in psoriatic tissue (32) showed that SP- and CGRP-containing neuropeptide nerve fibers are denser in psoriatic epidermis than in uninvolved epidermis. In a majority of studies, direct measurement of neuropeptides by radioimmunoassay have shown increased levels of substance P and/or VIP in biopsies from psoriatic lesions (33–36). However, there are contradictory reports. Wallengren et al. reported reduced VIP level in a suction blister raised from psoriatic plaques (36), Pincelli et al. (35) reported reduced levels of substance P in chronic psoriatic plaques, and Anand et al. (33) found no difference between SP levels in the psoriatic plaques and normal skin. These conflicting results may be due to several factors, in particular the fact that we do not know when SP and VIP become manifest and where they are located in the developing lesion and that neuropeptide levels are difficult to measure because they are readily metabolized. In their study on the dynamics of neuropeptides in tape-strip–induced evolving psoriatic lesions and mature psoriatic plaques, Naukkarinen and coworkers (37) found that in control skin, nonlesional skin, and Koebner-negative psoriatic skin, very few nerves contained SP, VIP, or CGRP. However, at the end of one week, SP-positive fibers were found in the papillary dermis in all the Koebner-positive lesions, VIP-positive fibers were observed around the capillaries in 66% of these lesions (37), and SP fibers were more abundant in mature psoriatic plaques. A subsequent study involving 28 psoriatics to identify SP, VIP, and CGRP in skin biopsies reported an increase in the number of SP-positive intraepidermal nerve fibers in lesional psoriatic skin specimens (2.8 nerves/mm biopsy) compared with nonlesional skin (0.01 nerves/mm biopsy) and normal skin (0.04 nerves/mm biopsy). The specimens from the psoriatic lesions also presented increased intraepidermal VIP- and CGRP-positive fibers (38).

There are other possible signs of neuropeptide involvement in the inflammatory and proliferative process in psoriasis. Keratinocyte hyper-proliferation, so important in psoriasis, can be triggered by VIP (39), CGRP acts synergistically with SP to stimulate keratinocyte proliferation (40), and both SP and VIP can enhance the mitogenic effect of leukotrine B_4 on human keratinocytes (41). Substance P can induce the degranulation and stimulate the increase in the number of mast cells (42,43) seen in early lesions of psoriasis (44). CGRP is a potent mitogenic factor for endothelial cells (45), and this might explain the angiogenesis observed in developing lesions of psoriasis (46). One of the earliest histological signs documented in psoriatic lesions is infiltration by leukocytes (47). Psoriatic skin shows increased adhesion of peripheral blood lymphocytes to the endothelium (48,49). And both SP and CGRP have been reported to enhance adhesion of lymphomononuclear cells (50,51). Furthermore, substance P has been shown to induce expression of endothelial leukocyte adhesion molecules (ELAM-1) on postcapillary dermal vessels (52), and it can promote neutrophil chemotaxis (53), stimulate IL-2 synthesis (54) in T cells, and induce IL-1 secretion from keratinocytes (55) and marked upregulation of E-selectin expression (56). All of these functions can contribute significantly to the pathogenesis of psoriasis.

Krogstad et al. (57) observed that local infiltration of psoriatic plaques with mepivacaine caused a 40% reduction of blood flow in the lesions, and surface anesthesia of UVB-induced erythema did not affect regional blood flow. The fact that cutaneous anesthesia can prevent vasodilatation induced by the axon reflex (58) supports the idea that a local neurogenic mechanism may be active in the psoriatic plaque. Studies in which peripheral nerve sectioning resulted in clearing of psoriatic plaques provide important evidence for the role of neurogenic inflammation in psoriasis. In various cases psoriatic lesions resolved at the site of anesthesia subsequent to damage of sensory nerves (59,60), and in one case a psoriatic lesion on the knee resolved and then reappeared upon the return of sensation (59).

These findings encouraged researchers to look for the cause of neural proliferation and upregulation of neuropeptides in psoriatic tissues. Since nerve growth factor plays a role in regulating innervation (61) and upregulating neuropeptides (62,63), the role of NGF was investigated in lesional and nonlesional psoriatic skin, skin from subjects with other inflammatory skin diseases, and normal skin from other subjects. Keratinocytes in lesional and nonlesional psoriatic tissue expressed high levels of NGF compared to that seen in controls (64). NGF is mitogenic to keratinocytes and protects keratinocytes from apoptosis (65,66), it recruits mast cells and promotes their degranulation (both early events in a developing lesion of psoriasis) (27), and it activates T lymphocytes and recruits inflammatory cellular infiltrates (67). NGF has also been observed to induce expression of a potent chemokine, RANTES, in keratinocytes. RANTES is chemotactic for resting CD4+ memory T cells and activated naive and memory T cells (68). In the case of psoriasis, the influx of mast cells and lymphocytes, which in turn initiate an inflammatory reaction contributing to the pathogenesis of the disease, is probably preceded by overexpression of NGF.

Many investigators consider psoriasis an autoimmune disease induced by an unidentified antigen (69), but T-cell activation alone does not clarify various salient features of psoriasis, including the Koebner phenomenon, the symmetrical distribution of psoriatic lesions, proliferation of cutaneous nerves, and the upregulation of neuropeptides in psoriatic tissue (21,29–31). Also, it does not explain why psoriatic lesions resolve at sites of anesthesia (59,60). It is well known that psoriasis frequently appears at sites of trauma and that a wound induces a reaction characterized by proliferation of keratinocytes, fibroblasts, vascular elements, nerves, and an accumulation of inflammatory cells. Reports suggest that NGF produced by keratinocytes plays a role in wound healing (70,71), and NGF promotes axonal regenera-tion and reinnervation of terminal cutaneous nerves. In non-psoriatics healing stops after a finite time, depending on the nature of the wound, and in psoriatics a wound frequently results in papulosquamous lesions.

Histologically, a psoriatic lesion is characterized by hyperkeratosis, parakeratosis, acanthosis, angiogenesis, neutrophilic microabscesses, lymphomononuclear cell infiltrates, and, discovered only in the last decade, hyperproliferation of cutaneous nerves (29,30). Several findings suggest that the increased expression of NGF in the keratinocytes of lesional and nonlesional psoriatic tissue may be an early event in the pathogenesis of psoriasis. Proliferation of keratinocytes induced by a wound will result in significantly higher levels of NGF in lesion-free skin compared to control skin. Elevated levels of NGF induce an inflammatory response, proliferation of nerves, and upregulation of neuropeptides such as SP and CGRP. Increased levels of neuropeptides and NGF, in addition to their proinflammatory effects, will induce keratinocyte proliferation (39,40,65,66), which, in turn, will result in increased expression of NGF. Thus, a vicious cycle of a proliferative and inflammatory process is established in one who is genetically predisposed to psoriasis. In subjects without psoriasis, the expression of NGF is three to four times less per square millimeter of epidermis than that seen in nonlesional skin in poriatics, thus, in the former, healing events do not generate the critical levels of NGF and neuropeptides necessary to initiate or maintain cascades essential for a chronic inflammatory reaction.

Some studies have shown that psychosocial stressful events result in increased levels of NGF in blood and NGF niRNA synthesis in the hypothalamus (72,24,25), and it is likely that the type of cascade of events mentioned above occurs in distressed psoriatics, indicating that NGF plays a crucial role in the development of an isomorphic lesion and is also responsible for exacerbation of psoriasis during stressful life events.

Currently the alleged role of an antigen in psoriasis is hypothetical; no specific antigen has yet been discovered for psoriasis. Wrone-Smith and Nickoloff (73) have reported that, in severe combined immune deficiency (SCID) mice, transplanted nonlesional psoriatic skin converts to a psoriatic plaque subsequent to intradermal delivery of activated T cells artificially activated with an antigen cocktail. Since an artificial antigen cocktail does not exist in psoriatic skin, it has been considered possible that substances in the epidermis and dermis, such as NGF and SP, may be responsible for lesional T-lymphocyte activation.

Other indirect evidence that supports the role of neuropeptides in psoriasis is the efficacy of neuropeptide-modulating drugs in healing or improving the lesions. Capsaicin, an SP depleter, has been reported to improve psoriasis, and peptide T, a VIP analogue, has been observed to be effective in the treatment of psoriasis. All these findings are consistent with the hypothesis that cutaneous nerves together with their neuropeptides play a key role in the pathogenesis of psoriasis (74,75).

ATOPIC DERMATITIS

Atopic dermatitis (AD) is another common skin disease characterized by chronic or chronically recurrent lesions. Individuals with this affection usually experience severe itching and present signs of scratching as well as eczematous papulovesicular lesions with crusting and lichenification. Exudative-eczematous lesions usually predominate in infants and toddlers, whereas in school-aged children and adults, pruritus, pruriginous lichenoid papules, and lichenification are prominent. The microscopic picture changes depending on the morphology of the lesions. Exudative lesions present spongiotic vesicles, acanthosis with hyperkeratosis and parakeratosis, and perivascular infiltration of lymphocytes and histiocytes with exocytosis. The lichenified areas of the epidermis are thickened, and the papillary body is hypertrophic, permeated by inflammatory cells (lymphocytes and histiocytes), and there are large numbers of mast cells, which explain the increased histamine content of chronically lichenified foci.

A typical, brief case history would be as follows. A family in which some member(s) has or has presented allergic asthma, hay fever, eczema (in bottle-fed babies), or cradle cap has a child who, usually at the age of about 3 months, presents with acute, often exudative and intensely itchy eczema on the cheeks and/or forehead and perhaps also on the forearms, diaper area, and the flexural regions in general. The lesions may extend to other areas and may become diffuse. The disease becomes chronic with practically no periods of remission in severe cases and alternate periods of relapse or improvement and exacerbation in other cases. In the most fortunate subjects, about 50%, the dermatitis pretty much disappears when the child is just over a year old, albeit with minor signs of delicate or dry skin and some itching or redness in flexural areas. In the other 50% the dermatosis persists, especially on the face (eyebrows, eyelids, around the mouth), the backs of the hands, and the cervical and malleolar regions. These children live their childhood, and subsequently adolescence, tormented by lichenified dermatitis. They usually have pale, grayish, cold, dry, anhydrotic skin with raised, keratotic follicles. The same characteristics persist in adulthood, but with more evident signs of lichenification in the most severely affected areas, particularly the flexural areas, the face, and the hands.

In the past AD was considered associated with neuropsychic factors, as evidenced by the nineteenth-century use of the term neurodermatitis; the term prurigo of Besnier, still used in Scandinavia, was based on the fact that this strange affection comports persistent itching, which is the most ambiguous and psychosomatic of all symptoms. Moreover, itching appears to be the leitmotif of the disease and may be the cause of its persistence (76,77).

Cutaneous stimulation appears to be an important factor for cell growth and differentiation and CNS maturation throughout infancy (78,79). In the rat model, handling and cutaneous stroking in early life appear to enhance humoral immunity later on (79); in preweaned rats, temporary interruption of active tactile stimulation or maternal deprivation is associated with reduced ornithine decarboxylase activity, a sensitive index of cell growth and differentiation and CNS maturation (78). Human preterm neonates who received tactile and kinesthetic stimulation were more alert, gained weight more rapidly, and exhibited more mature neurological reflexes than controls (80). And, in his long famous experiences with monkeys, Harlow (81) showed that deprivation of touch or contact comfort in early life leads to the development of inappropriately aggressive behavior and other psychological problems. All these findings underline the relevance of cutaneous perception and stimulation in physical and psychological development. Awareness of the psychobiological unity of the human being and the impossibility of considering the child's development separate from his environment obliges us to evaluate not only factors concerning the child alone, but also those related to the parent-child system with the goal of creating interactive semeiotics. Thus, investigators and physicians must try to bring out the most positive, significant, and functional choices of the child and family in that particular environment and moment.

Obermayer (11), one of the fathers of psychosomatic dermatology, pointed out that many babies were traumatized by early separation from their mother's breast, resulting in severe damage to their emotional stability. The psychodynamics of the mother-child relationship is often altered in the case of a child with AD. The extreme example is the mother's refusal to touch her child; this leads to anger, anxiety, or hostility on the part of the child toward the mother herself and/or mother substitutes. There are reports that in the 1950s up to 98% of children with AD had rejecting mothers, whereas few children in a non-AD control group experienced maternal rejection (76,77,82).

Such maternal rejection may be a reaction to the child's dermatitis (83,84), and the disturbed parent-child relationship further aggravates the skin lesions. (83). The child makes himself ugly (thus, unlovable, unworthy of love) by scratching and self-excoriation; the excoriations modify the individual's self-image and are also the result of disobeying the regular request not to scratch. According to Slany (84), many children with AD are in conflict with an unattentive, unaffectionate, and inadequate mother; this provokes an unconscious triggering of the psychosomatic mechanism that leads to onset of the disease. The progression of events would be that a small child or infant, who is unable to defend himself from psychic conflict except by removal, experiences internal tension and develops feelings of anguish, depression, and hostility followed by conversion and regression. There is a hypothesis that in the phase of detachment from the mother, the subject with AD does not invent or find a transitional object; the dermatitis substitutes the missing object, meaning that the child's difficulty or inability to progress along the normal path of development is expressed in the form of a somatic cutaneous pathology (76,77,85).

In general, subjects with AD experience more emotional upsets than normal subjects, and it has been claimed that there are frequent episodes of parental separations, psychiatric illness, and skin disorders in the family history. In addition, these subjects also tend to be more irritable, resentful, guilt-ridden, and hostile than persons who do not have eczema (86).

Various reports refer specifically to the personality of the infant with AD, an infant who is typically irritable, demanding, and unhappy, who needs more cuddling and skin contact than the average baby. The parents' pride and joy in their offspring is challenged by the persistent, ugly, very visible eczematous eruption. The combination of the need to follow a complicated medical regimen and the fact that the child is difficult and unattractive provokes some degree of parental resentment and embarrassment, and withdrawal occurs. This is the beginning of a difficult interpersonal relationship between the child and the parent(s) and, subsequently, the rest of the world, and the infant responds to unmet needs with self-stimulation and abusive scratching (83). A vicious cycle is created: anxiety provokes itching, and itching and scratching aggravate the anxiety.

As the child grows older, the problems associated with AD increase. In cases of severe eczematous lesions other persons tend to avoid the child, perhaps fearing contamination (the leper effect), and development of peer relationships suffer. School-related problems include increased absences and bad performance because of lack of sleep, and the child may have difficulty concentrating due to self-consciousness (87).

The individual with cutaneous atopy is often tense, insecure, and aggressive and may present many of the following characteristics: feelings of inferiority and inadequacy, repressed hostility toward parental figures, affective hypersensitivity, emotional instability, sexual difficulties with masochistic tendencies and cutaneous eroticism, and a fairly high level of intelligence (88), but no specific personality type is a constant in subjects with AD (89). What has been noted throughout all the investigations is that most of these individuals present some type of emotional disturbance (11,90), and they are usually repressed persons who internalize their problems and express their anxious and hostile emotional conflicts by scratching (83,91). Whitlock (92) and Champion and Parish (93) have indicated that atopic subjects have "conflicting" personality profiles.

Atopic subjects are more likely than others to experience itching in response to relatively minor signals and stimuli, and some of those signals are more profoundly significant in psychodynamic terms than would appear on the surface (83). Excitability and arousal of the CNS from an emotional upset can intensify the vasomotor and sweat responses in the skin and lead to the itch-scratch response, and these findings concur with the observation that many patients experience an emotionally disturbing event before an attack of AD (92). The emotional upset lowers the itch threshold and triggers the scratch response (94).

Excessive anxiety is known to correlate with ease of conditioning, and patients with AD are conditioned more readily to scratch responses than are their matched control counterparts (95,96). There may be some relationship with the fact that many normal persons also tend to scratch at sites that are typically affected by AD in moments of frustration or embarrassment.

On the other hand, AD alters the personality. The difficulties encountered in personal relationships are understandable given the unsightly skin lesions that may lead to discrimination. Nighttime awakening because of violent itching also takes its toll on the patient's disposition and personality (83). The pathway from the emotional phenomena, which the authors have tried to describe, to the triggering of the various phases of the disease phenomenon typical of AD still remains to be clarified. However, the acquisitions of modern psychoneuroendocrinimmunology are beginning to shed light on some of these pathways, and its multifactorial pathogenesis makes AD a good model for the preparation of an integrated hypothesis of biological psychosomatics (5–7,14,74–77).

Various experimental studies have led to the identification of neuropeptides and their receptors, documenting their involvement in the CNS and peripheral organs, including the skin, furnishing important background information on the relays between psyche-emotion-stress (5–7,14,74–77). The most significant findings regarding AD in this field are presented in Figs. 2–6. Figure 2 shows a hypothetical outline of the possible relationship between the pathogenesis of AD and emotional stress (dotted lines), which we presented in 1984 (85). Figure 3 illustrates the presumed influence of SP in the pathogenesis of AD (see also previous lists for functions of SP, CGRP, VIP, and NPY); SP has been found in the lichenoid infiltrate in the perivascular papillary dermis of AD subjects. Figure 4 shows the presumed influence of CGRP on the pathogenesis of AD. CGRP-like immunoreactivity is observed constantly as free endings in the papillary dermis close to the dermoepidermal junction; the same pattern and staining intensity are observed in AD and control subjects. Figure 5 illustrates the possible presumed influence of VIP on the pathogenesis of AD; VIP levels are increased in the lesional skin of AD patients. Figure 6

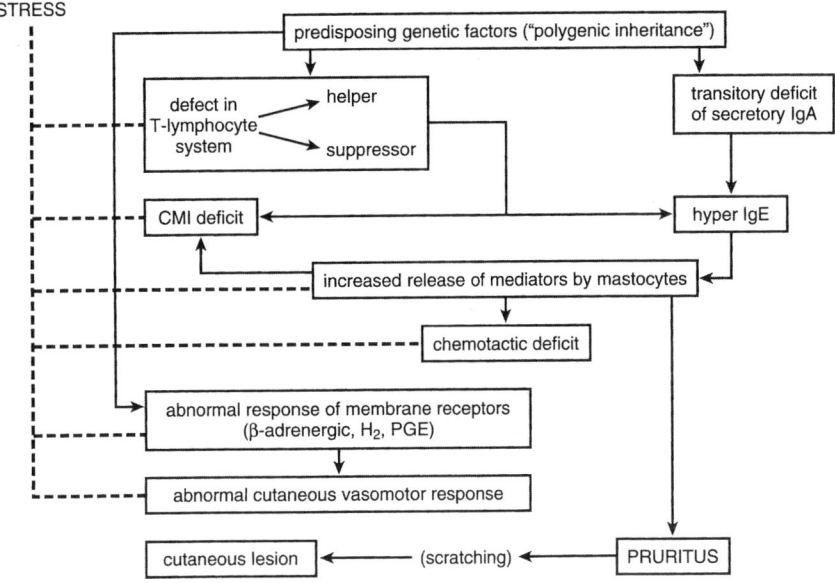

FIGURE 2 Hypothetic outline of the pathogenesis of AD correlated with the possible influence of emotional stress (dotted lines). CMI: cell-mediated immunity; H_2: type 2 receptors for histamine; PGE: prostaglandin E. (From Ref. 14.)

shows how NPY could influence the pathogenesis of AD; NPY-like immunoreactivity has been detected in Langerhans cells in 6 of 11 patients with AD, but not in normal control subjects (97–99).

Other peptides, such as the endorphins and somatostatin, may play a role in AD, but to date there is no experimental evidence to support their involvement. Endorphins could exercise various effects in different phases of the hypothetical outline shown in Fig. 2, and the endogenous opioids would represent the neuropeptidergic system that is involved in the emotion-related pleasure/pain axis, fundamental to survival. Further acquisitions in the field of neuroimmunological research will fill in the dotted lines of the diagram in Fig. 2, but for now the activities of the neuropeptides discussed here constitute a first step in explaining and understanding the biological psychosomatics of certain skin diseases.

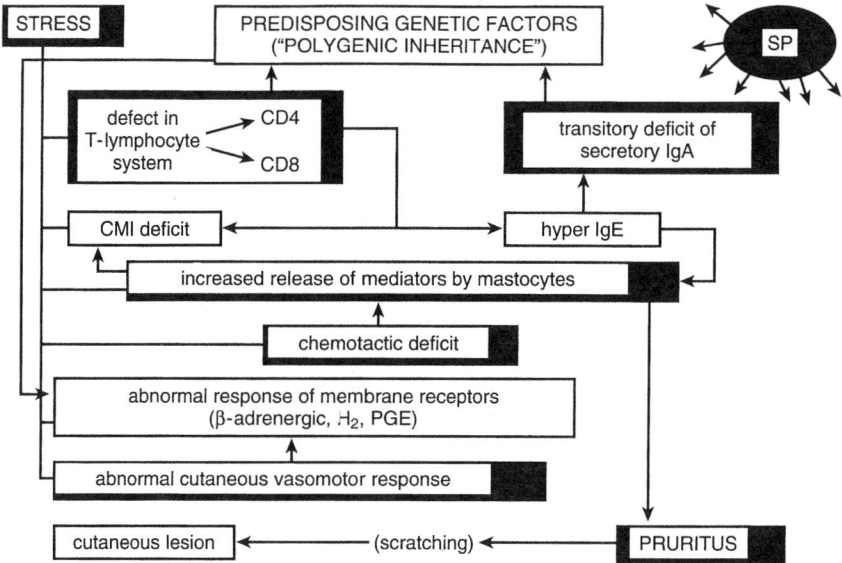

FIGURE 3 SP and AD. The possible points where SP may play a role are marked in black. (From Ref. 14.)

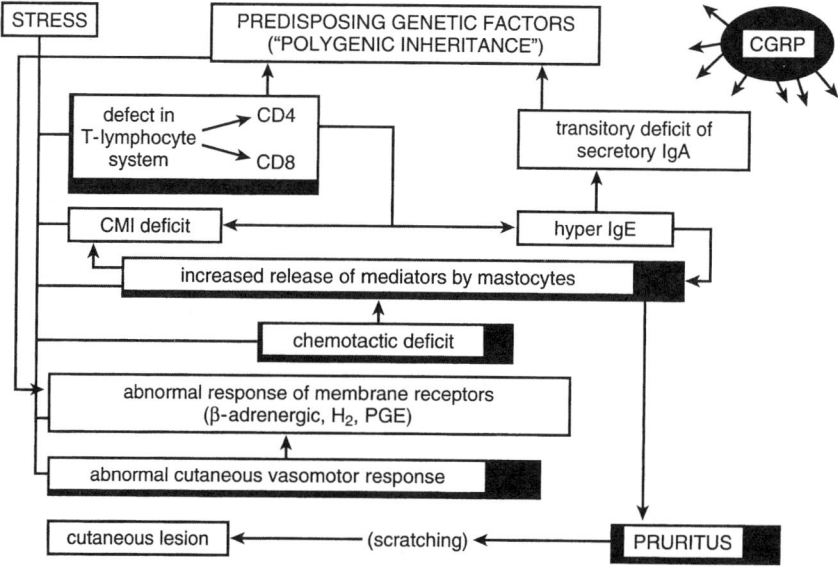

FIGURE 4 CGRP and AD. The possible points where CGRP may play a role are marked in black. (From Ref. 14.)

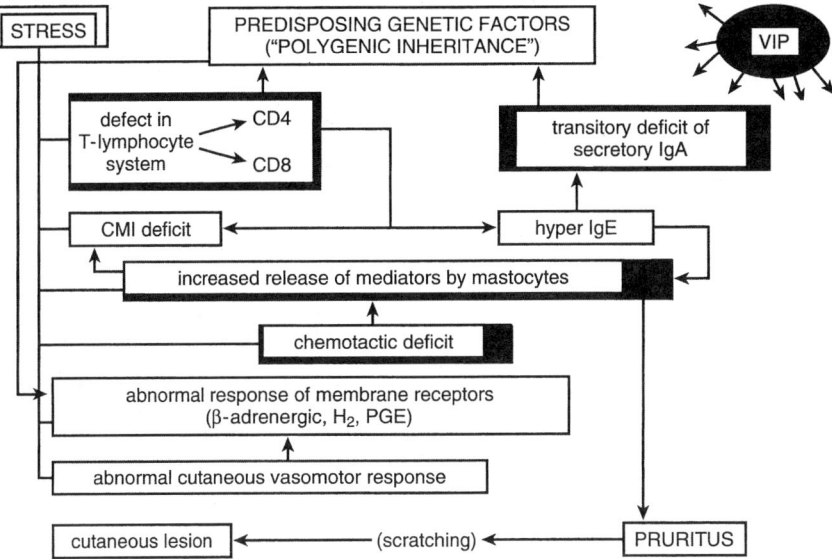

FIGURE 5 VIP and AD. The possible points where VIP may play a role are marked in black. (From Ref. 14.)

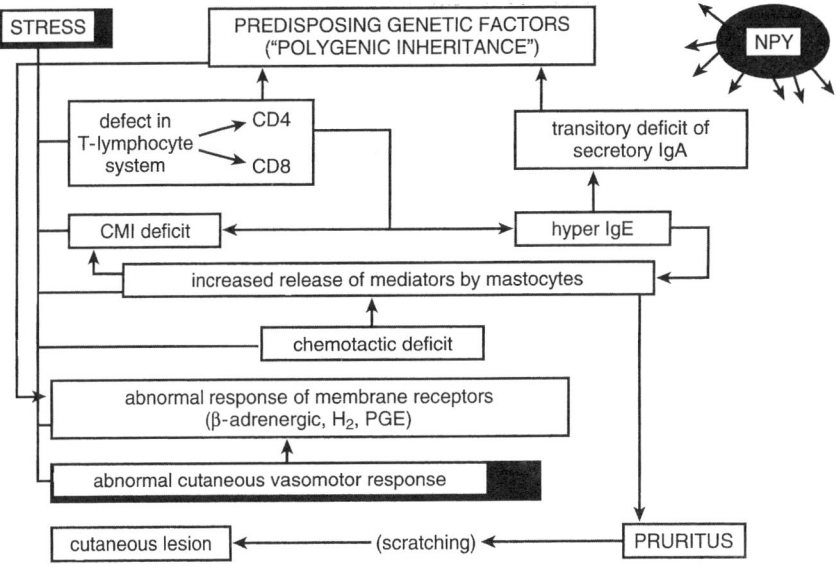

FIGURE 6 NPY and AD. The possible points where NPY may play a role are marked in black. (From Ref. 14.)

REFERENCES

1. Panconesi E, Hautmann G. Stress, stigmatization and psychogenic purpura. Int Angiol 1995; 14:130–137.
2. Panconesi E. Commentary. In: Panconesi E, ed. Stress and Skin Diseases: Psychosomatic Dermatology. Philadelphia: JB Lippincott, 1984:VIII–XIV.
3. Lewis T. Observation upon reaction of vessels in human skin to cold. Heart 1930; 15:177.
4. Jancso N, Jancso-Gabor A, Szolcsanyi J. Direct evidence for neurogenic inflammation and its prevention by denervation and by pretreatment with capsaicin. Br J Pharmacol 1967; 31:138–151.
5. Lotti T, Hautmann G, Panconesi E. Neuropeptides and skin. J Am Acad Dermatol 1995; 33:482–496.
6. Panconesi E, Hautmann G. Neuropeptides in psychosomatic dermatology. In Burgdorf WHC, Katz SI, eds. Dermatology: Progress and Perspectives. The Proceedings of the 18th World Congress of Dermatology, New York, June 12–18, 1992, pp 904–907.
7. Panconesi E, Hautmann G, Lotti T. Neuropeptides in skin: the state of the art. J Eur Acad Dermatol Venereol 1994; 3:109–115.
8. Blalock JE, Bost KL, Smith ME. Neuroendrocine peptide hormones and their receptors in the immune system production, processing and action. J Neuroimmunol 1985; 10:31–40.
9. Ironside W. Eczema, darkly mirror of the mind. Aust J Dermatol 1974; 15:5–9.
10. Rook A, Wilkinson DS. Psychocutaneous disorders. In: Rook A, Wilkinson DS, Ebling FJG, eds. Textbook of Dermatology. Oxford: Blackwell Scientific Publications 1979:2023–2035.
11. Obermayer ME. Psychocutaneous Medicine. Springfield, IL: Charles C Thomas, 1955.
12. Medansky RS, Handler RM. Dermatopsychosomatics: classification, physiology, and therapeutic approaches. J Am Acad Dermatol 1981; 5:125–136.
13. Eckert J. Diffuse hair loss and psychiatric disturbance. Acta Derm Venereol (Stockh) 1975; 55:147–149.
14. Panconesi E, Hautmann G. Psychophysiology of stress in dermatology. Dermatol Clin 1996; 14:399–421.
15. Arnetz BB, Fjellner B, Eneroth P, et al. Stress and psoriasis: psychoendocrine and metabolic reactions in psoriatic patients during standardized stressor exposure. Psychosom Med 1985; 47:528–541.
16. Farber EM, Nall ML. The national history of psoriasis in 5600 patients. Dermatologica 1974; 148:1–18.
17. Braun-Falco O, Burg G, Farber EM. Psoriasis: Eine Fragebogen-Studie bei 536 Patienten. Münch Med Wochenschr 1972; 114:1–15.
18. Fava CA, Perini CI, Santonastaso P, Fornasa CV. Life events and psychological distress in dermatological disorders: psoriasis, chronic urticaria, and fungal infections. Br J Med Psychol 1980; 53:277–282.
19. Seville RH. Psoriasis and stress. Br J Dermatol 1977; 97:297–302.

20. Raychaudhuri SP, Gross J. Psoriasis risk factors: role of lifestyle practices. Cutis 2000; 66:348–352.

21. Farber EM, Nickoloff BJ, Recht B, Fraki JE. Stress, symmetry, and psoriasis: possible role of neuropeptides. J Am Acad Dermatol 1986; 14:305–311.

22. Vaupel R, Jarry H, Schlomer HT, Wuttke W. Differential response of substance P containing subtypes of adrenomedullary cells to different stressors. Endocrinology 1988; 123:2140–2145.

23. Farber EM, Rein C, Lanigan SW. Stress and psoriasis. Psychoneuroimmunologic mechanisms. Int J Dermatol 1991; 30:8–12.

24. Luppi P, Levi-Montalcini R, Bracci-Laudiero L, Bertolini A, Arletti R, Tavernari D, Vigneti E, Aloe L. NGF is released into plasma during human preganancy: an oxytocin-mediated response? Neuroreport 1993; 4:1063–1065.

25. Maestripieri D, De Simone R, Aloe L, Alleva E. Social status and nerve growth factor serum levels after agonistic encounters in mice. Physiol Behav 1990; 47:161–164.

26. Aloe L, Levi-Mantalcini R. Mast cells increase in tissues of neonatal rats injected with the nerve growth factor. Brain Res 1977; 133:358–366.

27. Pearce FL, Thrompson HL. Some characteristics of histamine secretion from rat peritoneal mast cells stimulated with nerve growth factor. J Physiol 1977; 372:379–393.

28. Weddell G, Cowan MA, Palmer E, Ramaswamy S. Psoriatic skin. Arch Dermatol 1965; 91:252–266.

29. Naukkarinen A, Nickoloff BJ, Farber EM. Quantification of cutaneous sensory nerves and their substance P content in psoriasis. J Invest Dermatol 1989; 2:126–129.

30. Al'Abadie MSK, Senior HJ, Bleehen SS, Gawkrodger DJ. Neurogenic changes in psoriasis. An imunohistochemical study (abstr). J Invest Dermatol 1992; 98:535.

31. Naukkarinen A, Harvima IT, Aalto ML, Harvima RJ, Horsmanheimo M. Quantitative analysis of contact sites between mast cells and sensory nerves in cutaneous psoriasis and lichen planus based on histochemical double staining technique. Arch Dermatol Res 1991; 283:433–437.

32. Jiang WY, Raychaudhuri SP, Farber EM. Double labeled immunofluorescence study of cutaneous nerves in psoriasis. Intern J Dermatol 1988; 37:572–574.

33. Anand P, Springall DR, Blank MA, Sellu D, Polak JM, Bloom SR. Neuropeptides in skin disease: increased VIP in eczema and psoriasis but not axillary hyperhidrosis. BJ Dermatol 1991; 124:547–549.

34. Eedy DJ, Johnston CF, Shaw C, Buchanan KD. Neuropeptides in psoriasis: an immunocytochemical and radioimmunoassay study. J Invest Dermatol 1991; 96:434–438.

35. Pincelli C, Fantini F, Romualdi P, Sevignani C, Lesa C, Benassi L, Giannetti A. Substance P is diminished and VIP is augmented in psoriatic lesions and these peptides exert disparate effects on the proliferation of cultured human keratinocytes. J Invest Dermatol 1992; 98:421–427.

36. Wallengren J, Ekman R, Sunder F. Occurrence and distribution of nueropeptides in human skin. An immunochemical study of normal skin and blister fluid from inflamed skin. Acta Dermatol Venereol (Stockh) 1987; 67:185–192.

37. Naukkarinen A, Harvima I, Paukkonen K, Aalto ML, Horsmanheimo M. Immunohistochemical analysis of sensory nerves and neuropeptides and their contacts with mast cells in developing and mature psoriatic lesions. Arch Dermatol Res 1993; 285:341–346.

38. Chan J, Smoller BR, Raychauduri SP, Jiang WY, Farber EM. Intraepidermal nerve fiber expression of calcitonin gene-related peptide, vasoactive intestinal peptide and substance P in psoriasis. Arch Dermatol Res 1997; 289:611–616.

39. Haegerstrand A, Jonzon B, Dalsgaard CJ, Nilsson J. Vasoactive intestinal polypeptide stimulates cell proliferation and adenylate cyclase activity of cultured human keratinocytes. Proc Natl Acad Sci USA 1989; 86:5993–5996.

40. Wilkinson DI. Mitogenic effect of substance P and CGRP on keratinocytes. J Cell Biol 1989; 107:509a.

41. Rabier M, Wilkinson DI. Neuropeptides modulate leukotrine B4 mitogenicity toward cultured keratinocytes. Clin Res 1991; 39:536a.

42. Brody I. Mast cell degranulation in the evolution of acute eruptive guttate psoriasis vulgaris. J Invest Dermatol 1984; 82:460–464.

43. Cox AJ. Mast cells in psoriasis. In: Farber EM, Cox AJ, eds. Psoriasis. Proceedings of the Second International Symposium. New York: York Medical Books, 1976:36–37.

44. Erjavec F, Lembeck F, Florjanc-Irman T, Skofitsch G, Donnerer J, Saria A, Holzer P. Release of histamine by substance P. Arch Pharmacol 1981; 317:67–70.

45. Haegerstrand A, Dalsgaard CJ, Jonzon B, Larsson O, Nilsson J. Calcitonin gene-related peptide stimulates proliferation of human endothelial cells. Proc Natl Acad Sci USA 1990; 87:3299–3303.

46. Pinkus H, Mehregan AM. The primary histologic lesion of seborrheic dermatitis and psoriasis. J Invest Dermatol 1966; 46:109–116.

47. Ragaz A, Ackerman B. Evolution, motivation and regression of lesions of psoriasis. Am J Dermatopathol 1979; 1:199–214.

48. Sackstein R, Falanga V, Streilein JW, Chin YH. Lymphocyte adheision to psoriatic dermal endothelium is mediated by a tissue-specific receptor/ligand interaction. J Invest Dermatol 1988; 91:423–428.

49. Le Roy F, Brown KA, Graes MW. Blood mononuclear cells from patients with psoriasis exhibit an enhanced adherence to cultured vascular endothelium. J Invest Dermatol 1991; 97:511–516.

50. Sung CP, Arleth AJ, Aiyar N, Bhatnagar PK, Lysko PC, Feuerstein C. CGRP stimulates the adhesion of leukocytes to vascular endothelial cells. Peptides 1992; 13:429–434.

51. Rein C, Karasek M. Effect of substance P on adhesion of a human monocyte cell line to fibronectin. Clin Res 1992; 40:45a.

52. Matis WL, Lavker RM, Murphy CF. Substance P induces the expression of an endothelial-leukocyte adhesion molecule by microvascular endothelium. J Invest Dermatol 1990; 94:492–495.

53. Tomoe S, Iwamoto I, Tomioka H, Yoshida S. Comparison of substance P-induced and compound 48/80 induced neutrophil infiltrations in mouse skin. Int Arch Allergy Immunol 1992; 97:237–242.

54. Calvo CF, Chavanel C, Senica A. Substance P enhances interleukin-2 expression in activated human T cells. J Immunol 1992; 148:3498–3504.

55. Ansel J, Perry P, Brown J, Damm D, Phan T, Hart C, Luger T, Hefeneider S. Cytokine modulation of keratinocyte cytokines. J Invest Dermatol 1990; 94:101S–107S.

56. Smith CH, Barker JN, Morris RW, MacDonald DM, Lee TH. Neuropeptides induce rapid expression of endothelial cell adhesion molecules and elicit granulocytic infiltration in human skin. J Immunol 1993; 151:3274–3282.

57. Krogstad AL, Swanbeck G, Wallin G. Axon-reflex mediated vasodilatation in the psoriatic plaque? J Invest Dermatol 1995; 104:872–876.

58. Wardell K, Naver HK, Nilsson CE, Wallin BC. The cutaneous vascular axon reflex in humans characterized by laser doppler perfusion imaging. J Physiol (London) 1993; 460:185–199.

59. Farber EM, Lanigan SW, Boer J. The role of cutaneous sensory nerves in the maintenance of psoriasis. Int J Dermatol 1990; 29:418–420.

60. Raychaudhuri SP, Farber EM. Are sensory nerves essential for the pathogenesis of psoriasis? J Am Acad Dermatol 1993; 28:488–489.

61. Wyatt S, Shooeter EM, Davies AM. Expression of the NGF receptor gene in sensory neurons and their cutaneous targets prior to and during innervation. Neuron 1990; 421–427.

62. Lindsay RM, Harmar AI. Nerve growth factor regulates expression of neuropeptides genes in adult sensory neurons. Nature 1989; 337:362–364.

63. Schwartz J, Pearson J, Johnson E. Effect of exposure to anti-NGF on sensory neurons of adult rats and guinea pigs. Brain Res 1982; 244:378–381.

64. Raychaudhuri SP, Jiang WY, Farber EM. Psoriatic keratinocytes express high levels of nerve growth factor. Acta Dermatol Venereol 1998; 78:84–86.

65. Pincelli C, Haake AR, Benassi L, Grassilli E, Magnoni C, Ottani D, Polakowska R, Franceschi C, Giannetti A. Autocrine nerve growth factor protects human keratinocytes from apoptosis through its high affinity receptor (TRK): a role for BCL–2. J Invest Dermatol 1997; 109:757–764.

66. Wilkinson DI, Theeuwes MI, Farber EM. Nerve growth factor increases the mitogenicity of certain growth factors for cultured human keratinocytes: a comparison with epidermal growth factor. Exp Dermatol 1994; 3:239–245.

67. Lambiase A, Bracci-Laudiero L, Bonini S, Bonini S, Starace G, D'Elios MM, De Carli M, Aloe L. Human CD4 + T cell clones produce and release nerve growth factor and express high-affinity nerve growth factor receptors. J Allergy Clin Immunol 1997; 100:408–414.

68. Schall TJ. Biology of the RANTES/SIS cytokine family. Cytokine 1991;3:165–183.

69. Chang JCC, Smith LR, Froning KJ, Kurland HH, Schwabe BJ, Blumeyer KK, Karasek MA, Wilkinson DI, Farber EM, Carlo DJ, Borstoff SW. Persistence of T-cell clones in psoriatic lesions. Arch Dermatol 1997; 133:703–708.
70. Ansel JC, Kaynard AH, Armstrong CA, Olerud J, Bunnett N, Payan D. Skin-nervous system interactions. Dermatol Found 1995; 29:1–12.
71. Diamond J, Holmes M, Coughin M. Endogenous NGF and nerve impulses regulate the collateral sprouting of sensory axons in the skin of the adult rat. J Neurosci 1992; 12:1454–1466.
72. Aloe L, Alleva E, De Simone R. Changes of NGF level in mouse hypothalamus following intermale aggressive behavior: biological and imniunohistochemical evidence. Behav Res 1990; 39:53–61.
73. Wrone-Smith T, Nickoloff BJ. Dermal injection of immunocytes induces psoriasis. J Clin Invest 1996; 98:878–887.
74. Hautmann G, Panconesi E. Psychoimmunology in dermatology. In: Ich und die Haut. Kongress Arbeitskreis Psychosomatische Dermatologie, Giessen, Germany, September 23–25, 1994.
75. Hautmann G, Lotti T, Panconesi E. Neuropeptides and skin inflammation. In: Getting in Touch. 6th International Congress on Dermatology and Psychiatry, Amsterdam (Olanda), April 20–22, 1995, Abstract Book, p 44.
76. Panconesi E, Hautmann G. Aspectos psychosomaticos de la dermatitis atopica. Monograf Dermatol 1992; 5:428–439.
77. Panconesi E, Hautmann G. Neuropeptides in psychosomatic dermatology. In: Burgdorf WHC, Katz SI, eds. Dermatology: Progress and Perspectives. The Proceedings of the 18th World Congress of Dermatology, New York, June 12–18, 1992, pp 904–907.
78. Pauk J, Kuhn CM, Field TM, et al. Positive effect of tactile vs kinesthetic or vestibular stimulation on neuroendocrine and ornithine decarboxylase activity in maternally deprived rat pups. Life Sci 1986; 39:2081–2087.
79. Field TM, Schanberg SM, Scafid F, et al. Tactive kinesthetic stimulation effects on preterm neonates. Pediatrics 1986; 77:654–658.
80. Solomon CF, Levine S, Kraft JK. Early experience in immunity. Nature 1968; 220:821–822.
81. Harlow HF. Primary affectional patterns in primates. Am J Orthopsychiatry 1960; 30:676–677.
82. Miller H, Baruch DW. A study of hostility in allergic children. Am J Orthopsychiatry 1950; 20:506–519.
83. Kirshbaum BA. Eczema and Emotions. Kalamazoo, MI: Upjohn, 1982.
84. Slany E. Kinderpsychotherapie im Rahmen der Dermatologie. Hautartz 1975; 26:419–422.
85. Panconesi E. Stress and Skin Diseases. Psychosomatic Dermatology. Philadelphia: JB Lippincott, 1984:94–179.
86. Jordan JM, Whitlock FA. Emotions and the skin. The conditioning of scratch responses in case of atopic dermatitis. Br J Dermatol 1972; 86:574–585.
87. Fritz GK. Psychological aspects of atopic dermatitis. Clin Pediatr 1979; 18:360–364.

88. Stokes JH. The personality factor in psychoneurogenous reactions of the skin (AMA). Arch Dermatol Syphilol 1940; 42:780–801.
89. Musgrove K, Morgan JK. Infantile eczema: a longterm follow-up study. Br J Dermatol 1976; 95:365–372.
90. Brown DC. Emotional disturbance in eczema: a study of symptom-reporting behavior. J Psychosom Res 1967; 11:27–40.
91. McLaughlin JT, Shoemaker RJ, Guy WB. Personality factors in adult atopic eczema. Arch Dermatol 1953; 68:506–516.
92. Wtithlock RA. Psychophysiological Aspects of Skin Disease. Philadelphia: WB Saunders, 1976.
93. Champion RH, Parish WE. Atopic dermatitis. In: Rook A, Wilkinson DS, Ebling FJG, eds. Textbook of Dermatology. Oxford: Blackwell Scientific Publications, 1979:349–361.
94. Beerman H. Etiology and mechanisms of development of neurodermatitis. In: Nodene JH, Mayer JH, eds. Psychosomatic Medicine. London: Henry Kimpton, 1962.
95. Garrie EV, Garrie SA, Mote T. Anxiety and atopic dermatitis. J Consult Clin Psychol 1974; 42:742.
96. Jordan JM. Atopic dermatitis: anxiety and conditioned scratch responses. J Psychosom Res 1974; 18:297–299.
97. Giannetti A, Girolomoni G. Skin reactivity to neuropeptides in atopic dermatitis. Br J Dermatol 1989; 121:681–688.
98. Girolomoni G, Giannetti A. Neuropeptidi e cute. G Ital Dermatol Venereol 1989; 124:121–140.
99. Pincelli C, Fantini F, Massimi P, et al. Neuropeptides in skin from patients with atopic dermatitis: an immunohistochemical study. Br J Dermatol 1990; 122:745–750.

6

Psychoneuroendocrinimmunodermatology
Pathophysiological Mechanisms of Stress in Cutaneous Disease

Lee Thomas Zane
University of California, San Francisco
San Francisco, California, U.S.A.

INTRODUCTION

The role of stress in its various forms has been investigated in relation to a great number of cutaneous diseases (1). Such diseases as psoriasis, atopic dermatitis, urticaria, seborrheic dermatitis, alopecia areata, telogen effluvium, herpesvirus infection, pemphigus, acne vulgaris, lichen planus, vitiligo, aphthae, and acne rosacea have been reported to be associated with stress-induced exacerbations. Unfortunately, much of the data suggesting this postulated association is derived from anecdotal evidence, case series, and unconventional investigations. Picardi and Abeni (2) reviewed much of the extant literature on stressful life events and their role in skin disease with an emphasis on examining the scientific rigor of the available evidence. Though they found that many of the studies' methods for stress measurement did not meet rigorous standards, the role of stress in exacerbating psoriasis, atopic dermatitis, urticaria, and alopecia areata appeared clear. On the other hand, the contribution of stressful events to the worsening of vitiligo, lichen planus, acne, pemphigus, and seborrheic dermatitis remained less clear. This chapter will describe some of the fundamental physiological events of the stress response and elucidate a few mechanisms by which the stress response may potentially exacerbate such cutaneous diseases as psoriasis, recurrent herpes infection, and atopic dermatitis.

STRESS AND ADAPTATION

The link between the neuroendocrine and immunological systems during episodes of stress has been recognized for more than 60 years. The "general adaptation syndrome" described by Selye (3) proposes that organisms have the ability to adapt to acute changes in homeostasis, but that unrelenting challenges to that equilibrium lead to exhaustion of adaptive mechanisms and ultimately disease. Psychological distress, initially manifesting as anxiety, may lead to fear, anger, frustration, and ultimately helplessness. Ironically, the state of learned helplessness, which represents ultimate failure of adaptation, is nevertheless a powerful elicitor of the physiological stress response.

Stressors come in a number of varieties, including environmental, psychological, behavioral, and biological. The manner in which stressful stimuli are perceived and interpreted by the individual can significantly influence the nature of the response (physiological or pathological) to those stimuli at a systemic, regional, and local level. This chapter will review some of the physiological events associated with the stress response and propose some potential pathophysiological mechanisms underlying the relationship between stress and skin disease.

THE SYSTEMIC RESPONSE TO STRESS

Psychoneuroendocrinimmunology

The systemic response to stress is a complex and integrated multisystem reaction, which can be conceptualized in four primary stages: central nervous system (CNS) recognition, neuroendocrine response, systemic reactivity, and adaptation. Each stage may also be further subdivided into smaller constitutive phases (Fig. 1) (4).

The first stage of the systemic response to stress is that of CNS recognition. The initial phase of this stage is sensory perception. Mediated primarily by afferent sensory pathways, sensory perception begins with peripheral receptor organs (e.g., free nerve endings, Meissner's corpuscles,

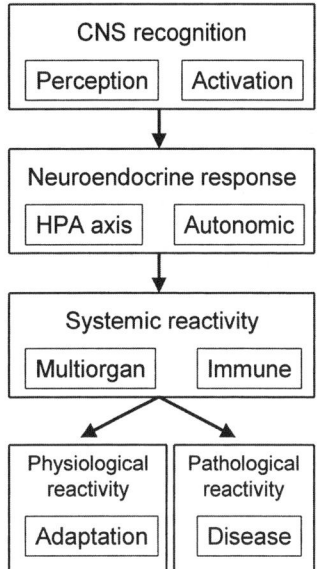

FIGURE 1 Stages of the systemic response to stress. HPA, hypothalamic-pituitary-adrenal axis. (Adapted from Ref. 4.)

retinal photoreceptors, Pacinian corpuscles) acquiring environmental stimuli. These stimuli are in turn relayed along the ascending spinal sensory pathways or cranial nerves to the appropriate areas of the sensory cortex.

Sensory information is then processed in the second element of the CNS recognition stage: the activation phase. Here, primary sensory stimuli are integrated with limbic input to produce active recognition of perceived sensations. While recognition can occur at either a subconscious or a cognitive level, stress is principally evoked by an organism's interpretation of an environmental stimulus as threatening, rather than by the character of the stimulus per se. That is to say, to one individual a particular stimulus may be perceived as a terrible threat, while to another that same stimulus may be seen as simply innocuous. Consider the example of a juvenile cheetah stalking through the grasslands of a savannah. While the nearby antelope perceives a life-threatening predator and prepares to spring away in a desperate dash for survival, the hulking rhinoceros remains largely unfazed by the cheetah's presence. In addition, the perception of stress may be largely dependent on the context in which the stimulus is presented. The sight of flashing police lights evokes a very different physiological response depending on whether one is seeing them in the rear view mirror of a speeding vehicle or one is noticing them coming to the aid of one's helplessly stalled vehicle.

Because a stimulus must be recognized as distressing in order to evoke a stress response, the idea of "mind over matter" becomes an inviting concept. That is, if an individual could be desensitized to stressful stimuli or trained to cope with adversity in an appropriate fashion so as to not interpret certain intense stimuli as threatening, would that empower the individual to avoid elicitation of the stress response? Certainly this is one of the aims of supportive psychotherapeutics, stress-coping workshops, and support groups (5).

The second stage of the systemic response to stress is the neuroendocrine response. At the heart of this response lies the hypothalamic-pituitary-adrenal (HPA) axis (reviewed in Ref. 6). When activated by such stimuli as perceived stress, parvicellular neurons in the hypothalamic paraventricular nuclei secrete corticotropin-releasing hormone (CRH) and arginine vasopressin (AVP) into the hypophyseal portal system down the pituitary stalk to the anterior pituitary. In the anterior adenohypophysis, corticotrophs are stimulated to release adrenocorticotropic hormone (ACTH) into the systemic circulation. Pituitary ACTH in turn stimulates the cells of the zona fasciculata of the adrenal cortex to secrete cortisol into the circulation. The increased levels of serum glucocorticoid serve a negative feedback function by inhibiting further production of ACTH by the anterior pituitary and CRH and AVP by the hypothalamic paraventricular nuclei.

Control of the HPA axis is also modulated by the autonomic nervous system, which may be activated concurrently during the neuroendocrine stage of the systemic stress response. The neurons of the locus ceruleus in the brain stem serve a key role in exerting control over these systems. In addition to maintaining reciprocal connections with the CRH- and AVP-secreting neurons in the paraventricular nuclei, the locus ceruleus also controls autonomic output by noradrenergic brain stem nuclei. In response to signals from these noradrenergic nuclei, paraspinal sympathetic ganglia are activated to produce norepinephrine and neuropeptides, while the adrenal medulla is stimulated to secrete catecholamines into the circulation.

In general, the autonomic stress system is activated by serotonergic and cholinergic input and inhibited by the γ-aminobutyric acid (GABA)/benzodiazepine (BDZ) system and proopiomelanocortin (POMC) peptides. POMC peptidergic neurons in the arcuate nucleus maintain reciprocal connections with the CRH-secreting neurons of the hypothalamic paraventricular nuclei as well as innervations to pain control areas of the hindbrain and spinal cord, thus exerting another level of modulation of the HPA axis as well as effecting the analgesic enhancement seen in periods of systemic stress.

This physiological surge of combined endocrine and autonomic output results in the third stage of the systemic stress response: multisystem reactivity. Increased sympathetic output shifts the physiology of a number of organ systems to a state of increased reactivity, producing the "fight-or-flight" response. In addition, the neuroendocrine component of the systemic stress response has profound effects on immune regulation. The immuno-modulatory effects of glucocorticoids, catecholamines, and neuropeptides, such as those elaborated in response to stress, will be discussed in greater detail in subsequent sections of this chapter.

The final stage of the systemic stress response can be referred to as adaptation. Representing the overall response of the organism to multi-system reactivity, adaptation is the product of appropriate physiological changes that result from having successfully endured the stress reaction. The adapted state increases the ability of the same organism to overcome subsequent stresses of a similar nature. On the other hand, inappropriate physiological responses and pathological reactivity to the stress response lead to exhaustion and the development or exacerbation of disease.

Thus, the systemic response to stress is a coordinated multistep process in which sequential events produce a multiorgan state of heightened activation. Initiated by the perception of a stimulus or set of stimuli as endangering, a stress response is elicited, producing a cascade of endocrine and neural signals leading to increased plasma cortisol and catecholamines. These soluble mediators act body-wide to produce a fight-or-flight response state as well as an altered immune microenvironment. These conditions can be overcome by physiological adaptation, or the organism can succumb to this state of adversity in a pathological fashion producing disease.

Trimodal Immunomodulation

Effects of the systemic stress response on the immune system appear to be variable. While it has generally been demonstrated that chronic stress tends to produce an immunosuppressive effect (7), it has been argued that acute stress actually leads to an enhanced level of skin immune function (8). In addition, several disease states in both humans and mice appear to be related to a dampened endocrine response to stress (9). Thus, modulation of the immune system during periods of duress may depend largely on both the chronicity and quality of the systemic stress response. It is therefore inviting to consider that the immune system can be modulated in a trimodal fashion dependent on the whether the nature of the stress response is acute, chronic, or blunted (Fig. 2).

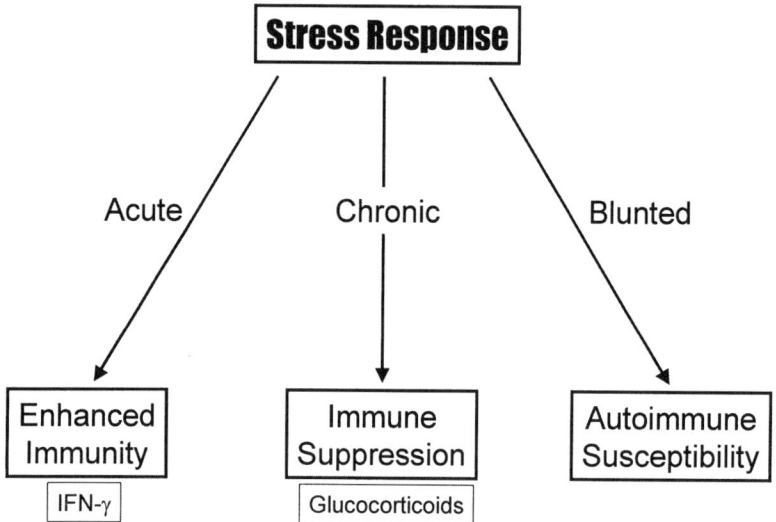

FIGURE 2   Trimodal immunomodulation by stress. Immunomodulatory effects may be dependent upon both the chronicity and character of the stress response. While acute stress appears to promote a state of immunoenhancement, likely mediated by IFN-γ, the immunosuppressive effects of chronic stress may be due in large part to the actions of glucocorticoids. In addition, organisms with blunted HPA axis function may exhibit yet a third type of stress-related immunomodulation that increases their susceptibility to autoimmune or inflammatory disease.

Acute Response: Immunoenhancement

Dhabhar and McEwen (10) investigated skin immune function during acute (1–4 hours) stress in rodents by examining their level of contact sensitivity in eliciting a delayed–type hypersensitivity (DTH) reaction. Animals subjected to acute stressors were found to demonstrate more intense contact sensitivity reactions than controls. Leukocyte recruitment, distribution, and migration to sites of inflammation were thought to be central to the observed immunoenhancement (11). Subsequent studies also supported the role of interferon (IFN)-γ in stress-induced skin immunoenhancement by comparing DTH responses in IFN-γ receptor–deficient knockouts with those in wild-type mice (12). IFN-γ receptor–deficient mice failed to show the stress-induced enhancement of skin DTH reactions seen in wild-type mice. Thus, according to this paradigm, acute stress hormones and catecholamines are postulated to potentiate the effects of IFN-γ on monocytes leading to enhanced cell-mediated immunity (CMI) functions such as antigen presentation, leukocyte recruitment, leukocyte activation, and effector cell function, producing overall immunoenhancement.

The concept of immunoenhancement during the acute stress response may help to reconcile two troubling paradoxes (10): 1) What evolutionary advantage is conferred by suppressing immune function during a period when survival is acutely threatened (e.g., risk of wounding by an assailant or predator)? and 2) If prior notions of acute stress being purely immunosuppressive were true, why are inflammatory immune-mediated diseases such as psoriasis and atopic dermatitis exacerbated during an acute stress reaction? The latter question is addressed later in this chapter.

Chronic Response: Immunosuppression

Unlike acute stress, chronic psychological stress is well known to have overall immunosuppressive effects, the key mediator of which appears to be endogenous glucocorticoids. The anti-inflammatory effects of glucocorticoids are wide-ranging at pharmacological and stress doses, suppressing such immune phenomena as 1) leukocyte adhesion, margination, and migration, 2) B-cell maturation and plasma cell antibody production, 3) macrophage activation and antigen presentation, and 4) T-cell activation, receptor expression, proliferation, differentiation, and cytotoxicity (9).

At physiological levels, glucocorticoids have been demonstrated to serve an immunomodulatory function as well, causing a shift in cytokine milieu from one promoting cell-mediated immunity (CMI; Th1) to one enhancing humoral (Th2) immunity (13). By way of review of this immunological dichotomy, T-helper lymphocytes are subclassified as Th0 (naive; non–antigen educated), Th1, and Th2 (Fig. 3). Th0 cells can be stimulated to differentiate into Th1 cells by interleukin (IL)-12. Th1 cells then secrete IL-2, IFN-γ, and transforming growth factor (TGF)-β, creating a cytokine milieu supportive of a CMI response, wherein cytotoxic T cells, natural killer (NK) cells, and activated macrophages are stimulated. IL-2 stimulates clonal expansion of Th1 cells, while IFN-γ and IL-12 serve the additional function of suppressing the antagonistic Th2 immune response. Th2 cells are the product of Th0 cells induced to differentiate by IL-4. This subset of cells in turn principally secretes IL-4, IL-10, and IL-13, a cytokine profile that promotes humoral immunity by stimulating B cells to undergo differentiation, immunoglobulin isotype switching (to IgE), and production of antibody. IL-4 and IL-10 also serve to antagonize the Th1 immune response. Glucocorticoids appear to mediate the switch from Th1 to Th2 by suppressing the effects of IL-12, the cytokine chiefly responsible for promoting the Th1 response and inhibiting the Th2 response. Glucocorticoids

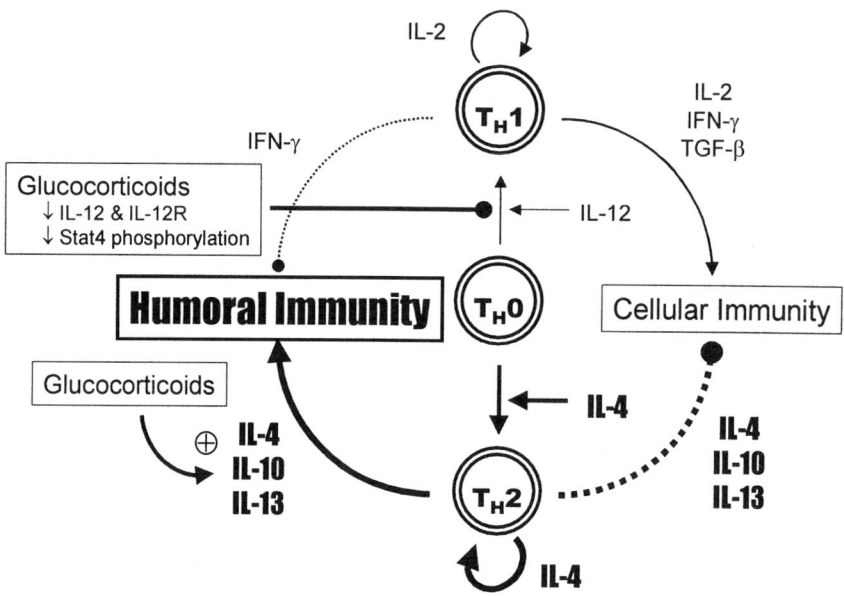

FIGURE 3 Glucocorticoids modulate a cytokine shift in favor of humoral immunity. Glucocorticoids inhibit the expression of interleukin (IL)-12 and its receptor (IL-12R) by T and natural killer (NK) cells and suppress IL-12–induced phosphorylation of Stat4, a key transcription factor in the expression such Th1 cytokines as interferon (IFN)-γ. Glucocorticoids also appear to potentiate the secretion of key Th2 cytokines, such as IL-10. Lines with round termini denote inhibitory action. TGF, transforming growth factor. (Adapted from Ref. 9.)

have been demonstrated to inhibit IL-12 production (13), downregulate IL-12 receptor expression by T and NK cells (14), and suppress IL-12–induced phosphorylation of Stat4, a key transcription factor in the expression such Th1 cytokines as IFN-γ (15). Further, glucocorticoids appear to potentiate the secretion of key Th2 cytokines, such as IL-10 (16). Catecholamines released during the sympathetic phase of the systemic stress response also appear to promote a shift in the cytokine profile from Th1 to Th2. Catecholamines are thought to elicit this shift via inhibition of IL-12 production and enhancement of IL-10 secretion, an effect believed to be mediated by β-adrenoreceptors on Th1 cells (17). Catecholamines are described to exert a tonic inhibition of Th1 immunity, with β-adrenoreceptor antagonists capable of releasing that suppression and hence promoting Th2 immunity (18).

Blunted Response: Altered HPA Axis Function

A third mode of immunomodulation in response to stress is seen in organisms with impaired HPA axis function, a condition that has been associated with increased susceptibility to inflammatory and autoimmune diseases. Animal studies have demonstrated a correlation between altered HPA axis responses and several inflammatory diseases in the chicken [spontaneous thyroiditis and avian scleroderma (19)], mouse [systemic lupus erythematosus, tuberculosis, and viral infections (20)], and rat [arthritis, experimental allergic encephalitis, and septic shock (21)]. Many of the rat studies have compared two particular inbred rat strains: the Lewis (LEW/N) rat, which has an impaired HPA axis and a blunted sympathetic noradrenergic response to inflammatory and stress stimuli, and the Fischer (F344/N) rat, which has an augmented HPA axis response and demonstrates relative resistance to developing inflammatory disease. The HPA axis defect in Lewis rats appears to lie in the hypothalamus as transplantation of hypothalamic tissue from Fischer rats into the third ventricle of Lewis rats restores their HPA axis responsiveness and abrogates their susceptibility to inflammatory disease (22).

Classes of human diseases that have been associated with depressed HPA axis function include allergic [asthma, atopic dermatitis (23)]; autoimmune [rheumatoid arthritis (24), systemic lupus erythematosus (25), Sjögren's syndrome (26)]; fatigue states [burn-out, posttraumatic stress disorder, fibromyalgia (27), chronic fatigue syndrome (28)]; and psychiatric (atypical depression) (reviewed in Ref. 29). How an impaired HPA axis figures into the pathophysiology of these disease states has not been fully elucidated, but animal and ex vivo studies suggest that resultant glucocorticoid receptor dysfunction on effector cells may contribute to the immune dysfunction (30,31).

Stress, Glucocorticoids, and the Skin Permeability Barrier

In addition to the immunomodulatory functions previously discussed, systemic glucocorticoids appear to have direct effects on cutaneous permeability barrier homeostasis. Denda et al. (32) demonstrated that hairless mice subjected to the stress of prolonged overcrowding exhibited altered skin barrier recovery kinetics as evaluated by tape stripping and measured transepidermal water loss. In a subsequent study, mice injected with corticosterone as well as those subjected to the stress of prolonged overcrowding were observed to have similar increases in serum cortisol levels and impairment of skin barrier recovery kinetics (33). Pretreatment of mice with the anxiolytic chlorpromazine prior to being placed in overcrowded conditions, however, dampened the production of serum cortisol and significantly reduced the adverse effects on skin barrier function, suggesting that the observed barrier impairment was due to psychological stress. When mice were pretreated with the glucocorticoid receptor antagonist RU-486 prior to either injection with corticosterone or exposure to an overcrowded environment, barrier impairment was blocked, suggesting that systemic glucocorticoids were responsible for producing the altered skin barrier function seen in prolonged psychological stress.

A similar phenomenon has been observed in humans during periods of psychological stress. Garg et al. (34) followed a cohort of health care students, measuring their stress levels and skin barrier recovery kinetics during various periods of the academic year. During the relatively low-stress period of winter vacation, baseline psychometric analyses and skin barrier studies were performed. These studies were repeated on the same students during the period of their final exams and demonstrated high levels of stress and skin barrier disruption, with impairment of barrier recovery kinetics paralleling psychological stress scores. Subsequently, when this same cohort was examined during their spring vacation, psychological stress scores returned to baseline and skin barrier recovery kinetics normalized. Cortisol levels were not examined in these subjects because previous studies had demonstrated that salivary and serum cortisol levels have not been well correlated to alterations in psychological stress despite clinically different outcomes (35).

Because such inflammatory skin diseases as psoriasis and atopic dermatitis are associated with impaired skin barrier function and exacerbation of clinical disease by psychological stress, these studies may offer adjunctive clues to elucidating the complex pathophysiology of these conditions and the role of psychological stress in their natural history.

NEUROPEPTIDES: LOCAL AND REGIONAL NEUROIMMUNOLOGICAL STRESS MEDIATORS

In addition to their function as the initial relay segment of the somatic afferent sensory pathway, cutaneous nerves also serve as an important source of peripherally secreted neuropeptides [reviewed extensively by Scholzen et al. (36)]. The predominant neuronal population responsible for the synthesis and secretion of skin neuropeptides is a subset of the afferent unmyelinated C fibers characterized as polymodal C nociceptors. In addition, a much smaller proportion of cutaneous neuropeptide is synthesized by small myelinated fibers, which function primarily as mechanoheat receptors, designated Aδ fibers (37). Epidermal nerves exhibit a different immunoreactivity profile of neuropeptide receptor from dermal nerves (38).

In addition to sensory neurons, there are a host of other sources of neuropeptides in the skin, including keratinocytes, melanocytes, endothelial cells, and a wide variety of immune cells (36). Neuropeptide-secreting immune cells include those resident to the skin (e.g., monocytes, macrophages) as well as those that infiltrate the skin under inflammatory conditions (e.g., lymphocytes, neutrophils, and eosinophils). The multitude of neuropeptide sources creates a complex interconnected network of cellular interactions which modulate tissue inflammation.

Neuropeptides themselves are a diverse group of small peptides fewer than 40 amino acids in length with diverse biological actions. Some of the best studied skin neuropeptides include the tachykinins [substance P (SP), neurokinin A (NKA), neurokinin B (NKB)], calcitonin gene–related peptide (CGRP), somatostatin, vasoactive intestinal peptide (VIP), neuropeptide Y (NPY), atrial natriuretic peptide (ANP), and proopiomelanocortin (POMC) peptides such as α- and γ-melanocyte–stimulating hormone (MSH) and β-endorphin.

The tachykinins are a class of peptides containing a conserved C-terminal sequence and include such neuropeptides as SP, NKA, and NKB. Derived from precursor preprotachykinin molecules, the tachykinins are primarily synthesized by neurons in the dorsal root ganglia (DRG) and conveyed out to the periphery by retrograde axonal transport. The sensory cutaneous nerves that secrete substance P in the skin appear to be those associated with dermal vessels and adnexae (39). Cutaneous mast cells, eosinophils, and macrophages also secrete substance P. A wide variety of soluble mediators appear to modulate the secretion of tachykinins, including interleukins, neurotrophic factors, and inflammatory stimulators such as lipopolysaccharide (40,41).

Tachykinins are recognized by G-protein cell-surface receptors, which modulate a number of biological effects. Largely secreted by nociceptive C-polymodal fibers, SP is classically associated with eliciting the cutaneous "triple response" in the skin (edema, pruritus, and erythema), achieving this largely through the stimulation of mast cells to release histamine and tumor necrosis factor alpha (TNF-α) (42). In addition to stimulating monocytes to secrete the proinflammatory and chemotactic interleukins 1, 6, and 8, SP also promotes inflammation by directly inciting the cutaneous microvasculature to undergo vasodilation, neovascularization, and increased expression of adhesion molecules, enhancing migration of circulating immune effector cells into the peripheral tissues (43–46). SP also has direct stimulatory effects on lymphocytes, activating T cells to proliferate via autocrine IL-2 (47–49) and inducing B cells to differentiate (50,51). Keratinocytes are stimulated by

SP in multiple ways, including upregulating their expression of neurotrophins (52) and proinflammatory cytokines (IL-1 and IL-8) (53,54) as well as enhancing their proliferation (54,55). SP also induces the proliferation and migration of dermal fibroblasts (56–58) and neovascularlization by endothelial cells (58). Thus, through the induction of multiple inflammatory cytokines, activation of lymphocytes, recruitment of immune cells to tissues, and promotion of cellular proliferation, SP plays a central role in producing and augmenting cutaneous neurogenic inflammation.

Neuronal stores of such neuropeptides as SP and CGRP can be depleted through the application of capsaicin, the active chemical in hot chili peppers. Capsaicin depolarizes sensory nerve terminals causing them to release these neuropeptides, producing an initially highly inflammatory state followed by an insensitive state where these same nerve terminals are desensitized to subsequent stimulation. It is believed that capsaicin exerts its effects on sensory nerves via the vanilloid receptor-1 (59).

α-CGRP is a 37-amino-acid peptide found predominantly in free nerve endings or sensory neurons associated with vascular smooth muscle in the skin. CGRP immunoreactivity is also exhibited by keratinocytes, Langerhans cells, melanocytes, mast cells, and Merkel cells. Elevated levels of CGRP are found in tissues following psychic stress and in psoriatic plaques (60,61).

CGRP is a potent vasodilator of both small and large vessels as well as a stimulator of neovascularization and IL-8 secretion by endothelial cells. Similar to SP, CGRP induces mast cell degranulation, leading to histamine release and TNF-α secretion. CGRP also impairs antigen presentation by dermal macrophages and dendritic Langerhans cells through the down-regulation of B7-2, the costimulatory molecule necessary for MHC-antigen recognition by T cells (62,63). In addition, Langerhans cells are stimulated by CGRP to secrete IL-10, a key mediator in the promotion of an "anti-inflammatory" Th2 cytokine milieu (63). CGRP is chemotactic for polymorphonuclear cells and mitogenic for both melanocytes and keratinocytes (64,65).

VIP is expressed by cutaneous nerve fibers associated with dermal vessels, adnexae, and Merkel cells. Receptors for VIP have been detected on keratinocytes, eccrine glandular epithelium, and immune cells (66). Like CGRP and SP, VIP contributes to the edema, erythema, and pruritus of neurogenic inflammation, a process believed to be mediated via mast cell histamine release and/or induction of nitric oxide synthesis by perivascular neurons (67). VIP is also mitogenic for keratinocytes (66) and is overexpressed in psoriatic plaque skin (68). In addition, VIP may serve a neurotrophic function, promoting nerve regeneration and growth (69,70).

Somatostatin has been localized to keratinocytes, Merkel cells, suprabasal Langerhans cells, dermal dendritic cells, and eccrine epithelium.

Somatostatin expression has been shown to be significantly decreased in skin from patients with atopic dermatitis (71). Much of the literature on somatostatin has focused on its inhibitory properties on exo- and endocrine secretion from gastrointestinal organs and its antiproliferative properties on cancer cells and T lymphocytes. In the skin, however, somatostatin may play a more stimulatory role, inducing the release of histamine by mast cells and the recruitment of monocytes to sites of inflammation (72).

Proopiomelanocortin is a large precursor peptide from which are derived such bioactive peptides as α-, β-, and γ-MSH, ACTH, and β-endorphin. POMC peptides are recognized by G-protein melanocortin receptors found on various cutaneous cells. Overall, the immunomodulatory effects of ACTH and α-MSH appear to be inhibitory in nature. They induce macrophages to secrete the Th2 cytokine IL-10 (73) as well as decrease their expression of B7-2, a necessary costimulatory molecule for antigen presentation and MHC recognition (74). α-MSH also appears to exert an anti-inflammatory effect via downregulation of NF-κB transcription of pro-inflammatory cytokines (75–77). Together, the POMC peptides impair contact hypersensitivity reactions. The cutaneous immunomodulatory functions of α-MSH are extensively reviewed by Luger et al. (78).

In summary, neuropeptides produced in response to stress appear to play a central role in mediating local neuroimmune reactions in the skin. Their varied cellular sources of secretion and multitude of biological functions allow for complex immunomodulatory interactions, which likely underlie much of the pathophysiology of several inflammatory skin diseases and their exacerbation by psychological stress.

STRESS AND RECURRENT HERPES SIMPLEX VIRUS INFECTION

The effects of stress on acute viral infections have been a common subject in the neuroimmunological literature [reviewed by Biondi and Zannino (79)]. Psychological stress has been shown to be associated with increased rates of rhinovirus infection as well as higher susceptibility to rates of influenza virus respiratory infection and clinical colds (80,81). One of the most well-studied associations of stress and viral infection is the link between psychological stress and recurrent herpes outbreaks.

There are three characteristic stages of herpes simplex virus (HSV) infection. The primary stage begins with inoculation of the skin with the herpes virus particle. The virus can form superficial vesicles teeming with viral particles, which can be shed. The virus migrates along sensory nerve fibers to take up residence in sensory ganglia, such as the dorsal root ganglia

(DRG). Once the host's CMI gains control of the peripheral infection, the skin manifestations clear and the infection enters the latent phase. During this phase, the virus remains quiescent in the DRG. Subsequently, in response to an inciting stimulus (e.g., psychological stress, sunlight), the infection enters the recurrent phase wherein the virus escapes from the DRG and migrates back out along nerve fibers to again infect the skin, forming vesicles and shedding viral particles into the environment.

The psychosocial factors implicated in triggering herpes recurrences are controversial and wide-ranging, including such precipitants as psychiatric illness [e.g. depression (82)], life events, unhappiness, and disgust (83). Psychological factors have also been found to be more predictive of the symptom severity of an outbreak than somatic indices such as duration of recurrences and number of lesions per recurrence (84). It has also been proposed that patient personality and coping methods are more important factors in the association between HSV and stress than the actual level of psychological stress itself (85). It also deserves mention that several studies point out exceptions to the link between psychosocial stress and recurrence of herpetic infection. Daily stress has been shown not to be predictive of genital herpes recurrences (86,87), and psychological stress does not appear to be associated with recurrences of ophthalmalogical HSV recurrences (88). Others assert that the causal relationship between stress and genital herpes recurrences is not a direct one. Instead, it has been proposed that psychosocial stress predisposes individuals to more generalized illnesses, which in turn permit recurrence (89). In either case, the psychological consequences of recurrent genital herpes are significant, and psychosocial management has been emphasized as important adjunctive therapy to biological treatments (90,91).

Several studies have examined the nature of the reaction by which stress appears to provoke recurrence of herpes infection. In one of the more compelling studies, Cohen and colleagues (86) prospectively examined the association of stress with recurrent genital herpes infection. A cohort of 58 women with a history of recurrent genital herpes were followed for a period of 6 months. These women were evaluated weekly for stress and mood variables and monthly for life change events. Participants were asked to maintain daily diaries to document any genital herpes recurrences, and, when possible, confirmatory medical examination was performed to verify patients' reported outbreaks (conducted in about 50% of cases). Examination of the association between stress and mood variables with the recurrences of genital herpes revealed several important findings. First, it was observed that recurrences occurred in the week following, not immediately after, the inciting psychological stressor. Second, the only stress or mood variable found to be significantly associated with genital herpes outbreak was persistent (>7 days duration) psychological stress (e.g., worry about a sister who is pregnant, single and alone; prolonged financial uncertainty; caring for an elder with Alzheimer's disease). The odds ratio correlated to an approximately 8% increased risk of recurrence in the subsequent week for each point increase in perceived psychological stress (on a 7-point scale). Short-term stress, mood, anger, anxiety, acute life change events, and menstrual period were not found to be predictive of recurrence in this study.

In an equally intriguing study, McKenna and colleagues (92) compared the immune responses between two cohorts of patients: those with frequent (>10 outbreaks per year) and those with infrequent (>4 outbreaks per year) orolabial herpes recrudescences. Through the examination of plasma and peripheral blood leukocytes in vitro, HSV-specific and nonspecific immune profiles were determined. Compared to those patients with infrequent outbreaks, patients who experienced frequent orolabial herpes recrudescences were found to produce more HSV-specific IgE, exhibit a blunted lymphocyte proliferation response, and secrete less IFN-γ following exposure to HSV in vitro. These findings support the notion that patients experiencing frequent orolabial herpes recurrences have a blunted Th1 (CMI/antiviral) immune response to HSV exposure.

From these studies, a potential paradigm for persistent stress-induced HSV recurrences emerges wherein the central mechanism is one of loss of antiviral control. As Cohen and colleagues demonstrated, persistent stress is predictive of herpes recurrence. Unlike short-term stress, persistent stress leads to a chronic stress response, largely mediated by endogenous corticosteroids. As mentioned previously, one of the fundamental immunomodulatory effects of chronic corticosteroids is induction of a cytokine profile shift from the cellular/antiviral Th1 state to one more supportive of humoral immunity (Th2). This shift leads to loss of antiviral control allowing for viral reactivation in the dorsal root ganglion. Subsequently, as McKenna and colleagues described, the host at risk for frequent herpes recrudescences can only mount a blunted CMI response, insufficient to contain the viral reactivation, ultimately allowing the virus to migrate to the periphery and produce cutaneous vesicles and viral shedding. While this proposed paradigm likely oversimplifies the intricate immunomodulatory signaling involved in the recurrence of herpes simplex viral infection, it provides a basic framework for loss of antiviral control, which is fundamental to the pathophysiology of viral reactivation and recurrent infection.

Several other actions of glucocorticoids may also be at work in eliciting HSV recurrence. In addition to their immunosuppressive effects, glucocorticoids may also promote reactivation of HSV on a molecular level by inducing cAMP-modulating adrenergic receptors or activating the HSV replication origin (oriL) (93). On the other hand, glucocorticoids also appear to play a protective role in reducing cytokine-mediated cell lethality in adrenalectomized mice during acute viral infection (94).

STRESS AND PSORIASIS

Psoriasis is a complex multifactorial disease, which is characterized by symmetrical, scaling, indurated plaques produced in large part by the activity of hyperproliferative keratinocytes. Stress and lifestyle practices have been described to play an important role in the variable clinical course of the disease (95,96).

Much of the recent literature has focused on the important role played by T lymphocytes in the pathogenesis of psoriasis, and rational modulation of T-cell activity has been the goal of many of the new biological therapeutic agents (144,145). This portrayal of psoriasis as an autoimmune inflammatory disease, however, is controversial and has led to much resistance from a few academic camps, which point to such etiologies as bacterial infection and neurogenic inflammation (97).

Farber and colleagues (98,99) have been the strongest proponents of the neurogenic inflammation hypothesis of psoriasis. They find that the T-cell paradigm of psoriasis alone fails to explain some of the most salient features of the disease, including the Köbner phenomenon, symmetrical distribution of lesions, increased nerve density in psoriatic lesions, increased neuropeptide expression in psoriatic plaques, and the clinical clearance of psoriatic plaques in anesthetic areas following sensory nerve injury.

Central to the neuroimmunological model of psoriasis is the role of nerve growth factor (NGF), a neurotrophic factor that is upregulated along with its receptor in both lesional and nonlesional keratinocytes of psoriatics (100,101). NGF is also produced in increasing amounts in response to stress (102). NGF is both neurotrophic (supportive of axonal growth) and neurotropic (providing directional guidance for axonal extension to targets) for neurons, and it exerts a variety of cellular effects in the skin. In addition to being directly mitogenic for keratinocytes (103), NGF is also capable of inducing the migration and degranulation of mast cells (104,105), a key proinflammatory step in the pathogenesis of neurogenic inflammation. Further, NGF has also been demonstrated to modulate T-cell activity in both a direct and an indirect fashion. In addition to stimulating T-cell proliferation through upregulation of IL-2 receptor (106), NGF has also been found to be overexpressed along with its high-affinity receptor in helper T-cell clones (107). Moreover, NGF has been demonstrated to induce keratinocytes to express the cytokine RANTES, which is activating and chemotactic for memory T cells, a subset of lymphocytes central to the T-cell paradigm of psoriasis (108,109).

A panoply of neuropeptides are also expressed in higher levels in psoriatic skin, including such key factors as substance P, CGRP, and VIP (61,68). Together with NGF, these neuropeptides exert cellular actions, which may help to explain the fundamental characteristic histological findings seen in psoriasis. The intracorneal collections of neutrophils (Munro microabscesses) may be produced by the chemotactic and activating action of CGRP on neutrophils either directly or through the expression of IL-8 (54,110,111). Similarly, NGF, substance P, CGRP, and VIP have all been demonstrated to be mitogenic for keratinocytes (55,103) and may also protect against apoptosis (112), potentially producing the high keratinocyte proliferation rate and epidermal hyperplasia seen in psoriatic skin. The vasoactive effects produced by NGF, substance P, and CGRP, either directly (43,113) or indirectly via mast cell degranulation, can account for the dilated vessels and edema seen in the papillary dermis of psoriatic plaques (114–116). Furthermore, the T-cell modulatory actions of NGF and substance P (chemotaxis, activation, proliferation, and TNF-α production) may produce the activated effector and memory T-cell infiltrates seen histologically in lesional skin (42,106,109).

Whatever the mechanisms may be which underlie stress-induced exacerbations of psoriasis, psychotherapeutic modalities are emerging as important adjunctive therapies in the management of psoriasis. Studies of hypnotherapy and cognitive-behavioral therapy with stress management have revealed significant clinical improvements when added to traditional dermatological therapy compared to standard treatments alone (117,118).

STRESS AND ATOPIC DERMATITIS

It is commonly held that psychological stress is associated with worsening of cutaneous lesions and symptom severity in atopic dermatitis. King and Wilson (119) used a diary technique to examine the nature of the relationship between psychological stress and the severity of atopic dermatitis. Their data suggest that this relationship may be a bi-directional one. That is, not only is psychological stress predictive of worsening atopic dermatitis, but exacerbation of atopic disease contributes significantly to a lowered stress threshold and heightened levels of psychological stress. The reciprocity of this relationship describes a circular pattern of worsening stress and disease. While some authors cite methodological shortcomings in limiting the interpretation of these data in regard to delineating causality

(120), they do not dispute that a clinical link exists between psychological stress and atopic dermatitis.

Nor is it disputed that the pathophysiology of atopic dermatitis is complex. Leung provides an excellent review of some of the proposed pathophysiological mechanisms of atopic dermatitis (121). The natural history of skin in atopic dermatitis can be described in pathological stages: uninvolved, acute, and chronic. Even in uninvolved skin of atopic patients, the cutaneous microenvironment maintains an immunological milieu that favors humoral immunity, rich in IgE, mast cells, eosinophils, and circulating Th2 lymphocytes. In the acute phase of atopic dermatitis, immune effector cells, already primed for humoral reactivity, are incited by the presence of antigen to elicit a considerable Th2 response. Antigen-exposed Langerhans cells present inciting antigen to circulating Th2 lymphocytes, which are activated to expand their populations, secrete Th2 cytokines [e.g., IL-4 and IL-5 (122)], promote IgE-mediated degranulation of mast cells, and recruit additional Th2 lymphocytes to sites of inflammation. As the inflammatory and irritative mechanical (scratching) stimuli persist, the reaction extends into the chronic phase. Here, macrophages, which have been accumulating in the inflamed tissues in response to epidermal chemokines, begin to secrete cytokines more supportive of a Th1 (CMI) response, especially IL-12. Thus, the acute and chronic stages of atopic dermatitis appear to be largely created by the dichotomatous nature of their cytokine profiles, with the acute phase predominantly Th2 and the chronic phase chiefly Th1. Hence, exacerbations of atopic dermatitis may largely represent a reversion of the cutaneous cytokine profile from the Th1 to the Th2 state, recapitulating the acute phase.

As discussed earlier in this chapter, one mechanism by which a Th1-to-Th2 shift can be educed is through the action of glucocorticoids. As also mentioned previously, atopic patients demonstrate abnormal regulation of their glucocorticoid regulation, exhibiting a blunted HPA axis response. Compared to controls, atopic patients display an altered 24-hour cortisol profile (123) and children with atopic dermatitis produce lower levels of cortisol in response to psychological stress tasks such as public speaking and mental arithmetic before an audience (23). Further, adult atopic patients injected with CRH were found to secrete attenuated levels of ACTH and cortisol compared to controls (124). In response to this blunted HPA axis reactivity and consequent lower circulating cortisol levels, one major physiological compensatory mechanism appears to be the upregulation of glucocorticoid receptors on peripheral leukocytes in atopic patients (125), resulting in effector cells which are potentially hyperreactive to glucocorticoid stimulation. Clinically, this may provide some physiological basis for the observed phenomena of atopic patients improving with lower doses of systemic steroids as well as their increased susceptibility to flares following withdrawal of the steroid. Thus, in spite of a blunted HPA axis response to stress, effector cells exquisitely sensitive to systemic glucocorticoid release may respond in a hyperreactive fashion to stress cortisol, accentuating the cytokine shift from the Th1 to the Th2 state, recreating the acute inflammatory stage characteristic of a dermatitic flare.

In addition to their effects on cytokine profiles, glucocorticoids also impair cutaneous barrier function homeostasis. As discussed earlier in this chapter, stress glucocorticoids can significantly alter the recovery kinetics of the skin barrier, resulting in increased susceptibility to cutaneous inoculation with environmental agents. This may play a significant role in the skin of atopic patients since pathogenic stimuli such as allergens (e.g., dust mites, dander), bacteria (e.g., *Staphylococcus aureus*), and viruses (e.g., HSV) have all been considered as potential precipitants of acute atopic dermatitis and elicitors of atopic flares.

Catecholamines and their metabolism may also play a significant role in atopic dermatitis. Atopic patients demonstrate a 2.5-fold higher mean concentration of plasma norepinephrine compared to controls as well as decreased levels of enzyme specific for the conversion of norepinephrine to epinephrine (126). Increased catecholamines have been shown to stimulate activity of intracellular type 4 phosphodiesterases (PDE4) via β_2-adreno-receptors, and young patients with atopic dermatitis have been demon-strated to have high levels of PDE4 activity (127). PDE4 degrades intracellular cAMP leading to secretion of IL-13 and IL-4 (128–131), potent Th2 cytokines. Blockade of PDE4 activity with specific inhibitors has likewise suppressed IL-13 secretion by peripheral blood mononuclear cells (132). Atopic patients display significantly enhanced levels of allergen-stimulated IL-13 secretion (133). Thus, the heightened catecholamine state in atopic patients, enhanced by sympathetic output from psychologic stress, may contribute significantly to the secretion of Th2 cytokines and exacerbation of disease.

The role of the cutaneous nervous system in atopic dermatitis is strongly suggested by one of the cardinal features of disease—pruritus, a sensation that can have multiple components in atopic disease (134). Modulated by unmyelinated sensory nerve fibers, the neurocutaneous mechanism of pruritus in atopic dermatitis is supported by the observed increased density and hypertrophy of immunoreactive nerve fibers in lesions of atopic dermatitis (135,136). The specific C-receptors for itch in human skin appear to have been identified by microneurography experiments on unmyelinated fibers in vivo (137). When activated, these histamine-sensitive unmyelinated C-fibers with slow conduction velocities and extensive innervation territories elicited local inflammatory reactions (axon reflex erythema). These local reactions are likely due in large part to antidromic axon potentials stimulating release of various neuropeptides, resulting in neurogenic inflammation of innervated tissues. Indeed, several neuropeptides, such as SP, CGRP, and VIP, have been identified in lesional skin of patients with atopic dermatitis (135,138,139).

The effects of sensory nerves on the neurocutaneous immune response have been partitioned into two phases: the acute vascular stage and the chronic cellular and regenerative stage (140). Much of the vasoactivity in the acute phase appears to be mediated by the effects of histamine released by tissue mast cells. Immobilization stress studies in rats have demonstrated that acute stress can trigger mast cell degranulation, a process mediated by such soluble factors as CRH, neurotensin, and SP (141). In addition to their ability to cause degranulation of mast cells, these neuropeptides also mediate effects on cutaneous vasculature, leukocyte adhesion and recruitment, antigen presentation, and lymphocyte differentiation and activation [reviewed by Scholzen et al. (36)]. In addition, VIP has mitogenic and immunomodulatory effects on keratinocytes, stimulating them to secrete such inflammatory cytokines as IL-6, IL-8, and RANTES (66). SP also appears to modulate production of such cytokines as IFN-γ and IL-4 in peripheral blood mononuclear cells isolated from patients with severe atopic dermatitis (142). As the role of neuropeptides and neurotrophins in atopic dermatitis gains importance in the pathophysiology of disease, attempts to correlate their levels to clinical disease have been made. Toyoda et al. (143) have found a strong positive correlation between plasma levels of SP and NGF with clinical disease severity as estimated by three different scoring systems compared to controls.

Thus, the mechanisms of stress induction of exacerbations of atopic dermatitis may be as complicated as those proposed for its natural pathophysiology. However, the role of stress glucocorticoids appears to be a central one, potentially mediating such effects as causing an overall shift in cytokine secretion from a Th1 to a Th2 profile as well as impairment of cutaneous barrier function homeostasis, promoting worsening pruritus and susceptibility to inoculation by allergens, bacteria, and viruses. These effects, coupled with the regional and local consequences of sympathetic catecholamines, neuropeptides, and neurotrophins, offer an attractive paradigm for the exacerbation of acute atopic dermatitis in response to psychological stress.

CONCLUSION

The association between psychological stress and the exacerbation of several dermatological conditions is well known. The stress response itself is a coordinated, multistep process, which challenges the physiological patterns of multiple organ systems, probably the most significant of which is the immune system. In the face of such systemic duress, an organism can either physiologically overcome the stress and adapt or succumb to physiological exhaustion, producing disease. The systemic, regional, and local reactions that comprise the stress response are interdependent and complex, but they offer some illuminating principles that may help to define the pathophysiology of stress-induced disease.

Although the extant literature has not yet crystallized the precise mechanisms by which psychoneuroendocrine modulation of the immune system affects dermatological disease, this research field is burgeoning with incisive questions and interdisciplinary potential. Studies that endeavor to draw causative associations between stress and disease face great methodological difficulties. Such challenges, however, provide just the sort of fertile ground that fosters the ingenuity necessary to develop truly innovative and creative research strategies. The field of psychoneuroendocrinimmunology holds tremendous promise and eagerly awaits additional mechanistic studies and rigorous clinical investigations. The field of psychocutaneous medicine may be the ideal setting for such breakthroughs to be realized.

REFERENCES

1. Al'Abadie MS, Kent GG, Gawkrodger DJ. The relationship between stress and the onset and exacerbation of psoriasis and other skin conditions. Br J Dermatol 1994; 130:199–203.
2. Picardi A, Abeni D. Stressful life events and skin diseases: disentangling evidence from myth. Psychother Psychosom 2001; 70:118–136.
3. Selye H. The general adaptation syndrome and the disease of adaptation. J Clin Endocrinol 1946; 6:117–230.
4. Panconesi E, Hautmann G. Psychophysiology of stress in dermatology. The psychobiologic pattern of psychosomatics. Dermatol Clin 1996; 14:399–421.
5. Spiegel D. Healing words: emotional expression and disease outcome. JAMA 1999; 281:1328–1329.
6. Chrousos GP. The hypothalamic-pituitary-adrenal axis and immune-mediated inflammation. N Engl J Med 1995; 332:1351–1362.
7. Agarwal SK, Marshall GD Jr. Stress effects on immunity and its application to clinical immunology. Clin Exp Allergy 2001; 31:25–31.

8. Dhabhar FS. Acute stress enhances while chronic stress suppresses skin immunity. The role of stress hormones and leukocyte trafficking. Ann NY Acad Sci 2000; 917:876–893.

9. Sternberg EM. Neuroendocrine regulation of autoimmune/inflammatory disease. J Endocrinol 2001; 169:429–435.

10. Dhabhar FS, McEwen BS. Stress-induced enhancement of antigen-specific cell-mediated immunity. J Immunol 1996; 156:2608–2615.

11. Dhabhar FS, Miller AH, McEwen BS, Spencer RL. Stress-induced changes in blood leukocyte distribution. Role of adrenal steroid hormones. J Immunol 1996; 157:1638–1644.

12. Dhabhar FS, Satoskar AR, Bluethmann H, David JR, McEwen BS. Stress-induced enhancement of skin immune function: a role for gamma interferon. Proc Natl Acad Sci USA 2000; 97:2846–2851.

13. Elenkov IJ, Chrousos GP. Stress, cytokine patterns and susceptibility to disease. Baillieres Best Pract Res Clin Endocrinol Metab 1999; 13:583–595.

14. Wu CY, Wang K, McDyer JF, Seder RA. Prostaglandin E2 and dexamethasone inhibit IL-12 receptor expression and IL-12 responsiveness. J Immunol 1998; 161:2723–2730.

15. Franchimont D, Galon J, Gadina M, Visconti R, Zhou Y, Aringer M, Frucht DM, Chrousos GP, O'Shea JJ. Inhibition of Th1 immune response by glucocorticoids: dexamethasone selectively inhibits IL-12-induced Stat4 phosphorylation in T lymphocytes. J Immunol 2000; 164:1768–1774.

16. Ramierz F, Fowell DJ, Puklavec M, Simmonds S, Mason D. Glucocorticoids promote a TH2 cytokine response by CD4 + T cells in vitro. J Immunol 1996; 156:2406–2412.

17. Hasko G, Szabo C, Nemeth ZH, Salzman AL, Vizi ES. Stimulation of beta-adrenoceptors inhibits endotoxin-induced IL-12 production in normal and IL-10 deficient mice. J Neuroimmunol 1998; 88:57–61.

18. Elenkov IJ, Chrousos GP. Stress hormones, Th1/Th2 patterns, pro/anti-inflammatory cytokines and susceptibility to disease. Trends Endocrinol Metab 1999; 10:359–368.

19. Wick G, Hu Y, Schwarz S, Kroemer G. Immunoendocrine communication via the hypothalamo-pituitary-adrenal axis in autoimmune diseases. Endocr Rev 1993; 14:539–563.

20. Lechner O, Hu Y, Jafarian-Tehrani M, Dietrich H, Schwarz S, Herold M, Haour F, Wick G. Disturbed immunoendocrine communication via the hypothalamo-pituitary-adrenal axis in murine lupus. Brain Behav Immun 1996; 10:337–350.

21. Jafarian-Tehrani M, Sternberg EM. Animal models of neuroimmune interactions in inflammatory diseases. J Neuroimmunol 1999; 100:13–20.

22. Misiewicz B, Poltorak M, Raybourne RB, Gomez M, Listwak S, Sternberg EM. Intracerebroventricular transplantation of embryonic neuronal tissue from inflammatory resistant into inflammatory susceptible rats suppresses specific components of inflammation. Exp Neurol 1997; 146:305–314.

23. Buske-Kirschbaum A, Jobst S, Psych D, Wustmans A, Kirschbaum C, Rauh W, Hellhammer D. Attenuated free cortisol response to psychosocial stress in children with atopic dermatitis. Psychosom Med 1997; 59:419–426.

24. Gutierrez MA, Garcia ME, Rodriguez JA, Mardonez G, Jacobelli S, Rivero S. Hypothalamic-pituitary-adrenal axis function in patients with active rheumatoid arthritis: a controlled study using insulin hypoglycemia stress test and prolactin stimulation. J Rheumatol 1999; 26:277–281.

25. Gutierrez MA, Garcia ME, Rodriguez JA, Rivero S, Jacobelli S. Hypothalamic-pituitary-adrenal axis function and prolactin secretion in systemic lupus erythematosus. Lupus 1998; 7:404–408.

26. Johnson EO, Vlachoyiannopoulos PG, Skopouli FN, Tzioufas AG, Moutsopoulos HM. Hypofunction of the stress axis in Sjögren's syndrome. J Rheumatol 1998; 25:1508–1514.

27. Crofford LJ, Pillemer SR, Kalogeras KT, Cash JM, Michelson D, Kling MA, Sternberg EM, Gold PW, Chrousos GP, Wilder RL. Hypothalamic-pituitary-adrenal axis perturbations in patients with fibromyalgia. Arthritis Rheum 1994; 37:1583–1592.

28. Demitrack MA, Dale JK, Straus SE, Laue L, Listwak SJ, Kruesi MJ, Chrousos GP, Gold PW. Evidence for impaired activation of the hypothalamic-pituitary-adrenal axis in patients with chronic fatigue syndrome. J Clin Endocrinol Metab 1991; 73:1224–1234.

29. Sternberg EM. Neural-immune interactions in health and disease. J Clin 1997; Invest 100:2641–2647.

30. Kellendonk C, Tronche F, Reichardt HM, Schutz G. Mutagenesis of the glucocorticoid receptor in mice. J Steroid Biochem Mol Biol 1999; 69:253–259.

31. Franchimont D, Louis E, Dupont P, Vrindts-Gevaert Y, Dewe W, Chrousos G, Geenen V, Belaiche J. Decreased corticosensitivity in quiescent Crohn's disease: an ex vivo study using whole blood cell cultures. Dig Dis Sci 1999; 44:1208–1215.

32. Denda M, Tsuchiya T, Hosoi J, Koyama J. Immobilization-induced and crowded environment-induced stress delay barrier recovery in murine skin. Br J Dermatol 1998; 138:780–785.

33. Denda M, Tsuchiya T, Elias PM, Feingold KR. Stress alters cutaneous permeability barrier homeostasis. Am J Physiol Regul Integr Comp Physiol 2000; 278:R367–372.

34. Garg A, Chren MM, Sands LP, Matsui MS, Marenus KD, Feingold KR, Elias PM. Psychological stress perturbs epidermal permeability barrier homeostasis: implications for the pathogenesis of stress-associated skin disorders. Arch Dermatol 2001; 137:53–59.

35. Malarkey WB, Pearl DK, Demers LM, Kiecolt-Glaser JK, Glaser R. Influence of academic stress and season on 24-hour mean concentrations of ACTH, cortisol, and beta-endorphin. Psychoneuroendocrinology 1995; 20:499–508.

36. Scholzen T, Armstrong CA, Bunnett NW, Luger TA, Olerud JE, Ansel JC. Neuropeptides in the skin: interactions between the neuroendocrine and the skin immune systems. Exp Dermatol 1998; 7:81–96.

37. Lawson SN. Peptides and cutaneous polymodal nociceptor neurones. Prog Brain Res 1996; 113:369–385.

38. Schulze E, Witt M, Fink T, Hofer A, Funk RH. Immunohistochemical detection of human skin nerve fibers. Acta Histochem 1997; 99:301–309.

39. Reilly DM, Ferdinando D, Johnston C, Shaw C, Buchanan KD, Green MR. The epidermal nerve fibre network: characterization of nerve fibres in human skin by confocal microscopy and assessment of racial variations. Br J Dermatol 1997; 137:163–170.

40. Bost KL, Breeding SA, Pascual DW. Modulation of the mRNAs encoding substance P and its receptor in rat macrophages by LPS. Reg Immunol 1992; 4:105–112.

41. Vedder H, Affolter HU, Otten U. Nerve growth factor (NGF) regulates tachykinin gene expression and biosynthesis in rat sensory neurons during early postnatal development. Neuropeptides 1993; 24:351–357.

42. Ansel JC, Brown JR, Payan DG, Brown MA. Substance P selectively activates TNF-alpha gene expression in murine mast cells. J Immunol 1993; 150:4478–4485.

43. Bowden JJ, Baluk P, Lefevre PM, Vigna SR, McDonald DM. Substance P (NK1) receptor immunoreactivity on endothelial cells of the rat tracheal mucosa. Am J Physiol 1996; 270:L404–414.

44. Quinlan KL, Naik SM, Cannon G, Armstrong CA, Bunnett NW, Ansel JC, Caughman SW. Substance P activates coincident NF-AT- and NF-kappa B-dependent adhesion molecule gene expression in microvascular endothelial cells through intracellular calcium mobilization. J Immunol 1999; 163:5656–5665.

45. Quinlan KL, Song IS, Bunnett NW, Letran E, Steinhoff M, Harten B, Olerud JE, Armstrong CA, Wright Caughman S, Ansel JC. Neuropeptide regulation of human dermal microvascular endothelial cell ICAM-1 expression and function. Am J Physiol 1998; 275:C1580–1590.

46. Quinlan KL, Song IS, Naik SM, Letran EL, Olerud JE, Bunnett NW, Armstrong CA, Caughman SW, Ansel JC. VCAM-1 expression on human dermal microvascular endothelial cells is directly and specifically up-regulated by substance P. J Immunol 1999; 162:1656–1661.

47. Rameshwar P, Gascon P, Ganea D. Stimulation of IL-2 production in murine lymphocytes by substance P and related tachykinins. J Immunol 1993; 151:2484–2496.

48. Calvo CF, Chavanel G, Senik A. Substance P enhances IL-2 expression in activated human T cells. J Immunol 1992; 148:3498–3504.

49. Santoni G, Perfumi MC, Spreghini E, Romagnoli S, Piccoli M. Neurokinin type-1 receptor antagonist inhibits enhancement of T cell functions by substance P in normal and neuromanipulated capsaicin-treated rats. J Neuroimmunol 1999; 93:15–25.

50. Pascual DW, Bost KL, Xu-Amano J, Kiyono H, McGhee JR. The cytokine-like action of substance P upon B cell differentiation. Reg Immunol 1992; 4:100–104.

51. Braun A, Wiebe P, Pfeufer A, Gessner R, Renz H. Differential modulation of human immunoglobulin isotype production by the neuropeptides substance P, NKA and NKB. J Neuroimmunol 1999; 97:43–50.

52. Burbach GJ, Kim KH, Zivony AS, Kim A, Aranda J, Wright S, Naik SM, Caughman SW, Ansel JC, Armstrong CA. The neurosensory tachykinins substance P and neurokinin A directly induce keratinocyte nerve growth factor. J Invest Dermatol 2001; 117:1075–1082.

53. Song IS, Bunnett NW, Olerud JE, Harten B, Steinhoff M, Brown JR, Sung KJ, Armstrong CA, Ansel JC. Substance P induction of murine keratinocyte PAM 212 interleukin 1 production is mediated by the neurokinin 2 receptor (NK-2R). Exp Dermatol 2000; 9:42–52.

54. Kiss M, Kemeny L, Gyulai R, Michel G, Husz S, Kovacs R, Dobozy A, Ruzicka T. Effects of the neuropeptides substance P, calcitonin gene-related peptide and alpha-melanocyte-stimulating hormone on the IL-8/IL-8 receptor system in a cultured human keratinocyte cell line and dermal fibroblasts. Inflammation 1999; 23:557–567.

55. Rabier MJ, Farber EM, Wilkinson DI. Neuropeptides modulate leukotriene B4 mitogenicity toward cultured human keratinocytes. J Invest Dermatol 1993; 100:132–136.

56. Parenti A, Amerini S, Ledda F, Maggi CA, Ziche M. The tachykinin NK1 receptor mediates the migration-promoting effect of substance P on human skin fibroblasts in culture. Naunyn Schmiedebergs Arch Pharmacol 1996; 353:475–481.

57. Katayama I, Nishioka K. Substance P augments fibrogenic cytokine-induced fibroblast proliferation: possible involvement of neuropeptide in tissue fibrosis. J Dermatol Sci 1997; 15:201–206.

58. Wiedermann CJ, Auer B, Sitte B, Reinisch N, Schratzberger P, Kahler CM. Induction of endothelial cell differentiation into capillary-like structures by substance P. Eur J Pharmacol 1996; 298:335–338.

59. Caterina MJ, Schumacher MA, Tominaga M, Rosen TA, Levine JD, Julius D. The capsaicin receptor: a heat-activated ion channel in the pain pathway. Nature 1997; 389:816–824.

60. Tsuchiya T, Kishimoto J, Granstein RD, Nakayama Y. Quantitative analysis of cutaneous calcitonin gene-related peptide content in response to acute cutaneous mechanical or thermal stimuli and immobilization-induced stress in rats. Neuropeptides 1996; 30:149–157.

61. Chan J, Smoller BR, Raychaudhuri SP, Jiang WY, Farber EM. Intraepidermal nerve fiber expression of calcitonin gene-related peptide, vasoactive intestinal peptide and substance P in psoriasis. Arch Dermatol Res 1997; 289:611–616.

62. Carucci JA, Ignatius R, Wei Y, Cypess AM, Schaer DA, Pope M, Steinman RM, Mojsov S. Calcitonin gene-related peptide decreases expression of HLA-DR and CD86 by human dendritic cells and dampens dendritic cell-driven T cell-proliferative responses via the type I calcitonin gene-related peptide receptor. J Immunol 2000; 164:3494–3499.

63. Fox FE, Kubin M, Cassin M, Niu Z, Hosoi J, Torii H, Granstein RD, Trinchieri G, Rook AH. Calcitonin gene-related peptide inhibits proliferation and antigen presentation by human peripheral blood mononuclear cells: effects on B7, interleukin 10, and interleukin 12. J Invest Dermatol 1997; 108:43–48.

64. Toyoda M, Luo Y, Makino T, Matsui C, Morohashi M. Calcitonin gene-related peptide upregulates melanogenesis and enhances melanocyte dendricity via induction of keratinocyte-derived melanotrophic factors. J Invest Dermatol Symp Proc 1999; 4:116–125.

65. Seike M, Ikeda M, Morimoto A, Matsumoto M, Kodama H. Increased synthesis of calcitonin gene-related peptide stimulates keratinocyte proliferation in murine UVB-irradiated skin. J Dermatol Sci 2002; 28:135–143.

66. Kakurai M, Fujita N, Murata S, Furukawa Y, Demitsu T, Nakagawa H. Vasoactive intestinal peptide regulates its receptor expression and functions of human keratinocytes via type I vasoactive intestinal peptide receptors. J Invest Dermatol 2001; 116:743–749.

67. Gonzalez C, Barroso C, Martin C, Gulbenkian S, Estrada C. Neuronal nitric oxide synthase activation by vasoactive intestinal peptide in bovine cerebral arteries. J Cereb Blood Flow Metab 1997; 17:977–984.

68. Jiang WY, Raychaudhuri SP, Farber EM. Double-labeled immunofluorescence study of cutaneous nerves in psoriasis. Int J Dermatol 1998; 37:572–574.

69. Waschek JA. Vasoactive intestinal peptide: an important trophic factor and developmental regulator? Dev Neurosci 1995; 17:1–7.

70. Fristad I, Jacobsen EB, Kvinnsland IH. Coexpression of vasoactive intestinal polypeptide and substance P in reinnervating pulpal nerves and in trigeminal ganglion neurones after axotomy of the inferior alveolar nerve in the rat. Arch Oral Biol 1998; 43:183–189.

71. Pincelli C, Fantini F, Massimi P, Girolomoni G, Seidenari S, Giannetti A. Neuropeptides in skin from patients with atopic dermatitis: an immuno-histochemical study. Br J Dermatol 1990; 122:745–750.

72. Church MK, el-Lati S, Caulfield JP. Neuropeptide-induced secretion from human skin mast cells. Int Arch Allergy Appl Immunol 1991; 94:310–318.

73. Redondo P, Garcia-Foncillas J, Okroujnov I, Bandres E. Alpha-MSH regulates interleukin-10 expression by human keratinocytes. Arch Dermatol Res 1998; 290:425–428.

74. Hedley SJ, Murray A, Sisley K, Ghanem G, Morandini R, Gawkrodger DJ, Mac Neil S. Alpha-melanocyte stimulating hormone can reduce T-cell interaction with melanoma cells in vitro. Melanoma Res 2000; 10:323–330.

75. Etemad-Moghadam B, Chen H, Yin P, Aziz N, Hedley ML. Inhibition of NF-kappaB activity by plasmid expressed alphaMSH peptide. J Neuroimmunol 2002; 125:23–29.

76. Ichiyama T, Okada K, Campbell IL, Furukawa S, Lipton JM. NF-kappaB activation is inhibited in human pulmonary epithelial cells transfected with alpha-melanocyte-stimulating hormone vector. Peptides 2000; 21:1473–1477.

77. Kalden DH, Scholzen T, Brzoska T, Luger TA. Mechanisms of the antiinflammatory effects of alpha-MSH. Role of transcription factor

NF-kappa B and adhesion molecule expression. Ann NY Acad Sci 1999; 885:254–261.

78. Luger TA, Scholzen T, Brzoska T, Becher E, Slominski A, Paus R. Cutaneous immunomodulation and coordination of skin stress responses by alpha-melanocyte-stimulating hormone. Ann NY Acad Sci 1998; 840:381–394.

79. Biondi M, Zannino LG. Psychological stress, neuroimmunomodulation, and susceptibility to infectious diseases in animals and man: a review. Psychother Psychosom 1997; 66:3–26.

80. Broadbent DE, Broadbent MH, Phillpotts RJ, Wallace J. Some further studies on the prediction of experimental colds in volunteers by psychological factors. J Psychosom Res 1984; 28:511–523.

81. Konstantinos AP, Sheridan JF. Stress and influenza viral infection: modulation of proinflammatory cytokine responses in the lung. Respir Physiol 2001; 128:71–77.

82. Dibble SL, Swanson JM. Gender differences for the predictors of depression in young adults with genital herpes. Public Health Nurs 2000; 17:187–194.

83. Buske-Kirschbaum A, Geiben A, Wermke C, Pirke KM, Hellhammer D. Preliminary evidence for herpes labialis recurrence following experimentally induced disgust. Psychother Psychosom 2001; 70:86–91.

84. Levenson JL, Hamer RM, Myers T, Hart RP, Kaplowitz LG. Psychological factors predict symptoms of severe recurrent genital herpes infection. J Psychosom Res 1987; 31:153–159.

85. Cassidy L, Meadows J, Catalan J, Barton S. Are reported stress and coping style associated with frequent recurrence of genital herpes? Genitourin Med 1997; 73:263–266.

86. Cohen F, Kemeny ME, Kearney KA, Zegans LS, Neuhaus JM, Conant MA. Persistent stress as a predictor of genital herpes recurrence. Arch Intern Med 1999; 159:2430–2436.

87. Rand KH, Hoon EF, Massey JK, Johnson JH. Daily stress and recurrence of genital herpes simplex. Arch Intern Med 1990; 150:1889–1893.

88. Psychological stress and other potential triggers for recurrences of herpes simplex virus eye infections. Herpetic Eye Disease Study Group. Arch Ophthalmol 2000; 118:1617–1625.

89. Hoon EF, Hoon PW, Rand KH, Johnson J, Hall NR, Edwards NB. A psycho-behavioral model of genital herpes recurrence. J Psychosom Res 1991; 35:25–36.

90. Longo D, Koehn K. Psychosocial factors and recurrent genital herpes: a review of prediction and psychiatric treatment studies. Int J Psychiatry Med 1993; 23:99–117.

91. Green J, Kocsis A. Psychological factors in recurrent genital herpes. Genitourin Med 1997; 73:253–258.

92. McKenna DB, Neill WA, Norval M. Herpes simplex virus-specific immune responses in subjects with frequent and infrequent orofacial recrudescences. Br J Dermatol 2001; 144:459–464.

93. Sainz B, Loutsch JM, Marquart ME, Hill JM. Stress-associated immunomodulation and herpes simplex virus infections. Med Hypotheses 2001; 56:348–356.
94. Ruzek MC, Pearce BD, Miller AH, Biron CA. Endogenous glucocorticoids protect against cytokine-mediated lethality during viral infection. J Immunol 1999; 162:3527–3533.
95. Raychaudhuri SP, Gross J. Psoriasis risk factors: role of lifestyle practices. Cutis 2000; 66:348–352.
96. Fortune DG, Richards HL, Griffiths CE, Main CJ. Psychological stress, distress and disability in patients with psoriasis: Consensus and variation in the contribution of illness perceptions, coping and alexithymia. Br J Clin Psychol 41 Part 2002; 2:157–174.
97. Nickoloff BJ, Schroder JM, von den Driesch P, Raychaudhuri SP, Farber EM, Boehncke WH, Morhenn VB, Rosenberg EW, Schon MP, Holick MF. Is psoriasis a T-cell disease? Exp Dermatol 2000; 9:359–375.
98. Farber EM, Nickoloff BJ, Recht B, Fraki JE. Stress, symmetry, and psoriasis: possible role of neuropeptides. J Am Acad Dermatol 1986; 14:305–311.
99. Raychaudhuri SP, Farber EM. Are sensory nerves essential for the development of psoriatic lesions? J Am Acad Dermatol 1993; 28:488–489.
100. Raychaudhuri SP, Jiang WY, Farber EM. Psoriatic keratinocytes express high levels of nerve growth factor. Acta Derm Venereol 1998; 78:84–86.
101. Raychaudhuri SP, Jiang WY, Smoller BR, Farber EM. Nerve growth factor and its receptor system in psoriasis. Br J Dermatol 2000; 143:198–200.
102. Aloe L, Alleva E, Fiore M. Stress and nerve growth factor. Findings in animal models and humans. Pharmacol Biochem Behav 2002; 73:159–166.
103. Wilkinson DI, Theeuwes MJ, Farber EM. Nerve growth factor increases the mitogenicity of certain growth factors for cultured human keratinocytes: a comparison with epidermal growth factor. Exp Dermatol 1994; 3:239–245.
104. Aloe L, Levi-Montalcini R. Mast cells increase in tissues of neonatal rats injected with the nerve growth factor. Brain Res 1977; 133:358–366.
105. Aloe L. Nerve growth factor and neuroimmune responses: basic and clinical observations. Arch Physiol Biochem 2001; 109:354–356.
106. Thorpe LW, Werrbach-Perez K, Perez-Polo JR. Effects of nerve growth factor on the expression of interleukin-2 receptors on cultured human lymphocytes. Ann NY Acad Sci 1987; 496:310–311.
107. Lambiase A, Bracci-Laudiero L, Bonini S, Starace G, D'Elios MM, De Carli M, Aloe L. Human CD4+ T cell clones produce and release nerve growth factor and express high-affinity nerve growth factor receptors. J Allergy Clin Immunol 1997; 100:408–414.
108. Raychaudhuri SP, Jiang WY, Farber EM, Schall TJ, Ruff MR, Pert CB. Upregulation of RANTES in psoriatic keratinocytes: a possible pathogenic mechanism for psoriasis. Acta Derm Venereol 1999; 79:9–11.
109. Raychaudhuri SP, Farber EM, Raychaudhuri SK. Role of nerve growth factor in RANTES expression by keratinocytes. Acta Derm Venereol 2000; 80:247–250.

110. Richter J, Andersson R, Edvinsson L, Gullberg U. Calcitonin gene-related peptide (CGRP) activates human neutrophils—inhibition by chemotactic peptide antagonist BOC-MLP. Immunology 1992; 77:416–421.

111. Sung CP, Arleth AJ, Aiyar N, Bhatnagar PK, Lysko PG, Feuerstein G. CGRP stimulates the adhesion of leukocytes to vascular endothelial cells. Peptides 1992; 13:429–434.

112. Pincelli C, Haake AR, Benassi L, Grassilli E, Magnoni C, Ottani D, Polakowska R, Franceschi C, Giannetti A. Autocrine nerve growth factor protects human keratinocytes from apoptosis through its high affinity receptor (TRK): a role for BCL-2. J Invest Dermatol 1997; 109:757–764.

113. Hong KW, Yoo SE, Yu SS, Lee JY, Rhim BY. Pharmacological coupling and functional role for CGRP receptors in the vasodilation of rat pial arterioles. Am J Physiol 1996; 270:H317–323.

114. Pearce FL, Thompson HL. Some characteristics of histamine secretion from rat peritoneal mast cells stimulated with nerve growth factor. J Physiol 1986; 372:379–393.

115. Columbo M, Horowitz EM, Kagey-Sobotka A, Lichtenstein LM. Substance P activates the release of histamine from human skin mast cells through a pertussis toxin-sensitive and protein kinase C-dependent mechanism. Clin Immunol Immunopathol 1996; 81:68–73.

116. Brain SD, Tippins JR, Morris HR, MacIntyre I, Williams TJ. Potent vasodilator activity of calcitonin gene-related peptide in human skin. J Invest Dermatol 1986; 87:533–536.

117. Tausk F, Whitmore SE. A pilot study of hypnosis in the treatment of patients with psoriasis. Psychother Psychosom 1999; 68:221–225.

118. Fortune DG, Richards HL, Kirby B, Bowcock S, Main CJ, Griffiths CE. A cognitive-behavioural symptom management programme as an adjunct in psoriasis therapy. Br J Dermatol 2002; 146:458–465.

119. King RM, Wilson GV. Use of a diary technique to investigate psychosomatic relations in atopic dermatitis. J Psychosom Res 1991; 35:697–706.

120. Buske-Kirschbaum A, Geiben A, Hellhammer D. Psychobiological aspects of atopic dermatitis: an overview. Psychother Psychosom 2001; 70:6–16.

121. Leung DY. Atopic dermatitis: new insights and opportunities for therapeutic intervention. J Allergy Clin Immunol 2000; 105:860–876.

122. Kagi MK, Wuthrich B, Montano E, Barandun J, Blaser K, Walker C. Differential cytokine profiles in peripheral blood lymphocyte supernatants and skin biopsies from patients with different forms of atopic dermatitis, psoriasis and normal individuals. Int Arch Allergy Immunol 1994; 103:332–340.

123. Heubeck B, Schonberger A, Hornstein OP. [Are shifts in circadian cortisol rhythm an endocrine symptom of atopic eczema?]. Hautarzt 1988; 39:12–17.

124. Rupprecht M, Hornstein OP, Schluter D, Schafers HJ, Koch HU, Beck G, Rupprecht R. Cortisol, corticotropin, and beta-endorphin responses to corticotropin-releasing hormone in patients with atopic eczema. Psychoneuroendocrinology 1995; 20:543–551.

125. Rupprecht M, Rupprecht R, Kornhuber J, Wodarz N, Koch HU, Riederer P, Hornstein OP. Elevated glucocorticoid receptor concentrations before and after glucocorticoid therapy in peripheral mononuclear leukocytes of patients with atopic dermatitis. Dermatologica 1991; 183:100–105.

126. Schallreuter KU, Pittelkow MR, Swanson NN, Beazley WD, Korner C, Ehrke C, Buttner G. Altered catecholamine synthesis and degradation in the epidermis of patients with atopic eczema. Arch Dermatol Res 1997; 289:663–666.

127. Delgado M, Fernandez-Alfonso MS, Fuentes A. Effect of adrenaline and glucocorticoids on monocyte cAMP-specific phosphodiesterase (PDE4) in a monocytic cell line. Arch Dermatol Res 2002; 294:190–197.

128. Chan SC, Brown MA, Willcox TM, Li SH, Stevens SR, Tara D, Hanifin JM. Abnormal IL-4 gene expression by atopic dermatitis T lymphocytes is reflected in altered nuclear protein interactions with IL-4 transcriptional regulatory element. J Invest Dermatol 1996; 106:1131–1136.

129. Chan SC, Li SH, Hanifin JM. Increased interleukin-4 production by atopic mononuclear leukocytes correlates with increased cyclic adenosine monophosphate-phosphodiesterase activity and is reversible by phosphodiesterase inhibition. J Invest Dermatol 1993; 100:681–684.

130. Essayan DM, Kagey-Sobotka A, Lichtenstein LM, Huang SK. Regulation of interleukin-13 by type 4 cyclic nucleotide phosphodiesterase (PDE) inhibitors in allergen-specific human T lymphocyte clones. Biochem Pharmacol 1997; 53:1055–1060.

131. Kanda N, Watanabe S. Intracellular $3', 5'$-adenosine cyclic monophosphate level regulates house dust mite-induced interleukin-13 production by T cells from mite-sensitive patients with atopic dermatitis. J Invest Dermatol 2001; 116:3–11.

132. Yoshida N, Shimizu Y, Kitaichi K, Hiramatsu K, Takeuchi M, Ito Y, Kume H, Yamaki K, Suzuki R, Shibata E, Hasegawa T, Takagi K. Differential effect of phosphodiesterase inhibitors on IL-13 release from peripheral blood mononuclear cells. Clin Exp Immunol 2001; 126:384–389.

133. Li Y, Simons FE, HayGlass KT. Environmental antigen-induced IL-13 responses are elevated among subjects with allergic rhinitis, are independent of IL-4, and are inhibited by endogenous IFN-gamma synthesis. J Immunol 1998; 161:7007–7014.

134. Darsow U, Scharein E, Simon D, Walter G, Bromm B, Ring J. New aspects of itch pathophysiology: component analysis of atopic itch using the 'Eppendorf Itch Questionnaire.' Int Arch Allergy Immunol 2001; 124:326–331.

135. Sugiura H, Omoto M, Hirota Y, Danno K, Uehara M. Density and fine structure of peripheral nerves in various skin lesions of atopic dermatitis. Arch Dermatol Res 1997; 289:125–131.

136. Tobin D, Nabarro G, Baart de la Faille H, van Vloten WA, van der Putte SC, Schuurman HJ. Increased number of immunoreactive nerve fibers in atopic dermatitis. J Allergy Clin Immunol 1992; 90:613–622.

137. Schmelz M, Schmidt R, Bickel A, Handwerker HO, Torebjork HE. Specific C-receptors for itch in human skin. J Neurosci 1997; 17:8003–8008.
138. Ostlere LS, Cowen T, Rustin MH. Neuropeptides in the skin of patients with atopic dermatitis. Clin Exp Dermatol 1995; 20:462–467.
139. Urashima R, Mihara M. Cutaneous nerves in atopic dermatitis. A histological, immunohistochemical and electron microscopic study. Virchows Arch 1998; 432:363–370.
140. Darsow U, Ring J. Neuroimmune interactions in the skin. Curr Opin Allergy Clin Immunol 2001; 1:435–439.
141. Singh LK, Pang X, Alexacos N, Letourneau R, Theoharides TC. Acute immobilization stress triggers skin mast cell degranulation via corticotropin releasing hormone, neurotensin, and substance P: a link to neurogenic skin disorders. Brain Behav Immun 1999; 13:225–239.
142. Kang H, Byun DG, Kim JW. Effects of substance P and vasoactive intestinal peptide on interferon-gamma and interleukin-4 production in severe atopic dermatitis. Ann Allergy Asthma Immunol 2000; 85:227–232.
143. Toyoda M, Nakamura M, Makino T, Hino T, Kagoura M, Morohashi M. Nerve growth factor and substance P are useful plasma markers of disease activity in atopic dermatitis. Br J Dermatol 2002; 147:71–79.
144. Krueger JG. The immunologic basis for the treatment of psoriasis with new biologic agents. J Am Acad Dermatol 2002; 46:1–23.
145. Ellis CN, Krueger GG. Alefacept Clinical Study Group. Treatment of chronic plaque psoriasis by selective targeting of memory effector T lymphocytes. N Engl J Med 2001; 345:248–255.

7

Psychophysiological Aspects of Atopic Dermatitis

Uwe Gieler, Volker Niemeier, Jörg Kupfer, and Burkhard Brosig
Justus-Liebig University
Giessen, Germany

INTRODUCTION

Atopic dermatitis can now be considered a typical psychosomatic disease in which there is interaction between genetic disposition, multifactorial eliciting circumstances, and psychosomatic factors in the exacerbation or in coping with the disease.

CLINICAL PATTERNS IN ATOPIC DERMATITIS

Atopic dermatitis can be described as a chronic or chronic-recurrent inflammatory dermatosis with severe itching, which varies widely in its morphological aspect and overall course and is generically determined (1). Other atopic diseases of the immediate type, like allergic rhinitis, allergic conjunctivitis, and allergic bronchial asthma, are frequently found in the patient or in the family. With atopic dermatitis, these form the so-called atopic disease group. The main symptoms of the disease are severe itching and dry skin. The course is unpredictable (2).

EPIDEMIOLOGY

Atopic dermatitis is a dermatosis occurring worldwide. It is estimated that about 1–3% of all adults and 5–20% of all children tend to the disease or suffer from it. An increasing incidence has been observed over the past 10 years. The disease manifests in about 60% of patients in the first year of life (usually after the first month) and in the subsequent 4 years in another 30% (3). Initial manifestation after puberty is relatively rare. Usually the disease heals in puberty. With a relatively late onset of disease after beginning school, persistence of the disease is observed more frequently. Both sexes are affected, but during the infantile phase, boys are somewhat more frequently afflicted than girls (4).

GENETICS

Atopic dermatitis presents with occurrence within families and is considered a genetic disposition disease. About two thirds of all patients with atopic dermatitis have a positive atopic family history. The probability of disease for children having one parent with atopy is estimated at 25–30%. If both parents suffer atopic disease, the probability is considerably greater at about 60% (1). The concordance rate in identical twins is 86%, in fraternal twins 30% (5). The genetic mode is not known in all details. Przybilla and Kaudewitz (6) postulate a polygenic, multifactorial heredity. Currently, evidence is growing for the existence of a mainly responsible atopy gene in chromosomal region 11q13 (3). There appears to be no influence by the HLA system. Leung (7) reported that more than 20 genes are involved in the development of allergic diseases. Chromosome 5q31–33, which contains several cytokine genes (IL-3, IL-4, IL-5, IL-13, and GM-CSF), is of particular interest. The disposition to atopic reaction is inherited. Beyond that, certain realization factors are necessary to elicit skin disease. Aeroallergens, sex hormones, climate, infections, food allergies, and emotional stress, as well as immunological characteristics (see below), play a decisive role (8).

CLINICAL SYMPTOMS

The clinical presentation of atopic dermatitis is extremely variable. It changes during the lifetime so much that differentiation between various age-related stages must be made. The main symptoms of atopic dermatitis are dry skin, itching, and eczematous skin inflammation (9). Increasing involvement of all skin areas may occur in all phases of the disease, reaching a generalized peak as atopic erythrodermia (see below). When the skin changes are extensive, reactive lymph node enlargement may occur— dermatopathic lymphadenopathy. Minor or hidden forms of atopic dermatitis may present, for example, as Dennie-Morgan folds (double lid folds), loss of the lateral eyebrows (Hertoghe sign), hyperlinear palmae, mamilla eczema, white dermographism, etc. (9).

Superinfections are observed, especially as complications. These may be bacterial (frequently coagulase-positive *Staphylococcus aureus* infection with impetiginization), viral (feared is the potentially life-threatening eczema herpeticatum, much rarer eczema vaccinatum), or occasionally mycotic. Erythrodermia exfoliativa is life threatening (6).

PATHOGENESIS

The cause of atopic dermatitis has not yet been completely clarified. There are various pathogenetic concepts, none of which appears alone able to explain the precise mechanism of the disease. It is certain that a disposition to atopic reaction is inherited. A multifactorial pathogenesis is assumed. On the one hand, there is impaired humoral immunity. Patients with atopy often react to contact with environmental substances (allergens) with sensitization of the immediate type (Type I, Coombs, and Gell). According to Leung (7), the main characteristic of atopic syndromes is increased production of IgE, the synthesis of which is controlled by T-cell cytokines, whereby interleukin (IL)-4 promotes synthesis of IgE and interferon inhibits it. Hanifin and Chan (10) point out that since 20% of patients with atopic dermatitis have normal serum IgE values, the role of IgE in this skin disease remains speculative. These forms of atopic dermatitis are also called "intrinsic atopic dermatitis," corresponding to asthma.

Patients with atopic dermatitis also appear to have impaired cellular immunity. The inflammation cells infiltrating the inflammation area, among others CD4 (t lymphocytes, are activated and synthesize IL-4 and IL-5, but hardly any interferon-) and are classified as Th2 cells (5). Hanifin and Chan (10) see an increased expression of IL-10 in skin lesions as a consistent result of studies.

In addition, interest for the past several years has focused on the pathogenetic role of the Langerhans cells in the Type IV reaction. Bruynzeel-Koomen et al. (11) showed that IgE binds to the high-affinity Fc receptors of the Langerhans cells. This appears relevant for the pathogenesis of the disease, since in addition to the release of mediators from the Langerhans cells via the Fc-IgE receptor network, binding of IgE can also serve to focus antigen uptake and thus permit presentation of the least quantities of allergens (12,13). Moreover, eosinophils and monocytes are increased. These may also possess low- or high-affinity IgE-Fc receptors by which the allergen can be bound, resulting in release of mediators from these cells.

A further disorder in the vegetative nervous system is found in patients with atopic dermatitis, which is expressed, among other ways, as white dermographism. Vascular contraction can be observed following mechanical skin stress in areas that appear healthy (14). Application of nicotinic acid ester does not result in reactive erythema, but in capillary contraction (white reaction).

One very important aspect is the disruption of cutaneous defense. Patients with atopic dermatitis present with marked skin colonization with *Staphylococcus aureus* and develop bacterial, fungal, or viral skin infections (15).

Finally, some other functional impairments of the skin occur in patients with atopic dermatitis: typical is reduced sebaceous gland production, or sebostasis (asteatosis). The skin is dry and sensitive and tends with frequent washing to further drying and itching. Sweating may be impaired, whereby subsequent sweating elicits severe itching.

STRESS AND ATOPIC DERMATITIS

Psychological factors seem to be important in atopic dermatitis as significant modulators of the disease. Stress increases atopic dermatitis symptoms depending on the severity of stress. In a very large population of 1457 patients questioned after the Japanese earthquake in Hanshin in 1995, Kodama et al. (16) showed that 38% of patients with atopic dermatitis in the most severely hit region and 34% in a moderately hit region reported exacerbation, compared to only 7% in a control group without earthquake stress. However, 9% and 5% in the respective earthquake regions and only 1% in the control region reported a marked improvement in atopic dermatitis. In a multiple regression analysis, subjective stress was the best indicator predicting exacerbation compared to genetic and treatment-related factors. The results of this study show that stress apparently has an immunological effect, which can, though to a slighter extent, exert an opposite inflammatory effect.

NEUROANATOMY

Atopy-relevant effector cells, such as mast cells and Langerhans cells, form a close anatomical relationship with nerve fibers staining positive for a number of neuroactive substances, for instance substance P, vasoactive peptide, or nerve growth factor (NGF). It seems possible that stress-induced stimulation of nerve fibers induces secretion of neuroactive substances. A growing number of studies indicates that atopic dermatitis patients show disturbances in the cyclic adenosine monophosphate (cAMP) system, suggesting an altered catecholamine responsiveness. This concept was introduced by Szentivanyi, who reported reduced responsiveness of β-adrenergic receptors in atopic dermatitis patients.

PSYCHONEUROENDOCRINOLOGY

Functional changes in the hypothalamus-pituitary-adrenal cortex axis are under discussion. Buske-Kirschbaum et al. compiled an overview of the psychobiological aspects of atopic dermatitis and confirmed by means of hypotheses the various endocrine, immunological, and psychophysiological influences on atopic dermatitis (17).

Pathophysiological studies follow the behavioral approach and address the pathophysiological reactibility of atopic dermatitis patients and conditioning as a means of influence. The following are among the parameters used: heart rate, electrical skin resistance, electromyographic activity, and skin temperature under defined stress situations. In addition, psychometric data, such as scores for anxiety and hostility and depressivity are measured.

The influence of serious events in life and of stressors of various degrees on the immune system is known. The autonomic nervous system acts as the connector between feelings and subsequent somatic response. Lymph nodes contain sympathic afferents; adrenergic and cholinergic fibers are found in the thymus; the lymphocytes also have adrenergic and cholinergic receptors.

Kupfer (18) examined the interaction between the severity of skin symptoms, the expression of individual emotions, and the excretion of salivary cortisol and salivary IgA. Aggression, depression, and anxiety were found to be emotions particularly related to skin symptoms.

The central immunoetological role of vasoactive mediators such as histamine and ECF-A (eosinophil-chemotactic factor of anaphylaxis) in atopic dermatitis patients have been delineated. The following factors were pointed out as the decisive influence of this mediator liberation: increased readiness of the basophiles to excrete histamines, so-called "leaky" mast cells, a β_2-adrenergic control defect among other things at the level of the intracellular cAMP-system, increased sensitivity to α-adrenergic, cholergenic stimuli demonstrated in vivo and in vitro, and elevated IgE levels. The histamine effect, besides its effect on the capillary-bronchial system, lies in a limitation of T-suppressor activity with consecutive IgE elevation. Increased sensitivity to histamine was found in nearly all atopics at the T-cell level.

PSYCHOSOMATIC ASPECTS OF ATOPIC DERMATITIS

Psychosomatic aspects must be considered, including disease-related stress in childhood, psychosocial stress of the parents, and special aspects of the parent-child relationships and, of course, of the mother-child relationship. Scratching as an interactional phenomenon and supportive interview with the parents must also be taken into account. The quality of life of atopic dermatitis patients is certainly most limited compared to that of other skin disease patients (19), so for that reason alone it is necessary to pay attention to its psychosomatic aspects.

DISEASE-RELATED STRESS IN CHILDHOOD

Genetically disposed atopic dermatitis has a central development–psychological influence on the personality development of the child, depending on the time of first manifestation. Even as an infant, before personality and body image are developed, the child with unhealthy skin constantly experiences two contradictory emotional stimuli in its skin: the loving attention from stroking and massaging with ointments, and at the same time the stimulus of pain and itching in the eczematous areas from too much pressure in massaging or from unpleasant external circumstances (20). The difficulty arises for the child of not being able to differentiate between loving attention and unpleasant irritations (21). Since the infant experiences the presence of the mother and the ointment that she applies as the only source of relief and comfort, the absence of the mother or reference figure is experienced as a threat, and fixation on the maternal object results. Separation from the mother is experienced by the child with unhealthy skin "not as though it was not being held, but rather as though he were being skinned" (20). Psychosomatic practitioners have conceived this psychodynamic structure model as an "allergic object relationship" (22,23).

The severe itching afflicts the sick child from its earliest childhood and alters its sleep rhythm to a considerable degree. Since the baby is uncomfortable when it is too warm, cuddling and rocking as the "most natural way of comforting the baby in its affliction" is forbidden to the mother (20). Frequently, the children are additionally stressed with special diets, in which they must avoid various foods (milk products, sweets, etc.), which are justified in only about 30% according to individual diagnostics.

Many parents are not capable of accepting the skin disease of their child and are thus ready to make many sacrifices to achieve improvement. Not infrequently the children become little "tyrants" because of the excessive protectiveness and indulgence of such parents. Small children attempt to compensate for the lack of security arising from a feeling of instability and disorientation with another form of safety, namely domination (24). At school, children with diseased skin usually suffer under their classmates, whether because they are teased or because of open rejection based on the appearance of the skin. Adolescents between 14 and 18 years in our atopic dermatitis training sessions, on being asked how they explain their atopic dermatitis to their classmates, say they explain first of all that the eczema is not contagious. Thus, contact difficulties arise in early childhood, which usually reach a first peak in puberty. Bryam (25) assumed that patients with asthma and atopic dermatitis have more sexual problems. In a comparative questionnaire for patients with atopic dermatitis and psoriasis, Niemeier et al. (26) could not confirm that sexuality is altered with respect to frequency of intercourse. However, the atopic dermatitis patients reported marked limitations and problems in touching and caressing.

PSYCHOSOCIAL STRESS OF THE PARENTS

The prevention of atopic diseases is an essential factor in the modern treatment of atopic dermatitis, especially since this disease is increasing in frequency. The earlier a child is treated and the earlier preventive measures are taken to hinder exacerbation of the disease, the better the prognostic outlook. Psychosocial stress, as a variable eliciting factor with given genetic disposition, is of decisive importance.

The fact that a child suffers from atopic dermatitis usually puts particularly high pressure on the parents. Repeatedly unsuccessful attempts, even with the most severe methods (like tying the hands or punishment), to reduce scratching and the skin symptoms may lead in individual cases to resigned despair, excessive devotion, or self-accusation or even aggression against the child. The parents, confronted with the requirements of providing the sick child with optimal care, repeatedly experience help-lessness in getting the disease under control. Many also feel guilty or fear they have not done enough. In addition, there is uncertainty in dealing with the disease and in deciding among the numerous therapeutic procedures and treatment suggestions. Moreover, there are frequently hints from the environment that this is a purely emotional problem of the mother, which leads to further despair and helplessness.

The parents' stress increases, especially during periods of disease activity. A study of 28 parent pairs whose children suffered acute atopic dermatitis showed that the groups differed significantly during an active phase compared to the subacute phase with respect to stress and well-being (27). The stress usually decreased again when the acute phase abated. However, the relationships among the family members can undergo lasting—sometimes negative—changes. The restless behavior of the children, their lack of frustration tolerance, and the high level of parental attention strains the family and partnership and potentiates sibling rivalry. If the child is permitted to sleep in the parents' bed at night to calm it, that usually disrupts the parents' sleep and may have a negative effect on their sexual relationship. Frequently, latent aggression and unconscious negative feelings result (28).

THE PARENT-CHILD RELATIONSHIP

Several studies of the parent-child relationship make clear the changes that must be expected due to chronic disease compared to physically healthy children and their parents.

Ring et al. (29) examined 55 children between 1 and 19 years of age with atopic dermatitis and compared them to 16 children suffering from nonatopic skin diseases. The Stapf scale was used to examine the parental style of raising the children; the characteristic "strictness" of the mother from the point of view of the atopic dermatitis children was significantly more pronounced than among the control children. There was no difference in the paternal childrearing style. In structured interviews with children and parents, it was noticed that the mothers of atopic children reacted less emotionally and spontaneously to the child's emotions than the mothers in the comparison group. Maternal affection appears to be limited mostly to hygiene rituals (such as applying cream to the skin) and fulfilling material wishes.

Ring et al. (29) emphasized that the findings of these studies do not permit description of a clear-cut "atopic mother" type, in the sense of a special personality structure. The mothers were neither "rejecting" nor "overprotective."

Solomon and Gagnon (30) performed a behavioral observation of mothers of 7-month-old infants with eczema. They observed that the mothers in the healthy control group had significantly more frequent and more positive contact to their children, while the mothers of the sick children reacted less sensitively and tended to react less frequently to expressions of discomfort by the children. Nevertheless, the behavior of the mothers to their children could not be described as either "too close" or "rejecting and impaired," as described in earlier studies.

These results give rise to the assumption that the observed limitations in communication between parents and child are a consequence of the disease. These are not specific to atopic dermatitis, but can be found in other comparable diseases in childhood.

Thus, Hermanns et al. (31) found disruptions in the parent-child relationships. The authors studied 25 asthmatic and 25 healthy children and their mothers. Initially, the mother was asked to describe her child to the study director in ~5 minutes (five-minute speech sample, FMSS); then the mother and child discussed a mutual problem. During the FMSS, significantly more mothers in the asthma group than in the control group showed a critical attitude toward the child and expressed significantly more criticism during the problem discussion. Overall, the communication between mother and child in the asthma group was characterized by more negative verbal interaction than in the control group. Wenninger et al. (32) report similarly finding more verbal and nonverbal negative behavior among mothers and children with atopic dermatitis than in a healthy control group

THE MOTHER-CHILD RELATIONSHIP

The importance of the early mother-child relationship in atopic dermatitis has repeatedly been the topic of studies. In early studies, Miller and Baruch (33) defined the rejecting mother as one "whose behavior toward the child is colored by the conscious or unconscious desire to be rid of the child and who considers it a burden." To test this definition, they performed a study to compare 63 allergic children with 37 nonallergic children and found that maternal rejection occurred in 9 of 37 of the families with nonallergic children but in 62 of 63 cases with allergic children. Another study by the same authors (34) of 90 allergic and 53 nonallergic children revealed that the allergic children were more inhibited in their ability to express aggression. Marmor et al. (35), in a study of 20 mothers of atopic dermatitis children, also concluded that the attitude of the mothers toward their children is characterized by rejection. They observed that in every case the onset of disease was preceded by a phase of rejection, negation, or necessary separation.

Assuming that maternal rejection can lead to the development and persistence of atopic dermatitis in children, Williams (36) performed interviews with mothers. Thirty-three mothers were instructed concerning the emotional needs of their children and shown possibilities for satisfying these needs. Of the children whose mothers received instruction, 45% were symptom-free after 7 months, as opposed to only 10% in the control group ($n = 20$), who received only conventional dermatological treatment.

More recent studies could not confirm maternal rejection in the sense of a pathogenic mother personality. Langfeldt and Luys (37) performed a pilot study to examine whether mothers of children with atopic dermatitis differ from mothers of healthy children with respect to overprotection and hostility. Twenty-five mothers of chronically ill children and 25 mothers of children recently afflicted with atopic dermatitis, as well as 31 mothers of healthy children, filled out a questionnaire on parental attitudes toward childrearing. Differences were found only in respect to the "hostile-rejecting childrearing attitude," whereby the mother of chronically ill children were more hostile than mothers of recently afflicted or healthy children. The authors conclude that the "hostile-rejecting attitude toward childrearing" can at best be interpreted "not as the cause of the onset of disease, but as its consequence," because of the temporal relationship. These studies make clear that changes must be anticipated because of the chronic disease itself compared to physically healthy children and their reference person. These are, by the way, not specific for atopic dermatitis, but can be observed also in other comparable diseases in childhood (diabetes, asthma, cancer, etc.). One characteristic of chronic diseases is that they overtax the adaptive capacity of the organism in their spontaneous course.

It is interesting in this connection to look at a special group of atopic dermatitis patients who present with special circumstances in their coping aspects.

Our team had the opportunity to examine children with cardiac transplantation who, when the transplantation was made before the first year of life, also developed atopic dermatitis overproportionally often (38). The conspicuous thing about these children and their parents was that, despite systemic therapy with cyclosporine, which is also used therapeutically in atopic dermatitis, the children developed atopic dermatitis. Moreover, compared to the atopic dermatitis outpatient department in a dermatology clinic, the fathers were relatively often present at the examinations, and the stress of the atopic dermatitis, measured with the questionnaire for parents of atopic dermatitis children (FEN), was considerably below the values in the calibration sample! Apparently, the subjective life-threatening heart transplantation results in development of positive coping among parents and children and they have no great problems with the symptoms.

SCRATCHING AS AN INTERACTIONAL PHENOMENON

Hünecke and Krüger (39) examined 30 mothers of children with eczema between 3 and 8 years of age and attempted to classify concepts for descriptions by the mother of the child's scratching using a cognitive-psychological approach. Four largely independent groups with different content could be formed: a "general uncontrollability," "inadequate attention from the mothers," "control intention of the mother," and "will and mood of the child." Moreover, the authors showed that of the 30 cause-attribution items, 17 showed important relationships to various emotions. The uncontrollability correlated especially to helplessness and to sensations of physical and nervous tension. Inadequate attention from the mother correlated especially to feelings of guilt and fear of failure; the control intention of the mother did not correlate to future hopes, but to sympathy and helplessness and the will/mood of the child with feelings of emotional and physical exhaustion.

The importance of attention from the parents in the occurrence of the child's scratching was pointed out many times in studies. Allen and Harris (40) described the case of a 5-year-old girl who suffered from an itching skin disease that was not specified. The mother of the child was instructed to ignore her daughter's scratching and to reward scratching-free phases. Within 6 weeks the child's skin eruptions abated entirely. Similar results were also reported by Bär and Kuypers (41) and by Walton (42). Increased attention from the reference person to the scratching is apparently an important factor for the scratching behavior of the child.

SUPPORTIVE INTERVIEW WITH THE PARENTS

Koblenzer and Koblenzer (28) conducted extensive therapeutic interviews with eight parent pairs whose children suffered from atopic dermatitis. Starting from the hypothesis that atopic dermatitis is an expression of a disrupted parent-child relationship, they attempted in cooperation with the parents to work out and discuss the difficulties in dealing with the children. They encouraged the parents to admit to negative feelings, to overcome feelings of guilt about the situation, and to set limits for the children. This change in behavior broke through the vicious circle of "skin symptoms–parental stress–unfavorable parental behavior–exacerbation of the skin symptoms." Rapid and long-lasting improvement of the skin condition and emotional development was the result in all of the children.

Broberg et al. (43) applied systematic training for parents of atopic dermatitis children with respect to 1) the patterns of atopic dermatitis, 2) local therapy of skin eruptions, and 3) influence of environmental factors.

This training also resulted in better therapeutic effects in the atopic dermatitis children than in the children of the control group.

Hünecke and Krüger (39) emphasize that the model of blaming the mother should be abandoned in favor of an interaction model in which the chain of action does not necessarily start with the mother but can begin with the disease. The authors make suggestions about how to approach the various aspects of the mother's responsibility during the interview. "Such an interview procedure can be viewed as a compensation or help toward self-help approach: the mothers are to correct problems—not ones which they have caused, but those caused by circumstances. The more pronounced such a solution-responsibility is, the more it is to be expected that the mother will not relinquish it. If the expert does not respect this internalized maternal responsibility and does not, contrary to the medical understanding of consultation, clearly limit himself to the expert's role, the expert-mother conflict is practically pre-programmed."

CONCLUSIONS FOR TREATMENT

Parents of children with atopic dermatitis are essentially involved in the treatment of the skin disease, since they provide the doctor with the main information and must provide for compliance with terms of treatment. In addition, the skin disease is stressful for the family, usually resulting in a change in everyday living. Frequently considerable disruption can be observed in the parent-child relationship. However, it has not yet been clarified whether these changes are the cause or the consequence of the skin disease.

On the one hand, a lack of parental affection could be the cause of scratching and thus persistence of the skin eruptions. Skin disease and scratching are one means for the child to obtain affection and attention from the parents. Scratching leads to greater attention from the parents and thus to a secondary profit of the disease.

On the other hand, the negative communication structures could also be a consequence of the chronic stress from the child's disease, with which the parents cannot cope. The skin symptoms are maintained or even exacerbated by unfavorable behavior. In most families a reciprocal potentiation of the two factors can probably be assumed.

Although an increasing number of children are afflicted with the skin disease atopic dermatitis, and although the positive effect of support and care has already been described, little help in coping with the problem is usually offered to the parents. Therapy is usually limited to prescription of care products and medications to suppress the itching, or even to dispensing well-meant suggestions for therapy, which often cause renewed disappointment when they are unsuccessfully applied. The uncertainty and confusion of the parents and their annoyance about doctors and therapeutic measures grow with every unsuccessful attempt at therapy. At the same time, these failures are another source of stress for the already-stressed family.

Parents are usually not able to cope with these conflicts alone. There is thus a danger that serious problems will arise early in the relationship to the reference person and to peers, which may have a detrimental effect on the child's self-confidence and emotional development. Support of the reference person with psychotherapy and training programs (44) are necessary to prevent such developments and to offer help to the afflicted parents and children in their current problems.

The question remains of the extent to which psychotherapeutic approaches lead to improvement or even freedom from symptoms in atopic dermatitis. Very few comparative studies have yet been performed. Bitzer et al. (45) found in a representative survey of atopic dermatitis patients in general practices, performed for a health insurance group, that patients reported satisfaction with psychotherapy to similar degrees as with cortisone therapy, although, considerably fewer patients had participated in psychotherapy than received treatment with cortisone. Other forms of therapy, like tar, light, and other topical treatments, were rated considerably poorer. There are no prospective studies yet on the effectiveness of deep psychological psychotherapy. In a catamnestic study, Williamson (46) examined 23 atopic dermatitis patients with psychodynamic psychotherapy in addition to routine dermatological treatment and 20 atopic dermatitis patients in a parallel control group who received exclusively dermatological care. About $1\frac{1}{2}$ years after conclusion of psychotherapy there was no difference in severity and coping with disease, but some (five) of the patients with additional deep psychological psychotherapy had event-free periods, while this was not reported in any case in the control group.

In presenting the psychotherapeutic possibilities for skin disease patients, the initiatives of the self-help groups in dermatology should not be forgotten. These groups are often able to offer very valuable psychotherapeutic assistance.

PSYCHOTHERAPY IN ATOPIC DERMATITIS

Suggested therapies in the literature refer mainly to behavioral therapeutic and depth psychological forms of therapy. In addition, there are numerous suggestions for combined therapy (47) (e.g., relaxation training, dermatological training). According to the depth psychology concept, psychotherapy can be performed with individual patients, with families, or even in groups. The treatment technique does not differ in these groups. The basis of the psychoanalytical-psychotherapeutic treatment is the creation of a viable therapeutic relationship via acceptance. On this basis, latent conflicts can be made accessible and conscious during the course of treatment. Correspondingly arising inner resistances and defense processes can be made accessible in order to be dealt with and overcome. This usually results in stabilization of the emotional balance and improved coping with the actual disease episodes. Supportive interventions alternate with revelatory interventions.

During in-depth psychological psychotherapy, special attention is paid to the affects (sadness, rage, etc.) and fantasies that arise during treatment. Making these affects and fantasies conscious should help the patient to obtain better insight into his own world and thus to attain altered coping ability in experiencing his disease.

An analytically oriented psychotherapeutic treatment may be indicated, especially in conjunction with chronic skin diseases, since stable and supportive family relationships appear to considerably improve the coping with disease in chronically ill patients.

STRESS IN CONNECTION WITH LIFE EVENTS

King and Wilson (48) examined 50 atopic dermatitis patients over a period of 14 days. In a subsequent meta-analysis, the calculated correlation coefficients revealed that the skin condition cross-correlated synchronously with values for anxiety/tension, interpersonal stress, depression, frustration, feelings of aggression, expressed aggression, and suppressed aggression (in that order). The authors showed that stress on the previous day correlated with the actual skin condition and the actual skin condition led to increased stress and elevated depression values on the following day.

Hospitalized atopic dermatitis patients were examined in a pilot study. An attempt was made to discover certain events that elicited the episodes. It was found that demonstrable psychosocial events (weekends, visits, discharge) were coupled significantly frequently with disease exacerbation. It was also able to demonstrate a number of cross-correlations between stress events and disease outbreak, as well as between emotional well-being and skin symptoms in a timed series study of six atopic dermatitis patients. Conversely, it was not possible to predict the skin condition on the subsequent day from the occurrence of stress events or any particular mood.

STATUS OF RESEARCH INTO THERAPEUTIC EFFECTIVENESS

Research into the effectiveness of psychotherapy in skin diseases, especially atopic dermatitis, is still largely in the beginning phase. To date, differential aspects in adult atopic dermatitis patients have only limited value with respect to prognostically relevant indication criteria, since the studies thus far refer usually to individual cases or very small numbers of patients. In general, clinical dermatology does not appear to have paid sufficient attention to psychological factors and psychotherapeutic possibilities.

A high level of motivation for therapy is considered prognostically positive, while early onset of disease and other additional atopical diseases are viewed as prognostically unfavorable. In a meta-analysis (49), various psychotherapeutic procedures were examined with respect to skin condition and subjective well-being. It was found that the psychotherapeutic procedures were clearly more effective than somatic-medical standard measures. The "atopic dermatitis personality" postulated in this study could not be confirmed, but the characteristics "anxiety," "depression," and "neuroticism" were significantly high. Of the 865 subjects examined, 553 were adult atopic dermatitis patients and 129 children. The effects of various combined psychotherapeutic interventions were examined. The skin symptoms improved significantly with all measures in the patients receiving psychotherapy. Their medication consumption and scratching frequency was also reduced.

Since skin diseases may be caused, according to psychoanalytical theory, by disruptions in early childhood development, other psychological therapy forms, like gestalt therapy or client-centered conversation (defined by Rogers), may be effective. However, no results with respect to atopic dermatitis have yet been published.

Atopic dermatitis has considerable influence on the patient's quality of life. The satisfaction with life is of central importance in experiencing and coping with disease. A number of stresses with corresponding psychosocial consequences make high demands on coping resources. It can therefore be assumed that various aspects of the disease will elicit various coping reactions, and they, in turn, may differ from the coping reactions in other stress situations. Chronic skin diseases like atopic dermatitis may lead to serious limitations in emotional well-being and are frequently coupled with social problems. It can be demonstrated that these stressing effects are underestimated in relation to other chronic diseases. Dermatological diseases like atopic dermatitis are particularly likely to be of considerable detriment to the self-image and to social relationships, since the symptoms are so visible. It happens frequently that patients with skin diseases experience negative social reactions from other persons, ranging from ambivalent reserve to distancing to open rejection. Occasionally, fear of contagion makes social contacts more difficult. Expectation of rejection and avoidance, for example, in public, leads to a consistent coping strategy of avoidance, which, however, in turn leads to generalization and exacerbation of the symptoms.

Itching is one symptom of atopic dermatitis. The intensive need to scratch is a serious limitation to well-being. Since itching can be elicited by external and internal stimuli, like heat, skin dryness, or simply imagining such sensations, it is a particularly stressful symptom. Likewise, the itching threshold can be lowered by stress. The scratching impulse to itching stimuli is a reflex that can be inhibited spinal by cortical structures. Scratching irritates the pain receptors. For a time, this reduces the sensation of itching, accompanied by a feeling of relief. With a slight delay, the itching threshold is reduced, which brings an increased sensation of itching and in turn increased scratching. When the skin is finally bleeding, it hardly itches—pain takes precedence over itching. In this constantly widening vicious circle, new skin damage arises and atopic dermatitis becomes chronic, with the known symptoms of thickening of the afflicted epidermis and coarsening of the skin structures. It has been demonstrated that even slight diffuse tensions or malaise can elicit scratching. Helplessness in the face of this vicious circle and guilt feelings of having failed in self-control give rise to additional emotional stress for the patients, which in turn can maintain the itching-scratching cycle. The ever-recurrent sequence of recurrences and freedom from episodes is also often accompanied by feelings of helplessness, of being thrown to the wolves, and by anxious-depressive moods. The stress of constant itching is also frequently underestimated. Sleep deficits and reduced ability to concentrate during episodes of the disease are frequent symptoms.

Due to disease-related habits like constant scratching or the experienced limitation of attractiveness, the negative aspects in communication increase. This, in turn, leads to additional unsolved problems in social relationships. The resultant increase in tension and aggression is expressed by more scratching and contributes to further exacerbation of the disease.

STATUS OF EMPIRICAL RESEARCH WITH ATOPIC DERMATITIS PREVENTION PROGRAMS

The effect of different combined psychotherapeutic interventions was investigated in several studies. A hydrocortisone therapy was compared alone with concomitant self-control strategies for the reduction of scratching, and another study investigated different topical applications including systemic steroids in comparison to a combined psychotherapy. The skin symptoms improved following all the methods, but significantly more so in patients with psychotherapy. The use of drugs decreased and systemic steroids were no longer used, even at one-month follow-up.

In methodically well-controlled studies (50), the effects of different forms of therapy were compared. Dermatological symptoms and scratching frequency were reduced by all the evaluated therapies studied, better by combined behavior therapy and scratching control techniques and in tendency better by behavior therapy compared with dermatological education and school medical therapy. In a further study the scratching frequency declined in one group while another group yielded better results with regard to itching, skin symptoms, and scratching frequency; in the first group the psychological variables "depressions," "fear of failure," "restrictions through atopic dermatitis," and "lack of self-assurance and attractiveness" were reduced; dermatological state and itching improved only in individual cases.

The psychological variables improved, especially following combined behavioral therapy and least in the control group. The fear tendency was most effectively reduced in the group with relaxation training and the combined behavior therapy group. The variable "anxiety" was in one study improved by dermatological teaching and combination therapy, but not significantly. The follow-up after 6 and 12 months showed that psychotherapeutical inverventions had more positive long-term effects on the course of the disease. The skin improved further following all psychological interventions. The combination of behavioral therapy and education (50) and the combined behavior therapy yielded marginally better results than the other forms of psychotherapy.

There are also studies concerning the effectivity of therapies in children with atopic dermatitis or their parents. In one study with children, complex dermatological therapy in a rehabilitation clinic was compared with an additional behavior therapy of 7 hours per week. At the end of the treatment, the skin was similarly improved in both atopic dermatitis groups.

In two recent controlled studies it was shown that educational measures were superior to routine therapy. Similar effects were observed in two groups, one of which underwent a direct training devised through to change behavior, while the other was schooled by videotapes. In a randomized study of 204 families it was shown that the quality of life of the mothers improved significantly in the invervention groups compared to the control group (44).

Atopic dermatitis is an important psychosomatic disease, and further studies should help to solve the problem of the missing link between affective state and psychoimmunological reactions.

REFERENCES

1. Braun-Falco O, Plewig P, Wolf H. Dermatologie und Venerologie. Heidelberg: Springer, 1996.
2. Jung EG. Dermatologie. Stuttgart: Hippokrates, 1998.
3. Fritsch P. Dermatologie und Venerologie: Lehrbuch und Atlas. Berlin: Springer, 1998.
4. Schmied C, Saurat JH. Epidemiology of atopic eczema. In: Ruzicka T, Ring J, Przybilla B, eds. Handbook of Atopic Eczema. New York: Springer, 1991.
5. Larsen FC, Holm NV, Henningsen K. Atopic dermatitis: a genetic-epidemiologic study in a population-based twin sample. J Am Acad Dermatol 1986; 1(15):487–494.
6. Przybilla B, Kaudewitz P. Ambulatory external treatment of psoriasis vulgaris: comparison of the effectiveness of a dithranol and glucocorticoid-containing preparation. Z Hautkr 1998; 61:60–62.
7. Leung DYM. Pathogenesis of atopic dermatitis. J Allergy Clin Immunol 1999; 104(suppl):99–108.
8. Werfel T, Kapp A. Environmental and other major provocation factors in atopic dermatitis. Allergy 1998; 53:731–739.
9. Merk H. Clinical symptoms of atopic eczema. In: Ruzicka T, Ring J, Przybilla B, eds. Handbook of Atopic Eczema. New York: Springer, 1991:27–30.
10. Hanifin JM, Chan S. Biochemical and immunologic mechanisms in atopic dermatitis: new targets for emerging therapies. J Am Acad Dermatol 1999; 41:72–77.
11. Bruynzeel-Koomen CA, van Wichen DF, Toonstra J, Berrens L, Bruynzeel PL. The presence of IgE molecules on epidermal Langerhans cells in patients with atopic dermatitis. Arch Dermatol Res 1986; 78:199–205.
12. Maurer D, Stingl G. Immunmechanismen der atopischen Dermatitis. Wien Klin Wschr 1993; 105:635–640.
13. Mudde G, van Rejsen FC, Boland GF. Allergen presentation by epidermal Langerhans cells from patients with atopis dermatitis is mediated by IgE. Immunology 1990; 69:335–341.
14. Szentivanyi A. The beta adrenergic theory of atopic abnormality in asthma. J Allergy 1968; 203–221.
15. Pichler WJ. In: Peter HH, Pichler WJ, eds. Klinische Immunologie. 2d ed. Munich: Urban & Schwarzenberg, 1996.
16. Kodama A, Horikawa T, Suzuki T, Ajiki W, Takashima T, Harada S, Ichihasha M. Effects of stress on atopic dermatitis: investigations in patients after the great Hanshin earthquake. J Allergy Clin Immunol 1999; 104:173–176.

17. Buske-Kirschbaum A, Geiben A, Hellhammer D. Psychobiological aspects of atopic dermatitis: an overview. Psychother Psychosom 2001; 70:6–16.

18. Kupfer J. Psychoimmunologische Verlaufsstudie bei Patientinnen mit atopischer Dermatitis. PhD dissertation, University of Gießen, Germany, 1994.

19. Augustin M, Zschocke I, Lange S, Seidenglanz K, Amon U. Lebensqualität bei Hauterkrankungen. Vergleich verschiedener Lebensqualitäts-Fragebogen bei Psoriasis und atopischer Dermatitis. Hautarzt 1999; 50:715–722.

20. Pines D. Skin communication: early skin disorders and their effect on transference and countertransference. Int J Psychoanal 1980; 61:315–323.

21. Gieler U, Detig-Kohler C. Nähe–Distanz bei Hautkranken. Psychotherapeutics 1994; 39:259–263.

22. Schur M. Comments on the metapsychology of somatization. Psychoanal Study Child 1955; 10:119–164.

23. Marty P. La relation objectale allergique. Rev Franc Psychoanal 1958; 22:5–35.

24. Prochazka P, von Uslar A. Die Machtverhältnisse in der Mutter-Kind Beziehung bei der Neurodermitis constitutionalis atopica (Atopische Dermatitis). Z Hautkr 1989; 64:863–866.

25. Bryam W. Sexual problems encountered with patients suffering from asthma and eczema. J Am Inst Hypnosis 1972; 13:26–34.

26. Niemeier V, Winckelsesser T, Gieler U. Hautkrankheit und Sexualität. Eine empirische Studie zum Sexualverhalten von Patienten mit Psoriasis vulgaris und Neurodermitis im Vergleich mit Hautgesunden. Hautarzt 1997; 48:629–633.

27. Hänsler B. Die Belastung und Befindlichkeit von Eltern, deren Kindern an atopischer Dermatitis erkrankt sind. Diplomarbeit am FB Psychologie, Universität Marburg, 1990.

28. Koblenzer C, Koblenzer P. Chronic intractable atopic eczema. Its occurence as a physical sign of impaired parent-child relationships and psychologic development arrest: improvement through parent insight and education. Arch Dermatol 1988; 124:1673–1677.

29. Ring J, Palos E, Zimmermann F. Psychosomatische Aspekte der Eltern-Kind Beziehung bei atopischen Ekzem im Kindesalter. II. Erziehungsstil, Familiensituation im Zeichentest und strukturierte Interviews. Hautarzt 1986; 37:560–567.

30. Solomon R, Gagnon C. Mother and child characteristics and involvement in dyads in which very young children have eczema. J Dev Behav Pediatr 1987; 8:213–220.

31. Hermanns J, Florin I, Dietrich M, Rieger C, Hahlweg K. Maternal criticism, mother-child interaction and bronchial asthma. J Psychosom Res 1989; 33/4:469–476.

32. Wenninger K, Ehlers A, Gieler U. Kommunikation von Neurodermitis-Patienten mit ihren Bezugspersonen—eine empirische Analyse. Zeitschr Klin Psychol 1991; 20:251–264.

33. Miller H, Baruch D. Psychosomatic studies of children with allergic manifestations. Psychosom Med 1948; 10:274.

34. Miller H, Baruch D. A study of hostility in allergic children. Am J Orthopsychiatry 1950; 20:506.

35. Marmor J, Ashley M, Tabachnik N, Storkman M, McDonald F. The mother child relationship in the genesis of neurodermatitis. Arch Dermatol Syphilol 1956; 74:599–605.

36. Williams D. Management of atopic dermatitis in children: control of the maternal rejection factor. Arch Dermatol 1951.

37. Langfeldt P, Luys K. Mütterliche Erziehungseinstellungen, Familienklima und Neurodermatitis bei Kindern—eine Pilotstudie. Praxis der Kinderpsychologie und Kinderpsychiatrie. Göttingen: Verlag Vandenhoeck & Ruprecht, 1993.

38. Passoth P. Das Auftreten einer Neurodermitisähnlichen Dermatitis bei Kindern nach Herztransplantation im ersten Lebensjahr unter Cyclosporin A. MD dissertation, Fachbereich Humanmedizin, Justus-Liebig-Universität, Gießen, 2001.

39. Hünecke P, Krüger C. Why is my child scratching? Ursachenverständnis von Müttern und dessen Konsequenzen. Unpublished, 1995.

40. Allen K, Harris F. Elimination of a child's excessive scratching by training the mother in reinforcement procedures. Behav Res Ther 1966; 4:79–84.

41. Bär L, Kuypers B. Behaviour therapy in dermatological practice. B J Dermatol 1973; 88:591–59.

42. Walton D. The application of learning theory to the treatment of a case of neurodermatitis. In: Eysenck H-J, ed. Behavior Research and Therapy and the Neuroses. New York: Pergamon Press, 1960:272–274.

43. Broberg A, Kalimo K, Lindblad B, Swanbeck G. Parental education in the treatment of childhood atopic eczema. Acta Derm Venereol (Stockh) 1990; 70:495–499.

44. Gieler U, Kupfer J, Niemeier V, Brosig B, Stangier U. Atopic eczema prevention programs: a new therapeutic concept for secondary prevention. Dermatol Psychosom 2000; 1:138–146.

45. Bitzer EM, Grobe TG, Dorning H. Die Bewertung therapeutischer Maßnahmen bei atopischer Dermatitis und Psoriasis aus der Perspektive der Patienten unter Berücksichtigung komplimentär medizinischer Verfahren. ISEG Studie Endbericht, 1997.

46. Williamson P. Psychotherapie bei Neurodermitis-Patienten—eine retrospektive Studie an 43 Neurodermitis-Patienten. Dissertation, Justus-Liebig-Universität Gießen, 2000.

47. Gieler U, Stangier U, Ernst R. Psychosomatische Behandlung im Rahmen der klinischen Therapie von Hautkrankheiten. In: Bosse K, Gieler U, eds. Seelische Faktoren bei Hautkrankheiten. Bern: Huber, 1986.

48. King RM, Wilson GV. Use of a diary technique to investigate psychosomatic relations in atopic dermatitis. J Psychosom Res 1991; 35:697–706.

49. Al Abesie, S. Atopische Dermatitis und Psyche. MD dissertation, Fachbereich Humanmedizin, Giessen, Germany, 2000.

50. Ehlers A, Stangier U, Gieler U. Treatment of atopic eczema: a comparison of psychological and dermatological approaches to relapse prevention. J Consult Clin Psychol 1995; 63(4):624–635.

8

Pathogenesis of Atopic Dermatitis
Integrating Physiological and Psychophysiological Data

Sandy Duyen Hong
UCLA Harbor Medical Center
Los Angeles, California, U.S.A.

John Y. M. Koo
University of California, San Francisco
San Francisco, California, U.S.A.

INTRODUCTION

Atopic dermatitis is a relapsing, chronic, inflammatory skin disorder that incurs significant morbidity and socioeconomical costs to patients and their families. The cause of atopic dermatitis (AD) is currently under investigation. The pathogenesis of AD is believed to be multifactorial, including genetic factors, immunological derangements, and allergenic environmental triggers (1). Increased psychological stress has clearly been shown to exacerbate or initiate the onset in a large proportion of AD patients (2–4). Psychological stress is clearly not an antigen, yet the majority of investigation about the pathogenesis of AD is focused on immunological and antigenic pathways, largely ignoring the role of the psyche and the nervous system. Although physicians have long recognized the role of psychological stress in the clinical exacerbation of AD, only a few studies have examined the psychoneuroimmunological pathogenesis of AD as a contributing etiological or exacerbating factor in AD. This chapter reviews recent studies that have investigated the neuroimmunological pathogenesis of psychological stress on AD and attempt to integrate this with current physiological explanations regarding the pathogenesis of AD.

METHODS

Two Medline literature searches were performed. One search included papers written in English, dated 1990–2000, using the key words atopic dermatitis and stress and pathophysiology. Original papers that discussed the pathophysiology of stress-induced/stress-related exacerbation of AD or how stress modulates the immune system are reviewed. The second search included reviews articles written in English, dated 1990–2000, using the key words atopic dermatitis with subheadings of etiology and pathogenesis.

RESULTS

Current Concepts in Atopic Dermatitis

Prior to reviewing how psychoneurological data integrate into the pathogenesis of AD, a short review of current concepts in AD is presented. Atopic dermatis is considered a chronic inflammatory disease of the skin. Its pathophysiology is believed to include genetic, immunological, environmental, skin barrier function, and psychological factors. Atopic dermatitis is an inflammatory disease characterized by pruritis, mild to severe erythema, scaling, excoriations, and, when chronic, the formation of lichenified skin. The majority of patients with AD are found to have elevated numbers of circulating eosinophils, serum IgE, and localization of mast cells in lesional skin (1). Both lesional and uninvolved skin of patients with AD have been found to have impaired barrier function with increased evaporative water loss, suggesting an intrinsic defect in the keratinocytes of patients with AD (5).

Epidemiology and Genetics

The prevalence of AD is increasing worldwide, with 0.7–2.4% of the U.S. population currently affected (6). The most important risk factor for the disease is the development of the "western lifestyle," although which factors of this lifestyle cause AD are unknown (5). Popular theories of why the western lifestyle is associated with increased atopy links early exposure to psychosocial stress from the fast pace of western life and also reduced microbial exposure. The "hygiene hypothesis" theorizes that reduced microbial exposure because of near-sterile food preparation and large-scale immunization affect the differentiation of T-cell populations to a more atopic profile of increased Th2 cells (7).

Genetic studies have attempted to find genetic polymorphism associated with common immune findings found in patients with AD such as elevated IgE levels and altered cytokine profiles. Thus far attempts to match specific gene polymorphism with phenotypes of AD have not been successful (5). Many genes are now thought to be involved in the development of AD. Currently, chromosome 5q31–33 is of great interest because it contains the genes responsible for cytokines interleukin (IL)-3, IL-4, IL-5, IL-13, and CM-CSF (1).

IgE and Allergens

IgE-mediated antigen presentation of allergens is considered a key event in the pathogenesis of AD. Following allergen presentation of IgE-allergen complexes to T cells, T cells are then activated to switch into Th1 or Th2 subtypes and B cells are activated to produce more IgE. Also found in the dermis of patients with AD are an increased number of Langerhans cells with high-affinity receptors that bind IgE and in turn also process IgE-binding allergens for presentation to T cells, amplifying the body's response to allergens (5). Foods such as egg, milk, and wheat have been implicated as allergens, as have aeroallergens such as ragweed pollen (1). Studies have shown that inhalation of dust mite and direct patch testing with allergens produces eczematous lesions. Autoallergens such as skin dander have also been shown to trigger reactions in the skin of patients with AD, suggesting a role for autoallergy (8).

Th1/Th2 Concept and the Link to IgE

In patients with AD there is systemic activation of T cells. Following activation, T-helper (Th) cells switch to become Th1 cells, producing IL-2 and interferon (IFN)-γ or Th2 cells producing cytokine IL-4 and IL-5 (5). In the dermis of patients with AD there are increased numbers of Th2 cells producing IL-4 and IL-5. Thus, associated with AD is an increased ratio of Th2 to Th1 cells. Th2 cytokines (IL-4 and IL-5) are believed to result in elevated IgE levels and eosinophilia often found in patients with AD (1).

Increased IgE levels in patients with AD is associated with an increased expression of type II T-helper cell (Th2) cytokines. Type II T-helper white blood cells are associated with secretion of cytokines IL-4 and IL-5, while type I T-helper cells (Th1) secrete IFN-γ (5). Th1 cells are associated with delayed-type hypersensitivity reactions, while Th2 cells are associated with humoral immunity. IL-4 is known to induce germline transcription switching, which promotes the maturation of plasma cells into IgE-producing B cells. IL-4 is also known to inhibit Th1 cytokines. IL-5 is associated with eosinophilic development, recruitment, and enhanced eosinophilic survival (1). There is an inverse correlation between IFN-γ levels and serum IgE levels of patients with AD, suggesting low Th1 activity. Current research has found evidence that expression of Th1 and Th2 cytokines changes over time. In acute AD the number of white blood cells in the skin expressing IL-4 is high and IFN-γ mRNA levels are low. In chronic lesions decreased IL-4 and increased IL-5 and IFN-γ levels are associated with infiltration of eosinophils and macrophages. IFN-γ is known to inhibit Th1 proliferation (1).

AD and Microbes

Staphylococcus aureus is found in more than 90% of AD skin lesions compared to 5% of healthy individuals. It is believed that this bacteria produces a supertoxin that acts as a superantigen, stimulating T-cell activation. Most patients with AD have IgE antibodies to these super-antigens, and clinical treatment with antistaphylococcal medication improves AD (1).

Phosphodiesterase Enzyme Activity

In patients with AD, mononuclear cells have increased cyclic AMP–phosphodiesterase (PDE) activity. In B cells this results in increased IgE synthesis and T cells increased IL-4 production. These monocytes also contribute to increased levels of pro-inflammatory PGE2, which inhibits the response of Th1 cells (9).

AD and Psychopathology: Mast Cells, Histamine, Neuropeptides, and Endorphins

Pruritis is a major symptom of AD. The mediators of pruritis so far identified include histamine, cytokines, leukotrienes, neuropeptides, and proteases. Cutaneous injection of these agents has been shown to cause pruritis. Histamines and cyclosporine, which block antihistamine release and decrease cytokine and leukotriene levels, have been shown to alleviate pruritis in AD patients (1).

Histamine levels of patients with AD are higher in both lesional and nonlesional skin compared to patients without skin disease. Histamine is released by mast cells and by basophils. Release of histamine causes vasodilation and stimulates cutaneous nerves, leading to the sensation of pruritis (1). Stimulation of the unmyelinated nerves causes the release of neuropeptides such as substance P and neurotensin, which acts on masts cells, amplifying the initial inflammatory response, potentiating histamine release by mast cells. Chronic itching and scratching by patients with AD leads to thickening and lichenification of the skin. These plaques have shown increased number of mast cells compared to nonlesional skin (10). In looking for an explanation of how psychological stress and trigger outbreaks of AD, Singh et al. (10) have investigated the reaction of mast cells to neuropeptides and neurohormones.

Corticotropin-releasing hormone (CRH) is released from the hypo-thalamus in response to stress. Cutaneous CRH injection has been shown to cause mast cell degranulation of histamine in the skin. Singh et al. looked for a direct correlation between stress and the exacerbation of AD by demonstrating that psychological stress increases mast cell degranulation (10). To establish the link between psychological stress and physiological changes, Singh et al. compared the amount of mast cell degranulation in mice that were psychologically unstressed versus those that were stressed. They stressed mice by immobilizing them in plexiglass containers for 30 minutes. Control mice were left in their cages. They then measured cutaneous mast cell degranulation by visually counting mast cells and estimating their degranulation in stressed mice exposed to anti-CRH antibodies. In stressed mice degranulation of mast cells was $40.7 \pm 9.1\%$ compared with $22.2 \pm 7.3\%$ in nonstressed mice ($p < 0.03$). However, for stressed mice pretreated with anti-CRH antibody, mast cell degranulation was comparable to nonstressed levels at $21.0 \pm 3.3\%$ ($p < 0.05$), despite being immobilized. Singh et al. also showed that mast cell degranulation in animals pretreated with capsaicin to prevent the production of neuropep-tides such as substance P was approximately 15% less than in untreated animals, suggesting that neuropeptides such as substance P have a role in the normal degranulation of mast cells. Pretreatment of stressed mice with neurotensin receptor antagonist also showed that mast cell degranulation was significantly decreased by approximately 12.5% (10).

Given that neuropeptides have mitogenic activity that is believed to modulate the immune system, Glinski et al. looked for differences in the opiate neuropeptide β-endorphin levels in patients with AD (11). Neuropeptides are found in dermal sensory type C fibers and small size–mediated nerve A-delta endings. β-endorphin is an opiate neuropeptide released by the pituitary and by inflammatory cells, in lesional skin, in response to stress. β-endorphin is known to diminish nociceptive sensation at the level of the sensory nerve so that the sensation of pain is lessened, although this is known to increase the sensation of pruritis. Glinski et al.

found that in AD patients with greater than 20% skin involvement, serum β-endorphin was on average 50% higher compared to controls (11).

AD and Psychopathology: IgE and Cytokines

Serum IgE is believed to play an important role in the pathogenesis of allergic diseases. IgE binds to mast cells, basophils, and Langerhans cells and, when cross-linked with allergens, can trigger activation of these cells, causing the subsequent release of histamine, proteases, and cytokines (12). Patients with AD are known to have increased levels of serum IgE compared to healthy patients (13). Researchers interested in the connection between the psychopathology of AD and its immunology have looked for links between known psychological traits associated with AD and immunological indices. Patients with AD are associated with psychological profiles that include increased anxiety and depression (96).

Scheich et al. (13) tested patients with AD using the Freiburg Personality Inventory and the State-Trait Anxiety Inventory. They found patients with AD to have increased traits of excitability and inadequate stress coping mechanisms. They then tested the serum IgE of these patients and found that patients with AD who have IgE levels greater than 100 IU/mL are more likely to have traits of excitability and inadequate stress coping compared to other patients with AD (13). However, given the small number of patients evaluated, the results of the study may be biased. Unfortunately, the investigators did not rate or record the severity of AD in these patients, which is another variable associated with serum IgE levels.

In a study that used the State-Trait Anxiety Inventory and a self-rating depression scale, patients with moderate to severe AD were found to have increased levels of depression and state/trait anxiety when compared to control patients (14). Hashiro and Okumura then looked at natural killer (NK) cell activity, IL-4, and IFN-γ levels as indices of the patients' immune function. They found that NK cell activity and IL-4 activity were lowered in depressive and/or anxious AD patients, while IFN-γ levels tended to be higher compared to normal controls. By analysis they found that a decrease in NK cell activity was strongly associated with patients who have higher anxiety levels, suggesting that anxiety most likely effects NK cell activity (14).

AD and Psychopathology: Impaired Glucocorticoid Response

Conventional investigation of the role of glucocorticoids in the pathogenesis of AD have focused on a subset of atopic patients with allergic rhinitis, asthma, or AD who are known to have poor responses to both topical and systemic therapy to treatment with glucocorticoids (GCs). Normally GCs act by binding to cytoplasmic GC receptors. The ligand-receptor complex then translocates into the nucleus and acts as a transcription factor to modulate cellular expression of cytokines. GC resistance and sensitivity has been mainly studied in patients with asthma, the results of which have important clinical implications to AD. Functional cellular abnormalities in GC-resistant patients such as persistent T-cell activation and failure of GCs to inhibit T-cell proliferation in vitro have been found. Recent research has suggested that increased levels of IL-2 and IL-4 may induce the expression of a defective T-cell GC ligand receptor, known as GCR-β. GCR-β has a decreased DNA-binding affinity, and so GCs bound to this receptor cannot effect the same cellular responses as GCs bound to normal T-cell GC receptors. Thus, current investigators postulate that increased levels of IL-2 and IL-4 from Th2-type cells may be responsible for derangements in response to endogenous and therapeutically administered glucocorticoids (1).

Psychoneurological research by many investigators has focused on the hypothalamic pituitary axis and the CRH glucocorticoid cascade. Rupprecht et al. (15) found that patients with AD have decreased ACTH and cortisol responses to CRH stimulation. Buske-Kirschbaum et al. (16) found that the cortisol response is blunted in children with atopic dermatitis exposed to stress, suggesting an altered hypothalamic-pituitary-adrenal (HPA) axis of patients with AD. They took children with AD who were currently in remission and compared their salivary cortisol response to a specific social stressor, such as public speaking, with control children who did not have AD. Following psychometric testing that did not show major differences in personality characteristics usually associated with AD, such as anxiety and depression, between the children with AD and controls, the authors found that children with AD had significantly blunted levels of salivary cortisol in response to the stress of public speaking (16).

Another paper that provides additional information about the HPA axis and stress is that of Tabata et al. (17). Dehydroepiandosterone (DHEA), another adrenal androgen regulated by the CRH and ACTH axis, is known to increase the production of Th1 lymphokines, IL-2, and IFN-γ. DHEA levels in animals have been shown to be decreased during stress (17). Tabata et al. looked for the action of DHEA in association with Th2-associated IL-4 and IL-5. IL-4 is known to increase serum IgE levels. The authors found that DHEA reduces IL-4 production by peripheral blood mononuclear cells. They also found that DHEA levels are reduced in patients with AD. DHEA levels are not correlated, however, to serum IgE levels.

DISCUSSION

The above studies that focus on the link between AD and neuropsycho-endocrinimmunology parallel studies of the pathogenesis of AD with a focus on four main areas: differences in mast cell function, alterations serum IgE level, a focus on cytokine profile variations, and the role of stress-released CRH and the HPA axis.

Psychological stress is viewed as an exacerbating factor that affects the inherent pathophysiological mechanisms involved in AD. Scheich et al. (13) found that patients with AD have increased personality traits of excitability and inadequate stress-coping mechanisms that were associated with levels of IgE > 100 IU/mL. Although they found no correlation between severity of acute skin condition and anxiety, the increased IgE levels in these patients may be a reflection of increased disease burden overall, resulting in psychological duress and inadequate coping mechanisms. A cause-and-effect relationship cannot be established, but the association of elevated IgE levels and increased patient anxiety is one that may be clinically useful, helping physicians to target specific patients for referral for anxiety or stress-coping therapy.

Hashiro and Okumura (14) found that in patients with AD who had increased levels of depression or anxiety, NK cell activity, IL-4, and IFN-γ levels were altered. They suggest that anxiety most likely affects NK cell activity. Unfortunately, they did not look at the NK cell activity of nonanxious patients with AD or stressed control patients, so that an understanding of whether NK function is affected by stress in all people or only in patients with AD was not reached. The mechanism by which stress directly or indirectly affects immune function was also not addressed in that study. Interestingly, the cytokine profile described in the AD patients with increased levels of depression and or anxiety matches those found in chronic lesional skin of AD patients. Hashiro's patients had moderate to severe AD. From these data one may infer that the cytokine profile observed in these patients is a reflection of their disease severity, which then affects their psyche. However, not all studies have found a correlation between the severity of AD and anxiety (18).

Glinski et al. (11) attempted to find direct links between the CNS and the factors involved in AD by studying neuropeptides released in the CNS and by inflammatory cells. They found that β-endorphins are increased in AD patients with up to 20% involvement skin involvement. The release of β-endorphins in lesional skin may be triggered by direct CNS to peripheral neural stimulation or through neuroendocrine stimulation with the release of CRH and direct or subsequent ACTH stimulation of endorphin release. Rupprecht's work (15), in which ACTH and cortisol levels were attenuated in response to CRH with no changes in β-endorphin levels, suggests that β-endorphins may be released locally either through direct peripheral neural stimulation or through another mechanism that does not include the CRH-ACTH pathway.

The work of Singh et al. (10) provides a clue to the link between psychological stress, the neuroendocrine system, and atopic dermatitis. By showing that CRH directly affects mast cell degranulation, Singh's work suggests that stress-released CRH from the hypothalamus can affect the pathogenesis of AD by increasing cutaneous levels of histamine. As expected, blocking neurotensin (NT) and substance P also decreased mast cell degranulation. Unfortunately, Singh et al. did not measure NT levels or substance P levels when anti-CRH antibody was administered in stressed mice. This would have provided information as to whether CRH has a direct effect on NT or substance P levels.

Other studies (15–17) strongly suggest that derangements in the HPA axis may be intrinsic in the pathogenesis of AD. The diminished levels of cortisol released in response to stress by children with AD suggest that patients with AD may have attenuated responses to CRH or ACTH or dysfunctional HPA feedback regulation. From the above studies we can postulate that exacerbations from psychological stress may be caused by CRH release in the hypothalamic-pituitary vasculature, which may transiently stimulate mast cell degranulation, triggering the inflammatory cascade and causing symptoms of pruritis and erythema. In patients with AD who have either lower cortisol and/or DHEA responses to hypo-thalamic/pituitary stimulation, an inappropriately vigorous immune response, which manifests itself as disease exacerbation, may occur because normal modulation of the immune response by cortisol and DHEA does not happen.

It is also possible, however, given the findings that increased levels of IL-4 and IL-2 from Th2 cells may cause an altered glucocorticoid response via induced expression of non–DNA-binding T-cell GC ligand receptors, that derangements in the HPA axis may be secondary to Th2 expansion. We can hypothesize that there is an inherent diathesis where, following an allergenic immune response that alters the body's intrinsic HPA axis via glucocorticoid dysregulation, the body continues to react inappropriately to psychological stress with loss of regular inhibitory signals.

SUMMARY

This chapter reviews recent studies that investigated the neuroimmunolo-gical pathogenesis of AD in conjunction with current pathophysiological understanding of AD. We found that CRH, neuropeptides, and the HPA axis may play key roles in the pathogenesis of AD, interacting with dysregulated immune function. However, future research in this area is needed to advance the integration between the "organic" and "psychodermatological" pathogenesis of atopic dermatitis.

REFERENCES

1. Leung DYM. Atopic dermatitis: new insights and opportunities for therapeutic intervention. J Allergy Clin Immunol 2000; 105(5):860–876.
2. Koblenzer CS. Psychosomatic concepts in dermatology: a dermatologist-psychoanalyst's viewpoint. Arch Dermatol 1983; 119:501–512.
3. Ginsburg J, Prystowsky J, Kornfeld D, Wolland H. Role of emotional factors in adults with atopic dermatitis. Int J Dermatol 1993; 32(2):656–660.
4. Gupta MA, Gupta AD. Psychodermatology: an update. J Am Acad Dermatol 1996; 134(6):1030–1046.
5. Wollenburg A, Bieber T. Atopic dermatitis: from the genes to skin lesions. Allergy 55:205–213.
6. Ehlers A, Stangier U, Gieler U. Treatment of atopic dermatitis: a comparison of psychological and dermatological approaches to relapse prevention. J Consult Clin Psychol 1995; 63(4):624–635.
7. Kalliomaki M, Salminen S, Arvilommi H, Kero P, Koskinin P, Isolauri E. Probiotic in primary prevention of atopic disease: a randomised placebo-controlled trial. Lancet 2001; 357:1057–1059.
8. Valenta R, Seiberler S, Natter S, Mahler V, Mossabeb R, Ring J, Stingl G. Autoallergy: a pathogenetic factor in atopic dermatitis? J Allergy Clin Immunol 2000; 5(3):432–437.
9. Hanfin J, Chan S. Biochemical and immunologic mechanisms in atopic dermatitis: new targets for emerging therapies. J Am Acad Dermatol 1999; 41(1):72–77.
10. Singh L, Pang X, Alexacos N, Letourneau R, Theoharides T. Acute immobilization stress triggers skin mast cell degranulation via corticotropin releasing hormone, neurotensin, and substance P: a link to neurogenic skin disorders. Brain Behav Immun 1999; 13:225–239.
11. Glinski W, Brodecka H, Glinska-Ferenz M, Kowalski D. Increased concentration of beta-endorphin in the sera of patients with severe atopic dermatitis. Arch Derm Venereol 1995; 75:9–11.
12. Leung D. Molecular basis of allergic diseases. Mol Gen Metab 1998; 63:157–167.
13. Scheich G, Florin I, Rudolph R, Wilhelm S. Personality characteristics and serum IgE level in patients with atopic dermatitis. J Psychosom Res 1993; 37:637–642.

14. Hashiro M, Okumura M. The relationship between the psychological and immunological state in patients with atopic dermatitis. J Derm Sci 1998; 16:231–235.

15. Rupprecht M, Hornstein O, Schluter D, Schafers H-J, Koch HU, Beck G, Rupprecht R. Cortisol, corticotropin, and beta endorphin responses to corticotropin-releasing hormone in patients with atopic eczema. Psychoneuroendocrinology 1995; 20(5):543–551.

16. Buske-Kirschbaum A, Jobst S, Wustmans A, Kirshbaum C, Rauh W, Hellhammer D. Attenuated free cortisol response to psychosocial stress in children with atopic dermatitis. Psychosom Med 1997; 59:419–426.

17. Tabata N, Tagami H, Terui T. Dehydroepiandosterone may be one of the regulators of cytokine production in atopic dermatitis. Arch Dermatol Res 1997; 289:410–414.

18. Linnet J, Jemech G. An assessment of anxiety and dermatology life quality in patients with atopic dermatitis. Br J Dermatol 1999; 140:268–272.

9

Practical Issues in the Management of the Delusional Patient

Sylvia Garnis-Jones and Barry Douglas Jones
McMaster University
Hamilton, Ontario, Canada

INTRODUCTION

Patients with certain psychiatric diagnoses seek dermatological care as a means of denying their psychopathology. In the majority of cases these patients have delusions. A delusion is a false, unshakeable idea or belief that is out of keeping with the patient's educational, cultural, and social background. The patient holds this belief with the same conviction and intensity as he holds other nondelusional beliefs about himself. Subjectively, a delusion is a belief. The deluded person is usually extremely irritated by any logical argument or evidence that is presented contrary to the belief (1). Therefore, these patients are usually difficult to assess and treat. This chapter focuses on 1) the symptomatology of delusional disorder as it relates to the dermatologist, 2) the differential diagnosis, 3) the approach to the patient, and 4) nonpharmacological and pharmacological treatment.

SYMPTOMATOLOGY

The chief presenting complaint can vary, but the content of the individual patient's delusion remains consistent over time. The most common complaints seen by dermatologists are as follows:

Delusions of parasitosis: The patient develops a fixed idea that his or her skin is infected by insects, internal parasites, or foreign bodies under the skin. This is usually associated with a compulsion to excoriate in an attempt to remove the offending substance. The patient usually brings in pieces of skin, paper, or articles of clothing as "specimens" to be analyzed in order to prove the existence of the problem (2). Delusions of parasitosis is discussed at length in another chapter.

Delusions of dysmorphosis: The patient is convinced that he or she is ugly, misshapen, or has an overprominent body part. These individuals seek the opinion of plastic surgeons in addition to dermatologists in attempts to rectify the abnormality. In some cases this is taken to an extreme, with the patient attempting to remove a "misshapen" body part themselves (3). Body dysmorphic disorder is discussed at length in another chapter.

Delusions of bromosis: The patient believes that he or she emits a foul odor from the skin or bowel or has severe halitosis (4).

Technically only delusions of parasitosis, dysmorphosis, and bromosis as discussed above are considered true delusional states in the psychiatric literature (5). However, we have included the following conditions within this discussion since from a dermatological viewpoint the differential diagnosis and the approach to the patient is similar.

Dysesthesias: The patient complains of burning, itching, dull ache, or throbbing pain of a body part such as the tongue or palate (glossodynia), palms or soles, or perivaginal (vulvodynia) or perirectal skin (6). Cutaneous sensory disorder is discussed at length in another chapter.

Factitial dermatitis: These patients present with multiple erosions or excoriations and in some cases ulcers, which can be localized or generalized on the surface of the skin that is within reach. Usually the lesions produced have a bizarre morphology with sharp angular borders since they are produced with pointed objects (7). Factitial dermatitis, also known as dermatitis artefacta, is discussed at length in another chapter.

Neurotic excoriations: Excoriating and picking behavior results in erosions on areas of the body that are within reach. The attempt is to remove "skin blemishes." An example would be the young female who cannot refrain from trying to remove any facial acne papule (acne excoriee de jeune filles) (8). Neurotic excoriation is discussed at length in another chapter.

Pruritus: Pruritus elicits the desire to scratch. Dermatologically these patients have linear erosions in areas they can reach. The complaint is of either a persistent sharp, localized sensation or an unpleasant diffuse itch with a burning quality. With localized itch, certain areas are involved with a greater frequency (e.g., perianal, vulvar, scrotal areas and scalp). If the condition has become chronic, one would also expect to see lichenified plaques and prurigo nodules (9).

DIFFERENTIAL DIAGNOSIS

The first task in evaluating the patient whose complaints suggest a psychogenic component is to exclude nonpsychogenic causes of the complaint. A differential diagnosis including metabolic problems is always a consideration. This will be discussed first, followed by a discussion of the psychiatric differential diagnosis.

Nonpsychogenic Causes

In the case of possible infestation, the effects of certain drugs can mimic a delusion. The most common offender is cocaine, which produces a perceptual disturbance in the form of tactile hallucinations referred to as "cocaine bugs" or "Magnan's sign" (10). Other drugs that have been implicated are amphetamines, methylphenidate, phenelzine, and anticholinergic agents (11). Alcohol withdrawal is another possibility (11). Metabolic conditions are also a consideration, in particular, multiple sclerosis, pernicious anemia, pellagra, hypothyroidism, diabetes mellitus, and polycythemia vera (12).

In terms of complaints regarding a feeling of ugliness or a distortion of body image, neurological disorders should be kept in mind. Unilateral spinal cord lesions, thrombosis of the posterior inferior cerebellar artery, multiple sclerosis, myasthenia gravis (13), and temporal lobe epilepsy (12) have been reported as producing "pseudodelusions." With respect to olfactory complaints, neurological problems, in particular temporal lobe epilepsy, should be considered (14).

In terms of the pain syndromes, dysesthesias of the mouth have been reported to be caused by poorly fitting dentures, moniliasis, vitamin B_{12} or iron deficiency, diabetes mellitus, and xerotomia secondary to Sjögren's syndrome (15). In terms of the palms and soles, peripheral neuropathies and nerve entrapment are a possibility. Grushka (16) and Coles (17) found that postmenopausal women had a higher incidence of dysesthesia and suggested that atrophic changes induced by menopause may play a role.

Neurotic excoriations and factitial disorder can both be considered self-mutilation syndromes (12). In both cases a disruption of the skin surface is the primary finding. The differential diagnosis includes an underlying peripheral neuropathy, which produces an unpleasant sensation resulting in the person scratching, rubbing, picking, or pulling at the skin in order to alleviate the sensation (18). Inherent biochemical anomalies can also result in self-mutilation as, for example, in the Lesch-Nyhan syndrome (18). Other considerations include the less common bacterial and fungal infections of the skin, septic infarcts, polyarteritis nodosa, pyoderma gangrenosum, inflammatory panniculitis, spider bites, Wegener's granulomatosis, and granulomatous vasculitis (18).

With generalized pruritus, the paucity of clinical findings is in sharp contrast to the symptoms. Lyell (19) reported that in 74 patients, 31% had pruritus due to an underlying dermatological problem, 25% had systemic illness, 31% were psychogenic, and in 10% an underlying cause could not be found. Beare (20) investigated 43 individuals with pruritus but no signs of excoriation. He found that only 16% had an underlying systemic cause. In terms of systemic disease, some information is available with respect to incidence. Eighty to 90% of patients with renal failure have pruritus (21). In liver disease, pruritus is present in 25% of jaundiced patients, virtually all patients with primary biliary cirrhosis, and 50% of patients with carcinoma. It is also present in 1.5–3% of pregnant women and in patients taking medication that can cause cholestasis, the primary offenders being phenothiazines, tolbutamide, anabolic steroids, estrogens, and progestins (22). In terms of hematological problems, 30–50% of patients with polycythemia itch (22). Hodgkin's lymphoma has associated itch in 30% of cases and thyrotoxicosis in 4–11% (22). With respect to diabetes, Gilchrest quotes an incidence of 3% (22).

In addition to the differential diagnosis for metabolic problems, an underlying dermatological problem is always of concern and should also be excluded before assuming the presenting problem is psychogenic. All of the following groups of skin disorders should be considered: sensitivity reactions to medication, infection, environmentally related skin disorders such as polymorphous light eruption, the endogenous and exogenous dermatoses such as atopic dermatitis and contact dermatitis, respectively, bullous eruptions, papulosquamous eruptions, and cutaneous neoplasm (12).

Psychogenic Causes

The differential diagnosis from the psychiatric perspective is broad. In patients where it can be determined that delusions are definitely present, the diagnosis can range from schizophrenia to psychotic depression in the absence of known organic etiology for the psychopathological symptoms. In patients where delusions can be ruled out as discussed in the section above, the underlying psychiatric disorder can be a nonpsychotic depressive disorder, obsessive-compulsive disorder, or factitious disorder. A discussion of the salient points of these psychiatric disorders follows, as they can be helpful to the dermatologist in deciding which route to follow with respect to further management and treatment.

Delusions Present

In the psychotic patient with delusions, he or she does not have any insight. They are convinced that their belief is absolutely true although no one in their immediate family or of their acquaintances share their belief. The belief is usually "encapsulated," in other words, the rest of their personality remains appropriate. However, the severity of the delusion is such that it takes over the person's lifestyle. He or she is driven to seek appropriate treatment for the imaginary physical ailment or infestation (23). A delusion may also be part of a more severe psychosis, schizophrenia, where the entire personality structure and thought process is affected. Their delusions tend to take on a bizarre quality, such as complaining that "lasers are destroying their organs" or "extraterrestrial influences are at work." Physicians should consider the possibility of schizophrenia when a young adult makes unusual persistent complaints that are not matched by physical findings (24). Delusions, however, can also be the only presenting psychiatric symptom, in which case the diagnosis is delusional disorder (24).

Depressive disorder can have associated delusions. This is termed "psychotic depression." In the early stages of depression, complaints of ill health overshadow the depression. These complaints often are vague, for example, fatigue, constipation, and nonspecific aches and pains. As the depression worsens, so do their delusions and complaints. They have vegetative symptoms, complaining of insomnia, weight loss, or loss of sexual libido. This occurs in association with ideas of hopelessness and self-blame (23).

Delusions are commonly seen in organic mental disorders brought on by substance abuse, but they are also relatively common in dementia such as Alzhheimer's disease (24). At first they can be exaggerations of an older person's obsession with health, but as the dementia worsens and memory abnormalities become more severe, the complaints become fragmented and vague and are mixed with other concerns. Patients with multi-infarct dementia can sometimes also become depressed and suicidal (24).

Delusions Absent

Obsessive-compulsive patients have an uncontrollable, repetitive thought with ideational content, which may be identical to that of a delusion but is not held with the same conviction. They are driven to remove actual or imaginary skin lesions. They may rationalize their behavior by stating that the skin lesion itches or burns. In terms of history taking, they do admit to manipulating the skin (25).

In contrast to the obsessive-compulsive disorder patient, the factitious disorder patient denies any possibility that the lesions are self-inflicted. They are usually produced for secondary gain, but in other instances they may be produced unconsciously to satisfy a psychological need that remains unconscious (25). In the latter case, patients tend to have serious psychiatric pathology and may present with factitious delusional symptoms that by definition are not true delusions (delusions are fixed false beliefs, factitious disorder patients do not believe in the delusional symptoms with which they present) (12). Finally, patients with milder disorders such as depression without psychosis and anxiety disorders may develop dermatological manifestations as a result of psychogenic causes (12).

APPROACH TO THE PATIENT

Establishing rapport and gaining the patient's trust are primary concerns before any treatment is initiated. With psychodermatological patients this may be difficult if their psychopathology is severe. In general, a physician who is empathetic and nonjudgmental will foster the relationship. It is important to realize as a physician that for the psychodermatological patient, skin problems are a means of seeking medical attention without coming to terms with what could be severe psychological problems (12). The following is an outline of the approach to such a patient:

1. Do not immediately bring up the possibility of psychiatric problems and the need to be seen by a psychologist or psychiatrist, as this will, at best, be viewed as unnecessary by the patient and, at worst, provoke hostility in the patient and will most certainly lead to the patient seeking another physician to deal with what they believe are true somatic complaints (26).

2. Listen noncritically to the history and perform a thorough dermatological exam. This is the best way to communicate to patients that their complaints are being taken seriously.

3. Metabolic problems should be excluded, and informing the patient that this is being done will further strength the doctor-patient relationship. Consequently, in assessing the patient the appropriate investigations for metabolic disease should include a complete blood cell count, liver function tests, a fasting serum glucose, thyroid-stimulating hormone, serum creatinine, and, if there is any suggestion of photosensitivity, an antinuclear antibody assay. With a history of substance abuse, vitamin B_{12} and folate levels are also of benefit. An x-ray of the spinal column may be of benefit if the complaints appear to be dermatomal.

4. An underlying dermatological disorder is always of prime consideration. Therefore, the following dermatological investigations may be of benefit: skin biopsy, fungal and bacterial cultures, and patch testing. A biopsy for immunofluorescence may also be needed in cases with a history of photosensitivity. If the patient brings in material which he or she believes is infested, have the specimens looked at by the pathologist.

5. The physician may have to spend several visits dealing with the patient on completely somatic terms before discussing any possibility of a psychological problem (12). If the results of the investigations are negative and the patient gradually realizes that he or she does not appear to have a severe dermatological illness, then he or she may gradually become more accepting of the physician bringing up the possibility that in fact there is a psychological component to their dermatological complaints.

6. Once the issue of treatment is raised, it is important to communicate clearly to the patient that the physician's goal is to help the patient in terms of relief of their symptoms. Whether they agree or not with the physician's assessment regarding the role of psychological factors, they may be willing to take psychotropic medication if it is offered in this manner and it is communicated to the patient that it is not the intent of the physician to cast judgment or stigmatize the patient (12).

7. If the patient continues to cling to a delusion, do not confront the patient, as this once again will only reinforce the delusion and the patient may become agitated and hostile. To deal with this patient, a physician could state "I have treated many patients with your problem in the past with this medication. Although we don't at this particular time know why you have this problem, we

do know that you don't have any evidence of internal disease and the medication I am going to suggest will be helpful in dealing with some of the unpleasant symptoms you are having" (26).

8. When the issue of psychotrophic medication is discussed with the patient, it is also important to provide symptomatic topical therapy for the dermatological problems. This will provide the therapeutic environment that will enable patients to keep follow-up appointments without feeling that their complaints have not been taken seriously by the physician. It is important for the physician to realize that accepting the patient's emotional pain at a somatic level enables him or her to continue treatment (26).

9. If the patient becomes argumentative, do not succumb to ordering unnecessary or repeated tests, as this only serves to reinforce the symptoms. In this case, the help of family members may be required. When the situation is explained, they will usually encourage the patient to take the medication offered on a trial basis.

10. Most of us as dermatologists have neither the time or expertise to engage in psychiatric care. Preparing the patient for psychiatric referral may take several visits, as mentioned previously. If the suggestion of a psychiatric referral is to be accepted by the patient, these visits can be used to obtain information about their feelings, which can then be used in such a way as to make a persuasive case. The patient can be reminded of other symptoms that have become evident during their frequent visits (e.g., anxiety, increased fatigue, changes in sleeping habits, difficulties in the workplace or at home). At the same time the patient should again be reminded that the somatic aspects of their presenting complaint have been investigated appropriately and symptomatic topical care has also been instituted. Empathize with the discomfort that the patient feels and point out how the discomfort and other symptoms are interfering with his or her ability to function normally. Help the patient to understand that by taking the time to see a psychiatrist, he or she will feel better in the sense that the emotional side of the illness will also be assessed (26).

11. Finally, if you have a patient who is not willing to accept your advice regarding psychiatric intervention and may be self-mutilating for secondary gain or is overtly psychotic, the family members should be informed. They may be of assistance.

TREATMENT

Initiation of treatment in the form of psychoactive medication in these patients may be difficult until some insight is gained by the patient. However, there are alternative therapies that may be beneficial and which the patient may be willing to try. These include hypnosis, behavior therapy, biofeedback, and supportive group therapy. These are discussed at length in another chapter.

In terms of psychopharmacology, the number of psychoactive agents available to the practitioner is enormous. As dermatologists, it is beneficial to become familiar with one or two agents within each class of drugs. This will enable the patient who is willing to take medication to begin therapy until he or she is seen by a psychiatrist.

For the patient who is anxious due to the nature of the skin lesions, two types of antianxiety medications can be suggested: the benzodiazepine family of antianxiety agents and buspirone. Alprazolam, which differs from the older benzodiazepines such as diazepam or chlordiazepoxide in that its half-life is short and predictable, may be preferable if a benzodiazepine is the drug of choice. Most of the previous dose is eliminated or inactivated by the body before the next dose is taken. Many of the older benzodiazepines have numerous active metabolites that contribute to a much longer half-life. However, with the new benzodiazepines, it is important to taper the medication when it is discontinued. Suddenly discontinuation may result in a rapid recurrence of the symptoms due to rapid metabolism and elimination of alprazolam. The doses of alprazolam used in a dermatological practice are usually 0.25 or 0.5 mg per os three or four times daily. Since situational stress usually resolves itself within 2–3 weeks and since there is a risk of drug dependence, the most cautious way of prescribing the drug is to restrict its use to 2–3 weeks and to begin dosing at 0.125 mg per os four times daily and slowly increase the dose until therapeutic benefit is achieved (27). If the patient requires long-term therapy, buspirone is a consideration since it does not cause dependence or sedation. The drawbacks are that therapeutic effect is not achieved for at least 2 weeks and it cannot be taken on an "as-needed" basis. The usual dosage ranges from 5 mg per os three times per day to 10 mg per os four times per day. The possible side effects are nausea, diarrhea, fatigue, restlessness, and dizziness (28).

The easiest way to determine if a patient would benefit from antidepressants is to ask: "Are you feeling sad?," "Have you lost weight?," and "Have you had difficulty sleeping?" Most patients who are depressed are glad that the questions were asked and can communicate their feelings. However, others can be in denial. If a physician encounters a patient who he or she feels is depressed but the patient denies any symptoms, it is generally unproductive to argue the point. It may be helpful to change the discussion to one regarding an appetite change or sleeping habits. The patient with depression would not suspect that the clinician is actually trying to make the diagnosis of depression (29). There are numerous antidepressants to choose from in order to treat the depression if the patient is willing to do so. The newer serotonin-reuptake inhibitors such as fluoxetine (Prozac), sertraline (Zoloft), and paroxetine (Paxil) are generally free of side effects and are much better tolerated than the older tricyclic antidepressants such as doxepin, desipramine, or amitriptyline. They have no activity against the muscarinic cholinergic receptor and therefore do not cause urinary retention, dry mouth, blurred vision, or constipation. They also do not have any activity against alpha-adrenergic receptors and therefore are not associated with orthostatic hypotension. The side effects of the serotonin reuptake inhibitors may be somnolence, insomnia, nervousness, and sexual dysfunction. These usually resolve after a few weeks. The recommended dosing is to begin at a low dose and increase slowly over several weeks. For fluoxetine, 10 mg per os daily would be an adequate starting dose, for sertraline 50 mg daily, and for paroxetine 10 mg daily. These newer antidepressants are also indicated for obsessive-compulsive disorder (27). Rare cases of increased suicidal thoughts have been reported while taking fluoxetine (30). It is therefore recommended that, in general, dermatologists not attempt to treat anyone with suicidal ideation, whether drug-related or due to depression (12).

Patients with obvious delusions benefit from antipsychotic medication. The treatment of choice in the past has been pimozide or Orap. The use of pimozide in dermatology is described in detail elsewhere. However, there are now new atypical antipsychotic medications such as olanzapine and risperidone that do not have the same risk of extrapyramidal side effects such as drug-induced parkinsonism, acute dystonic reactions, and akathisia. All of these side effects can occur abruptly but tend to be dose related. However, the atypicals such as olanzapine have been shown to have extrapyramidal side effects at no higher frequency than placebo. The pathophysiology of psychotic disorders for which olanzapine has been shown to be effective include overactivity in several specific regional dopamine systems. Dopamine receptor binding is regarded as being predictive of clinical and pharmacological potencies of antipsychotic drugs. Olanzapine and other atypicals have also been demonstrated to antagonize the serotonin-2 receptor. This activity may protect against motor side effects. Interaction with serotonin receptors may also be important in those patients who are receiving antidepressant medication. Olanzapine may potentiate antidepressant action, and this has been observed in patients with treatment-resistant depression (31). One final action that olanzapine possesses that the other atypical antipsychotis such as risperidone do not is antihistaminic activity. Such activity may potentiate the ability of the drug to control scratching and secondary inflammatory responses that result from manipulation of the skin. This medication can therefore be safely prescribed by dermatologists for the psychotic patient and also in the treatment of severe unexplained itch, dysesthesia, and self-mutilation when the patient is not psychotic. The dosing of olanzapine in dermatology is low relative to the dose used to treat schizophrenia (10–20 mg per os daily). It is recommended that dosing be initiated at 1.25 mg per os nightly for olanzapine and 0.25 mg for risperidone and slowing increased every 2 weeks to the point where the symptoms are alleviated. One possible side effect of olanzapine is weight gain, which is less of a problem with risperidone (32).

CONCLUSION

It has been reported that somatizing patients lack the psychological means for communicating emotional distress and therefore are not amenable to psychotherapeutic intervention (33). However, with a nonjudgmental approach on the part of the physician who is at the same time empathetic, these difficult-to-treat patients can gain trust in their physician and begin a therapeutic alliance that will eventually lead to symptom relief with the appropriate therapy.

REFERENCES

1. Anderson EW, Trethowan WH. Psychiatry. London: Bailliere and Tindall, 1973:22.
2. Lyell A. Delusions of parasitosis. Br J Dermatol 1983; 108:485–499.
3. Koblenzer CS. The dysmorphic syndrome. Arch Dermatol 1985; 121:780–784.
4. Sneddon IB. The mind and the skin. Br Med J 1949; I:472–475.
5. Bishop ER Jr. Monosymptomatic hypochrondriasis. Psychosomatics 1980; 21:731–747.
6. Engel GL. "Psychogenic" pain. Med Clin North Am 1958; 42:1481–1496.
7. Fabisch W. What is dermatitis artefacta? Int J Dermatol 1981; 20:427–428.
8. Adamson HG. Acne urticaria and other forms of "neurotic excoriations." Br J Dermatol 1915; 27:1–12.
9. Cormia FE. Basic concepts in the production and management of the psychosomatic dermatoses. Br J Dermatol Syph 1951; 63:83–92.
10. Siegel RK. Cocaine hallucinations. Am J Psychiatry 1978; 135:309–314.
11. Bishop ER Jr. Monosymptomatic hypochondriacal syndromes in dermatology. J Am Acad Dermatol 1983; 9:152–158.

12. Koo JYM. Psychodermatology: a practical manual for clinicians. Curr Prob Dermatol 1995; 6:199–234.
13. Critchley M. The body image in neurology. Lancet 1950; i:335–341.
14. Horowitz MJ. A cognitive model of hallucinations. Am J Psychiatry 1975; 132:789–795.
15. Basker RM, Sturdee DW, Davenport JC. Patients with burning mouths. Br Dent J 1978; 145:9–16.
16. Grushka M. Burning mouth: a review and update. Ont Dent 1983; 60:56–61.
17. Coles RB. Glossodynia—a psychosomatic problem. Trans St. John Hosp Derm Soc 1966; 52:79–83.
18. Koblenzer CS. Psychocutaneous disease. Orlando, FL: Grune & Stratton, 1987:94–98.
19. Lyell A. The itching patient: a review of the causes of pruritus. Scot Med J 1972; 17:334–347.
20. Beare JM. Generalized pruritus. A study of 43 cases. Clin Exp Dermatol 1976; 1:343–359.
21. Young AW, Sweeney EW, David D. Dermatologic evaluation of pruritus in patients on hemodialysis. NY State J Med 1973; 73:2670–2674.
22. Gilchrest BA. Pruritus. Review article. Arch Intern Med 1982; 142:101–105.
23. Munro A. Dealing with hypochondriacal delusions. Can J Diagnosis Oct 1990; 111–125.
24. Munro A. Delusional parasitosis: a form of monosymptomatic hypochondriacal psychosis. Semin Dermatol 1983; 2:197–202.
25. Nemiah JC, Uhde TW. Obsessive-compulsive disorder. In: Kaplan HI, Sadock BJ, eds. Comprehensive Textbook of Psychiatry. Baltimore: Williams & Wilkins, 1989:985–1000.
26. Koblenzer CS. Psychocutaneous disease. Orlando, FL: Grune & Stratton, 1987:116–128.
27. Garnis-Jones S. Psychological aspects of rosacea. J Cut Med Surg 1998; 2(suppl 4):16–19.
28. Koblenzer CS. Safe and successful use of psychotropic drugs for dermatologists. In: Burgdorf WHC, Katz SI, eds. Dermatology. Progress and Perspectives. New York: Parthenon, 1993:914.
29. Koblenzer CS. Psychosomatic concepts in dermatology: a dermatologist-psychoanalyst's viewpoint. Arch Dermatol 1983; 119:501–512.
30. Tollefson GD. Fluoxetine and suicidal ideation. Am J Psychiatry 1990; 147:1691–1693.
31. Zarate CA Jr, Narendran R, Tohen M. Clinical predictors of acute response with olanzapine in psychotic mood disorders. J Clin Psychiatry 1998; 59:24–28.
32. Garnis-Jones S, Collins S, Rosenthal D. Treatment of self-mutilation with olanzapine. J Cut Med Surg 2000; 4:160–162.
33. Brown HN, Vaillant GE. Hypochondriasis. Arch Intern Med 1981; 141:723–726.

10

Delusional Parasitosis

M. Musalek
University of Vienna
Vienna, Austria

INTRODUCTION

Since the first description of delusional parasitosis by Thiebièrge and Perrin, scientific work on the unshakable belief of being infested by parasites has been published under various terms. Thiebièrge himself called the syndrome acarophobia (1). Perrin entitled his 1896 case-report "De névrodermies parasitophobiques" (2). Other terms often found in the scientific literature are parasitophobia, entomophobia, delusions of infestation, monosymptomatic hypochondriacal psychoses, and Ekbom syndrome (3–8).

Patients suffering from delusional parasitosis claim that they are infested by parasites when from a dermatological or parasitological point of view there is no evidence of such an infestation. Most patients report that they feel the bugs in, on, or under the skin; in some cases they feel the parasites entering the body. Some patients report seeing them, and some even bring the parasites for further examination. Usually textile fibers, hair, and pieces of skin are maintained for parasites. According to parasitological knowledge—or, more accurately, nonknowledge—the bugs are referred to by exotic terms or simply called lice or fleas (9,10). The characteristics of the parasites are, on the one hand, that their number increases rapidly and that they are difficult to find at physical examinations; on the other hand they are, of course, totally resistent to dermatological treatment.

Epidemiological data concerning the occurrence of delusional parasitosis are still lacking, but observations in dermatological, psychodermatological, and parasitological units indicate that delusional parasitosis is a relatively common syndrome in dermatology and parasitology, whereas this clinical picture is very rarely seen in psychiatry (11–13).

DEFINITION AND DIAGNOSIS

According to the diagnostic criteria of Karl Jaspers (14), delusions are defined as ideas characterized by an unshakable conviction (*unvergleichlich hohe subjektive Gewißheit*) and its incorrigibility (*Unkorrigierbarkeit*). Delusional parasitosis therefore is defined as the incorrigible conviction of being infested by parasites. The third Jasperian criterion, the impossibility of content (*Unmöglichkeit des Inhaltes*), is only an accessory sign but not an indispensable requirement for the diagnosis of a delusion (15,16). This means that the delusional content can also be part of the real world; e.g., it is possible to suffer from both a delusional parasitosis and a real parasitic infestation.

Reviewing literature on delusional parasitosis, delusions are often mixed up with phobias and obsessive-compulsive disorders. Sometimes the terms "delusional parasitosis" and "parasitophobias" are even used synonymously in dermatological publications (1,17,18). In psychopathology we strictly distinguish between phobias, obsessive-compulsive disorders, and delusions. Phobias are defined by pathological fear and avoidance behavior, obsessive-compulsive disorders by recurrent, intrusive thoughts and compulsive, stereotyped, repetitive behaviors or cognitions (19), whereas the term delusion is only used in case of an incorrigible conviction. The accurate distinction between these three psychopathological phenomena is not only of theoretical interest but also of great practical importance, especially with respect to psychotherapy. Because totally different dynamics, intentions, and problems are the reason and the effect of these symptoms, different therapy strategies are needed in order to plan effective treatment.

PATHOGENESIS

Considering delusional parasitosis as a psychopathological phenomenon with a particular content defined by the high certainty and incorrigibility of belief, two types of questions arise in pathogenesis research: 1) What are the factors that might explain the choice of a specific delusional theme? Why do some patients suffer from delusions of parasitosis and others from HIV delusions or dysmorphic delusions? 2) Which factors play an important role in the delusional fixation? What causes the incorrigible conviction?

During the last decades numerous empirical studies have been carried out in order to answer these questions. The results of these studies indicate that the choice of the particular delusional theme is caused by a complex interaction of factors: age, gender, social situation, and so-called "key experiences" (11,20,21). In delusional parasitosis patients—typically elderly, socially isolated women—tactile phenomena constitute such key experiences. The vast majority of patients feel sensations of movements in and under the skin, which make them believe they could be caused by parasites. For the fixation of a particular theme—the incorrigible conviction—other factors are responsible: cognitive disorders in the frame of organic or schizophrenic psychoses and emotional disorders as observable in the course of affective psychoses (11). There is some evidence that in some cases personality disorders and social isolation may be of importance in connection with the development of delusional fixation, but further studies will be necessary to clarify their role in the pathogenesis of delusions. We may conclude that various psychic and social factors become effective in the choice of a particular delusional theme, whereas physical factors such as cognitive and emotional disorders are the indispensable basis for the occurrence of the incorrigible conviction.

According to recent studies, delusions in general and delusional parasitosis in particular cannot be considered as static psychopathological manifestations once established and therefore persisting forever. Delusions have to be considered as a dynamic process that will only persist if disorder-maintaining factors become effective. These disorder-maintaining factors may be the same cognitive and emotional deviations mentioned above. Some additional factors may prolong a delusional conviction, two of which are especially important in the pathogenesis of delusions: the "self-dynamics" of delusions and the meaning of delusions (22).

The term self-dynamics indicates that the behavoir as well as the social isolation and alienation of the deluded patients induce a particular reaction from those communicating with the patient. Avoidance behavior by one person usually induces avoidance behavior in others; the avoidance behavior of the people surrounding the patient serves then as an argument for the delusional belief of the patient and enhances the paranoia, which itself enhances again the avoidance behavior of the relatives. Such enhancement circles may act as promotors in intensifying and prolonging delusional convictions.

Every illness exists not only in its "pathos," or its symptomatology, but also in its "nosos," or the meaning or significance of the disorder (*das Wesen der Krankheit*). Every psychiatric disorder has its particular meaning—and that applies especially to delusions; suffering from delusions is the paragon of being crazy. As shown in previous psychopathological analyses, this fact alone can make patients defend their ideas with all the arguments they may find (23). But delusions have a particular meaning not only for the patients, but also for the people surrounding them. Patients with delusions often suffer greatly from the prejudice of their relatives, friends, colleagues, etc.—and such prejudices in the social network of the patient may enhance and prolong the delusional ideas as disorder-maintaining factors. In this context we should not forget that medical doctors and therapists are part of the social network of the patient, and therefore may also become a disorder-maintaining factor. Considering the results of studies on the origin of delusions, the pathogenesis of delusions has to be considered as a multifactorical process in which psychic, physical, and social circumstances are acting as disorder-predisposing, -triggering, and -maintaining factors.

NOSOGRAPHY

Summarizing the literature on the nosological theory of delusional parasitosis, we are confronted with various opinions. Assumptions have ranged from an independent nosological entity to the attribution to a certain disorder (as, for example, to organic psychoses or schizophrenic or affective disorders) and to multicategorical classification models (3,24–26). In summary, delusions may occur in all kinds of psychiatric disorders. Therefore, they have to be considered today as nosological nonspecific syndromes (27,28). The question as to whether delusions may also occur without any other psychiatric disorder ("primary delusions") remains unanswered. In recent polydiagnostic studies it was shown that the diagnosis of a primary delusion or delusional disorder was much more an artificial product of particular diagnostic algorithms in contemporary classification systems than a reflection of observable reality (28).

Monosymptomatic Hypochondriacal Psychoses

Since the studies of Riding and Munro (7) in the late 1970s, many researchers consider delusional parasitosis as a particular manifestation of monosymptomatic hypochondriasis or a monosymptomatic hypochondriacal disorder. The discussion as to whether delusional parasitosis is a hypochondriacal delusion or a special kind of persecutory delusion goes back to the beginning of the twentieth century. Leroy, in 1905 (29), was the first to posit that delusional parasitosis is due to paranoia. Later, Callieri and Priori (30), Janzarik (31), and Dumas et al. (32) shared his view. In contrast, Thiebièrge (1) and Perrin (2) and, later, Borel and Ey (33), Reilly and Beard (34), and Bishop (35) emphasized the hypochondriacal character of the psychopathological feature. The results of an empirical psychological study of a sample of delusional parasitosis patients carried out in Vienna as well as psychopathological analyses of a large number of single cases indicate that delusional parasitosis syndromes cannot be considered in total as hypochondriacal psychoses (11,36). There are three subgroups of delusional parasitosis:

1. Patients with predominantly hypochondriacal traits, convinced that they suffer from a severe physical illness that is incurable. This form is referred to as "hypochondriacal delusions of parasitosis" or simply "delusional parasitosis in a narrower sense." Some such cases—if not due to other forms of psychoses, e.g., affective, organic, or schizophrenic psychoses—may be attributed to the group of monosymptomatic hypochondriacal psychoses.
2. Patients with paranoid symptoms and without hypochondriacal apprehensions. These patients usually fight against their parasites, which impair their existence. This is referred to as "delusions of infestation." Patients suffering from this kind of delusion usually consult entomologists, parasitologists, and pest control companies and are seldom seen in dermatological practices.
3. Patients with signs of both hypochondriacal as well as paranoid delusions, referred to as "hypochondriacal delusions of infestation." Like patients from the first group, they usually go from one dermatologist to the next ("doctor shopping") often hopelessly trapped in their beliefs.

An accurate distinction between the three groups is not only of scientific interest but also of practical importance—for the development of psychotherapy strategies it is of utmost importance to distinguish between paranoid and hypochondriacal forms (37). The third form represents a major problem in psychotherapy: when a therapist succeeds in treating the hypochondria (e.g., improvement of the dermatological symptoms), the patient focuses on the paranoid concerns (e.g., increasing number of parasites); when the paranoid conviction is successfully treated (e.g., decreasing number of parasites), the patient turns to the hypochondriacal part of the delusion (e.g., few parasites, each of which is much more virulent).

Shared Delusions of Parasitosis

A particular nosological problem is the group of induced or shared delusions of parasitosis (38). Induction of psychiatric disturbances is a well-known phenomenon in psychiatry. Scharfetter (39) found a preponderance of blood relatives, indicating that genetic aspects may be of importance in the development of induced psychoses. In a study of the frequency of shared delusions in delusions of infestation (40) carried out on 107 personally investigated patients with delusional parasitosis, the phenomenon of shared delusions was found in 9%, wherein a greater number of females (ratio of females to males $= 3.5{:}1$) induced others. The relative rare occurrence of shared delusions (in contrast to the high percentage of induced pruritus) as well as psychopathological single-case analyses led to the assumption that delusional transference only occurs if the potential recepient displays a paranoid predisposition based on physical, psychic, and/or social constellations of conditions. Since the ratio of blood relations to nonblood relations was only 1:2.3, genetic factors seem to play a minor role compared to the relationship of deluded patients to their environment. Only if paranoid preconditions exist does a shared delusion become possible; if not, the ideas of the recipient will remain restricted to the apprehension or supposition of being affected.

TREATMENT

Most patients with delusions are more or less reluctant to seek psychiatric treatment and care. It is crucial in the treatment of such patients, therefore, to establish contact and to build up stable relationships based on trust. A possible solution to the problem of reluctance exists in the Viennese model (11,23). In this model, the patient is referred from a cooperating dermatological department to the liaison psychiatry outpatient clinic of the department for dermatology. At first contact the patient is seen by a psychiatrist together with a dermatologist. The patient is referred to specialists for the particular disorder or problem without further specification of the profession of the specialists. At this stage the patient is not aware that he or she is also to be seen by a psychiatrist. Nevertheless, it is not necessary to deny this fact, which is of great importance for further psychiatric treatment. This mode of referral enables the psychiatrist to become acquainted with the patient. After three or four sessions, the patient usually agrees to be treated by a psychiatrist, particularly if the establishment of a confidential relationship has been successful. Major mistakes that could be made in this first phase of treatment are, on the one hand, informing the patient too early that he is suffering from delusional ideas and, on the other hand, confirming his delusional ideas. We suggest accepting totally the complaints of the patient as an experienced reality and leaving open the correctness of his or her interpretations of the experiences.

When a stable relationship based on confidence is built up, the next step is a careful differential diagnosis. This differential diagnosis should include all physical, psychic, and social circumstances that may play a major role in the pathogenesis of the delusion as predisposing, triggering, and maintaining factors. Such a careful differential diagnosis then provides information for planning treatment strategies, including medication and psychotherapeutic and sociotherapeutic methods. The ability to coordinate and integrate methods is essential, because a combination of all three kinds of therapy may become necessary. The psychopharmacological treatment should be chosen according to the basic psychiatric symptomatology (11). This means that if depression is the underlying disorder, the patient should be treated with antidepressants. In cases in which an effective treatment of the basic disorder is not (yet) available, the patient may be treated with (atypical) antipsychotics (41,42). This kind of psychopharmacological agent helps the patient to gain distance from the delusional ideas and provides the basis for psychotherapeutic interventions, which are the indispensable basis of an effective treatment.

As mentioned above, a large number of delusional parasitosis patients are resistant to psychiatric care in general and to psychotherapy in particular. Therefore, in most cases a stable relationship based on trust between the patient and the therapist can only be obtained by an intensive emotional engagement by the therapist. This means that those forms of psychotherapy requiring more or less distance from the patient are not appropriate for the treatment of delusional parasitosis patients. Good results could be reached by applying psychotherapeutic interventions based on the theory of client-centered psychotherapy enlarged by system-oriented aspects (37,43). After establishing a trusting relationship by accepting the patient's physical complaints and gaining a deep understanding of the patient's cognitive and emotional world, the first step in psychotherapy of the delusional symptomatology should be to become aware of the various aspects of the problem and to reach, together with the patient, strategies to solve the problem. In this context the therapeutic relation's function will provide fertile ground for the self-healing forces of the patient.

All of us are social beings—we are closely related to and highly dependent on members of our social network. It is of utmost importance for effective treatment to focus intensively and extensively on the various interactional problems occurring in the frame of the delusions or even provoking and catalyzing them. A major problem is the often observed social isolation and alienation of the patients, which makes sociotherapeutic measures necessary in most cases (44).

As shown in a treatment study of delusional parasitosis patients, an improvement in delusional symptomatology can be expected in about two thirds of patients if an integrative treatment approach including psychopharmacological, psychotherapeutic, and sociotherapeutic methods is followed (37,45). These study results indicate that the implementation of an integrative treatment approach, based on a multidimensional differential diagnosis including all the predisposing, triggering, and disorder-maintaining factors, improves the prognosis and outcome of delusional parasitosis significantly.

REFERENCES

1. Thibièrge G. Les acarophobes. Rev Gén Clin Thér 1894; 32:373–376.
2. Perrin L. Des névrodermies parasitophobiques. Ann Dermatol Syphil 1896; 7:129–138.
3. Hopkinson G. Delusions of infestation. Acta Psychiatr Scand 1970; 46:111–119.
4. Pethö B, Szilagyi A. Von der nosologischen Lage des Ekbom Syndroms. Beitrag zur Weiterentwicklung der Symptomatologie körperlich begründbarer Psychosen. Psychiatr Clin 1970; 3:296–319.
5. Eller JJ. Neurogenic and psychogenic disorders of the skin. Med J Rec 1929; 129.
6. Waldron WG. The role of the entomologist in delusory parasitosis. Bull Ent Soc Am 1962; 8:81–83.
7. Riding JBE, Munro A. Pimozide in the treatment of monosymptomatic hypochondriacal psychosis. Acta Psychiatr Scand 1975; 52:23–30.
8. Koo J, Gambla C. Delusions of parasitosis and other forms of monosymptomatic hypchondriacal psychosis: general discussion and case illustrations. Dermatol Clin 1996; 14:429–438.
9. Lyell A. Delusions of parasitosis. Br J Dermatol 1983; 108:485–499.
10. Hamann K, Avnstorp C. Delusions of infestation treated by pimozide: a double blind cross over clinical study. Acta Derm Venereol 1982; 62:55–58.
11. Musalek M. Der Dermatozoenwahn. Stuttgart: Thieme, 1991.
12. Ohtaki N. Delusions of parasitosis: report of 94 cases. Nippon-Hifuka-Gakkai-Zasshi 1991; 101:439–446.
13. Trabert W. 100 years of delusional parasitosis: meta-analysis of 1,223 case reports. Psychopathology 1995; 28:238–246.
14. Jaspers K. Allgemeine Psychopathologie. 8th ed. Berlin: Springer, 1975.
15. Berner P. Psychiatrische Systematik. Bern: Huber, 1982.

16. Berner P, Musalek M. Schizophrenie und Wahnkrankheiten. In: Handbuch der Gerontologie. Vol 4. Neurologie und Psychiatrie. Stuttgart: Fischer, 1989:297–317.

17. Olkowski H, Olkowski W. Entomophobia in the urban ecosystem: some observations and suggestions. Bull Entomol Soc Am 1976; 22 313–317.

18. Wilson WJ. Delusions of parasitosis (acarophobia): further observations in clinical practice. Arch Dermatol Syphil 1952; 66:577–585.

19. Jun Ayd FJ. Lexicon of Psychiatry, Neurology and the Neurosciences. Baltimore: Williams & Wilkins, 1985.

20. Musalek M, Berner P, Katschnig H. Delusional theme, sex, and age. Psychopathology, 1989.

21. Kretschmer K. Der sensitive Beziehungswahn. 4th ed. Berlin: Springer, 1966.

22. Musalek M, Hobl B. Der Affekt als Bedingung des Wahns. In: Mundt C, Fuchs T, eds. Affekt und affektive Störungen, 2001.

23. Musalek M, Hobl B, Mossbacher U, Zoghlami A. Delusions in dermatology. In: Grimalt F, Cotteril J, eds. Dermatologia y Psiquiatria: Historias, Clinicas, Comentadas. Madrid: Aula Médica, 2001.

24. McLaughlin JA, Sims A. Coexistence of the Capgras and the Ekbom syndromes. Br J Psychiatry 1984; 145:439–443.

25. Berrios GE. Delusional parasitosis and physical disease. Compr Psychiatry 1985; 26:395–404.

26. Munro A. Delusional parasitosis: a form of monosymptomatic hypochondriacal psychosis. Semin Dermatol 1983; 2:197–202.

27. Skott A. Delusions of Infestation. Kungälv: Gotab, 1978.

28. Musalek M, Bach M, Passweg V, Zadro-Jaeger S. The position of delusional parasitosis in psychiatric nosology and classification. Psychopathology 1990; 23:115–124.

29. Leroy EB. Les délires du parasitiférisme. Rev Neurol 1905; 13:871.

30. Callieri B, Priori R. Contributo allo studio dell'esperienza psicotica dermatozoica, zooptica et zoopatica. Arch Psicolog Neurol Psychiat 1962; 23:108–148.

31. Janzarik W. Über das Kontaktmangelparanoid des höheren Alters und den Syndromcharakter schizophrenen Krankseins. Nervenarzt 1973; 44:515–526.

32. Dumas M, et al. Manifestations neurologiques et psychiatriques des parasitoses. Rapport de Neurologie, Congr Psichat Neurol. Le Mans. Paris: Masson, 1986.

33. Borel J, Ey H. Obsession hallucinatoire zoopathique guérie par psychothérapie. Ann Méd Psychol 1932; 90:181–185.

34. Reilly TM, Beard AW. Monosymptomatic hypchondriasis. Br J Psychiatry 1976; 129:191–192.

35. Bishop ER. Monosymptomatic hypchondriasis. Psychosomatics 1980; 21:731–747.

36. Musalek M, et al. Zur Psychopathologie des Dermatozoenwahnkranken. Nervenarzt 59, 1988.

37. Musalek M. Psychotherapie von Wahnsyndromen. In: Strobl R, ed. Schizophrenie und Psychotherapie. Edition pro mente, 1996.

38. Trabert W. Shared psychotic disorder in delusional parasitosis. Psychopathology 1999; 32:30–34.
39. Scharfetter W. Symbiontische Psychosen. Bern: Huber, 1970.
40. Musalek M, Kutzer E. The frequency of shared delusions of parasitosis. Eur Arch Psychiatr Neurol Sci 1989; 239:263–266.
41. DeLeon OA, et al. Risperidone in the treatment of delusions of infestation. Int J Psychiatry Med 1997; 27:403–409.
42. Yorston G. Treatment of delusional parasitosis with sertindole. Int J Geriatr Psychiatry 1997; 12:1127–1128.
43. Rogers CR. Client Centered Therapy: Its Current Practice, Implications and Theory. Boston: Houghton Mifflin, 1951.
44. Musalek M. Die Bedeutung des Wahns in unserer Gesellschaft. In: Zapotoczky HG, Fabisch K, eds. Paranoia und Diktatur. Linz: Universitätsverlag Rudolf Trauner, 2000.
45. Musalek M. Les indicateurs psychopathologiques et biologiques pour la thérapeutique des délires chroniques. Psychol Méd 1989; 21:1355–1359.

11

Body Dysmorphic Disorder*

Katharine A. Phillips
Brown Medical School and Butler Hospital
Providence, Rhode Island, U.S.A.

Raymond G. Dufresne, Jr.
Brown Medical School and Rhode Island Hospital
Providence, Rhode Island, U.S.A.

INTRODUCTION

Body dysmorphic disorder (BDD), also known as dysmorphophobia, is a relatively common yet underrecognized psychiatric disorder that often presents to dermatologists (1–3). Although the symptoms may sound trivial, in more severe cases individuals with this disorder may be unable to work, socialize, or leave their house, and some commit suicide (1–3). These patients, especially those with more severe BDD, can be challenging to treat. As one dermatologist stated, "I know of no more difficult patients to treat than those with body dysmorphic disorder" (4).

Although BDD remains underrecognized by dermatologists and mental health professionals alike, it has been described for more than a

---

*Adapted with permission from Phillips KA, Dufresne RG Jr. Body dysmorphic disorder: a guide for dermatologists and cosmetic surgeons. Am J Clin Dermatol 2000; 1:235–243.

century and reported around the world (1). BDD is included as a separate diagnosis in DSM-IV, psychiatry's diagnostic manual, where it is classified as a somatoform disorder (5). As defined in DSM-IV, BDD consists of a preoccupation with an imagined defect in appearance; if a slight physical anomaly is present, the person's concern is markedly excessive. The preoccupation causes clinically significant distress or impairment in social, occupational, or other important areas of functioning.

The dermatology literature contains many descriptions of patients with BDD, often under such rubrics as dysmorphophobia (6,7), dysmorphic syndrome (8,9), dermatological hypochondriasis (10), dermatological nondisease (6), and monosymptomatic hypochondriasis (delusions of dysmorphosis) (7). Monosymptomatic hypochondriasis and delusions of dysmorphosis are equivalent to the delusional form of BDD, in which patients are completely convinced (as opposed to having some insight) that their view of the "defect" is accurate and undistorted. Patients with BDD who compulsively pick their skin are often referred to as having "psychogenic excoriation" (11,12).

The dermatology literature notes that the treatment outcome of patients with BDD is often poor, with patients often voicing dissatisfaction with an outcome that is objectively acceptable. In some cases, the patient is satisfied with the appearance of the treated body part but then focuses his or her dissatisfaction on another body area (1,4,6,8,13).

This clinically focused chapter provides an overview of BDD for dermatologists. It describes BDD's clinical features and prevalence, its treatment response, and how to recognize and diagnose BDD. We also offer practical suggestions for dermatologists who encounter these often difficult-to-treat, high-risk patients.

CLINICAL FEATURES

Appearance Preoccupations

Individuals with BDD are preoccupied with the thought that some aspect of their appearance is unattractive, deformed, or "not right" in some way (1–3). These preoccupations commonly involve the face or head, although any body part can be the focus of concern (2,14). The most common areas of concern are the skin and hair (14–16). Patients often present with worries about acne, scarring, facial lines, marks, pale skin, thinning head hair, or excessive body hair. In reality, the body area appears normal or the flaw is quite minimal (e.g., not noticeable at conversational distance). These minimal or nonexistent appearance flaws are perceived by the patient to be very unattractive, distressing, and the cause of much anxiety. "Muscle dysmorphia" is a type of BDD in which individuals (usually men) worry that their body build is small and puny, when in reality they are typically large and muscular (17).

BDD preoccupations are distressing, time consuming, and usually difficult to resist or control. Most patients have poor insight or are delusional, not recognizing that the flaw they perceive is actually minimal or nonexistent (18). When the clinician reassures them that they look fine or attempts to talk them out of their belief about the perceived deformity, most patients are not swayed from their view. A majority of individuals have ideas or delusions of reference (2,18); that is, they think that other people take special notice of the supposed defect and perhaps talk about it or mock it. For example, one man who sang in a choir thought the entire audience was staring at a barely visible scar on his neck.

Repetitive Behaviors

Although repetitive behaviors are not included in BDD's diagnostic criteria, presented above, nearly all patients with the disorder engage in one or more repetitive, often time-consuming, and compulsive behaviors (2,3,14). The usual purpose of such behaviors is to examine, improve, or hide the perceived defect. The behaviors include excessively checking the perceived appearance flaw in mirrors and other reflecting surfaces, such as car bumpers and the backs of spoons. Many patients also excessively groom; for example, comb, style, wash, or cut their hair for hours a day. A majority camouflage the perceived deformity with hair, makeup, body position, or clothing (e.g., wearing a hat to hide "balding"). To avoid looking "pale," some individuals excessively tan, even to the point of severely burning and damaging their skin. Other common behaviors include comparing their appearance with that of other people, seeking reassurance about how they look (usually without believing the reassurance provided), or compulsively and repeatedly requesting dermatological treatment or cosmetic surgery.

Skin picking is a BDD symptom that is of particular relevance to dermatologists. Approximately one third of patients compulsively pick at their skin, trying to remove minor blemishes or to otherwise clear or perfect their skin (11,14). A growing literature documents how time consuming and problematic this behavior can be. Some patients, for example, report spending 8 or 12 hours a day picking at their skin. They may use their fingers, pins, needles, staple removers, razor blades, or knives (11). This behavior can cause considerable skin damage, and this is the one subgroup of BDD patients who may not look normal. In more extreme cases the behavior can be life threatening (11,19), as in the case of a woman who picked with tweezers at a pimple on her neck, exposing her carotid artery and requiring emergency surgery (19).

Complications

Both the psychiatry and dermatology literatures emphasize that BDD causes considerable distress and impairment in functioning (1,4,6,8–10,13,16). Preoccupations and related behaviors can impair concentration and consume large amounts of time. Many individuals avoid work, relationships, and social situations because they worry that they look ugly or that others are laughing at or talking about them. BDD can cause severe depression and anxiety and can lead to unemployment or dropping out of school. Being housebound and requiring psychiatric hospitalization are relatively common. Level of functioning is variable, however (3). Individuals with milder symptoms may, with effort, function well despite their distress, although usually below their capacity. Individuals with severe BDD may be completely incapacitated by their symptoms. Patients with BDD also have an unusually poor quality of life. The only published study of this issue found that they have poorer mental health–related quality of life than has been reported for patients with other severe illnesses, such as type II diabetes, a recent myocardial infarction, or depression (20).

It should be emphasized that patients with BDD, especially those with more severe symptoms, are at risk of suicide. In the largest series of patients with DSM-IV–defined BDD, approximately one quarter of patients had attempted suicide (14). Suicide risk is also emphasized in the dermatology literature. Cotterill, for example, reported on several patients with BDD ("dermatologic nondisease") who committed suicide (6). In a more recent study, the same author found that in a series of dermatology patients who had committed suicide, most had acne or BDD (21).

Demographic Features and Course of Illness

The reported sex ratio of BDD varies, with some studies reporting a preponderance of men (16) and others a preponderance of women (15,22). In the largest published series in a psychiatric setting, 51% were men (14). In a study in a dermatology setting, 9.9% of men and 12.8% of women screened positive for BDD (a statistically nonsignificant difference) (23). Nearly three quarters of patients have never been married (14). BDD usually begins during adolescence and can occur in childhood (24). The disorder appears to usually be chronic (18), although patients who receive appropriate psychiatric treatment appear to have a generally favorable course (25). Prospective studies are needed to confirm these retrospective findings.

Associated Psychiatric Disorders

Most patients with BDD who are seen in psychiatric settings have other psychiatric disorders (2,14). The most commonly co-occurring disorders are major depression, substance abuse and dependence, social phobia, and obsessive-compulsive disorder (2,14). In addition, available data indicate that a majority of patients with BDD have a personality disorder (15,26,27).

Case Example

The following case illustrates many of BDD's clinical features.

Ms. A., a 27-year-old single white female, was referred to the first author by a dermatologist, who stated, "I'm referring you a patient with perfect skin." The patient presented with a chief complaint of "I see a lot of skin doctors." She had seen dozens of dermatologists, to no avail. Ms. A. was convinced that she had severe acne, scars, and "veins" on her face. She frequently checked mirrors, applied makeup for hours a day, and picked at her skin. She also frequently asked other people, including her dermatologists, whether her skin looked okay. She stated that because she so incessantly sought reassurance from her doctors, most of the dermatologists in Boston were probably seeing therapists.

As a result of her BDD symptoms, Ms. A. had dropped out of school, was unemployed, and was completely socially isolated and housebound; she had attempted suicide and been psychiatrically hospitalized. Treatment with numerous antibiotics and isotretinoin had not diminished Ms. A.'s appearance concerns. An antipsychotic and a tricyclic antidepressant (desipramine) were also ineffective. However, she had a good response to fluoxetine (Prozac) 40 mg/day, with a significant decrease in her preoccupation, distress, picking behavior, and suicidality, as well as significant improvement in functioning.

PREVALENCE

BDD appears relatively common but underdiagnosed in psychiatric settings (28,29). In cosmetic surgery settings, rates of 6% (30), 7% (31), and 15% (32) have been reported. In the dermatology literature, BDD has been noted to be relatively common yet underrecognized (6,7,9,10,13). To our knowledge, we have conducted the only prevalence study in a dermatology setting. In this study of 268 patients presenting for dermatological treatment, 11.9% (95% C.I. 8.0–15.8%) of patients screened positive for BDD (23), with similar rates in a community general dermatology setting and a university cosmetic surgery setting. Most patients had concerns about the appearance of their skin, and a sizable percentage reported experiencing severe or extreme distress or functional impairment as a result of these concerns.

TREATMENT RESPONSE

Surgical, Dermatological, and Other Nonpsychiatric Medical Treatment

A majority of BDD patients seen in a psychiatric setting have sought and received nonpsychiatric treatment (2,15,16,52). Dermatological treatment is most often received (52). The largest study to date ($n = 250$ adults with BDD) found that 55% had sought, and 45% had received, dermatologic treatment (52). From an anecdotal perspective, the dermatology literature notes that individuals with "dermatological hypochondriasis" (10) or "dermatological non-disease" (6) often seek dermatologic treatment, including laser therapy, dermabrasion, or transplant, even when such treatment is not warranted.

Although prospective treatment outcome studies with nonpsychiatric treatment have not been done, BDD has been described in the dermatology literature as difficult to treat (4,6,8,13). This literature notes that these patients may consult numerous physicians and pressure dermatologists to prescribe unsuitable and ineffective treatments (8,9). Some patients sue or threaten to harm their dermatologist (4). These patients are said to often have a poor response to dermatological treatment (4,6,8). The surgery literature similarly suggests that the treatment outcome of BDD patients is generally poor (1). Cosmetic surgery in men has been cited as sometimes generating aggression toward the surgeon, even triggering murder (33,34).

Most patients with BDD who are seen in a psychiatric setting retrospectively report that nonpsychiatric treatment (e.g., dermatological or surgical) was not beneficial or that it even made them worse (15,18). In the previously noted study ($n = 250$), 20% of patients who received dermatologic treatment reported that this treatment improved their concern with the treated body area, but only 10% reported that their overall BDD symptoms improved (some, for example, developed a new concern with another body area); 8% reported a worsening of overall BDD symptoms. Multiple procedures may be received in the search for a cosmetic solution to this psychiatric problem. Some patients treat themselves—e.g., attempting to smooth their skin with a razor blade. Prospective studies are needed to confirm these empirical findings and clinical impressions.

Pharmacotherapy

Available data indicate that serotonin-reuptake inhibitors (SRIs) are often effective for BDD (35–39). These medications are antidepressants that, unlike other antidepressants, also decrease obsessions and repetitive behaviors. SRIs currently marketed in the United States are fluvoxamine (Luvox), fluoxetine (Prozac), paroxetine (Paxil), citalopram (Celexa), escitalopram (Lexapro), sertraline (Zoloft), and clomipramine (Anafranil).

The best studied SRIs in BDD are fluoxetine, fluvoxamine, clomipramine, and citalopram. In the only placebo-controlled pharmacotherapy study in BDD ($n = 74$), fluoxetine was significantly more effective than placebo, with a response rate of 53% to fluoxetine versus 18% to placebo (36a). In a double-blind cross-over study of 29 randomized patients, clomipramine (an SRI) was superior to desipramine (a non-SRI tricyclic antidepressant) (39). In an open-label study of fluvoxamine, 19 (63%) of 30 subjects with BDD responded (36). In another open-label study of fluvoxamine, two-thirds of 15 subjects responded (38). And in an open-label study of citalopram, 11 of 15 subjects (73%) improved, as did psychosocial functioning and quality of life (53).

Although fluoxetine, fluvoxamine, citalopram, and clomipramine are the best studied SRIs, clinical experience suggests that all SRIs are effective for BDD (18,37). A growing literature suggests that SRIs are also often effective for compulsive skin picking (11,19,40,41). For an individual patient, one SRI may be more effective than another, although the SRI that is most effective for a given patient must be determined by trial and error and cannot be predicted. Of note, available data suggest that SRIs are also effective for patients with delusional BDD (i.e., those who are completely convinced that their view of the "defect" is correct) (18,36,39). Furthermore, delusional patients appear to not respond to antipsychotics (including pimozide) when used as single agents (18). Non-SRI psychotropic medications have been less well studied for BDD; however, available data indicate that while some may be useful as adjunctive treatments with SRIs, they are generally ineffective for BDD when used as single agents (2,18,39,42,43).

Cognitive-Behavioral Therapy

Cognitive-behavioral therapy (CBT) also appears to be effective for BDD. CBT is a here-and-now kind of treatment that focuses specifically on BDD symptoms. The therapist is quite active in the treatment, and homework is prescribed. CBT consists of elements known as exposure and response prevention. Exposure consists of having patients expose the perceived defect in social situations (e.g., going to avoided restaurants or stores without a hat or heavy makeup or sitting in a crowded waiting room). Response prevention consists of helping patients avoid performing repetitive behaviors (e.g., stopping excessive mirror checking, limiting grooming time, and stopping use of excessive makeup and reassurance seeking). Cognitive restructuring helps patients change their erroneous beliefs about their appearance and the importance attributed to appearance. Behavioral experiments may be used to empirically test hypotheses based on the patient's erroneous beliefs (e.g., testing the hypothesis that 80% of people in a video store will recoil from the patient with a look of horror on their face and walk away from them within 5 seconds).

Case series and studies using no-treatment wait-list controls have found that CBT is effective for a majority of patients with BDD. In a report of five patients with BDD, four improved using such approaches in 90-minute sessions 1 or 5 days per week (with the total number of sessions ranging from 12 to 48) (44). A report of 13 patients found that BDD significantly improved in 12 90-minute group therapy sessions (45). In another study, exposure and response prevention plus cognitive techniques were effective in 77% of 27 women who received this treatment in eight weekly 2-hour group sessions (22). Subjects in the treatment group improved more than those in a no-treatment waiting-list control group. In a pilot study of 19 patients (primarily women) who were randomly assigned to a CBT group or a no-treatment waiting-list control group, there was significantly greater improvement in BDD symptoms in the group that received CBT (46). One small study ($n = 10$) found that patients who participated in an intensive behavioral therapy program, including a 6-month maintenance program, maintained their improvement at up to 2 years (47).

Although the efficacy of other types of therapy for BDD has not been well studied, available evidence suggests that supportive psychotherapy, insight-oriented psychotherapy, and counseling are generally ineffective for BDD (2,18).

RECOGNIZING AND DIAGNOSING BODY DYSMORPHIC DISORDER

Because of the morbidity associated with BDD as well as the potential for a poor treatment outcome, it is important to identify BDD in dermatology settings (13). BDD is diagnosed by asking questions that determine whether the DSM-IV diagnostic criteria (presented above) are met. Questions that can be asked to determine this are listed in Table 1 (48). Clues to the presence of BDD are listed in Table 2. Dermatologists who encounter patients presenting with one or more of these clues should ask the diagnostic questions listed in Table 1 to determine whether BDD is present.

Practical Suggestions for Dermatologists

The following suggestions are based on available data and the authors' clinical experience. These recommendations may change over time as more is learned about BDD.

1. Provide psychoeducation about BDD. Psychoeducation is an important element of any treatment. In the case of BDD, we suggest approaching patients in the following way:

> Tell them that they appear to have a body image problem (or disorder) known as body dysmorphic disorder. Tell them that BDD is a known and treatable disorder that many people have.
>
> Recommend reading material on BDD so that patients can learn more about their condition. Several books and websites contain information on BDD for the layperson (3,17,49,50).
>
> For patients who repeatedly seek reassurance about how they look, explain that reassuring them generally isn't helpful and that a more effective approach is to obtain appropriate treatment for their body image concerns.
>
> Don't discount or disparage patients' appearance concerns. Doing so can be devastating to them. Keep in mind that these patients suffer tremendously. Explain that rather than having a significant dermatological problem, they have a body image problem consisting

---

TABLE 1 Diagnostic Questions for BDD

1.	Are you very worried about your appearance in any way? If yes: What is your concern? Do you think (body part) is especially unattractive? If yes: What about the appearance of your face, skin, hair, nose, or the shape or size or other aspect of any other part of your body?
2.	Does this concern preoccupy you? That is, do you think about it a lot and wish you could worry about it less?
3.	What effect has this concern had on your life? Has it caused you a lot of distress or interfered with your functioning in any way?

These questions are a guide to diagnosing BDD. BDD is diagnosed if the criteria presented in the introduction are met. In addition, for BDD to be diagnosed, the appearance concerns should not be better accounted for by an eating disorder.

TABLE 2 Clues to the Presence of BDD

---

1. Excessive concern with, or distress over, minor or nonexistent appearance flaws
2. Difficulty functioning—e.g., problems at work or social avoidance
3. Skin picking
4. Camouflaging—e.g., wearing heavy makeup or a hat
5. Other BDD-related behaviors, such as excessive tanning, reassurance seeking, or excessive grooming
6. Referential thinking—i.e., thinking that others are taking special notice of them because of how they look
7. Dissatisfaction with previous dermatological or surgical treatment
8. Unusual or excessive requests for cosmetic procedures
9. Belief that the procedure will transform the individual's life or fix his or her problems

---

of being overly concerned about and affected by how they think they look.

If clinically appropriate for a particular patient, it may be helpful to educate family members and significant others about BDD.

2. It is generally ineffective to try to talk patients out of their concern or to tell them to stop picking their skin. Because most patients with BDD think that their view of their appearance is accurate, it is usually fruitless to try to convince them—especially delusional patients—that their beliefs are irrational, that their defect is "imagined," or that they look normal. You might tell them that your view of how they look differs from theirs, but trying to convince them that you are right and they are wrong is likely to be unsuccessful and frustrating. An exception to this pertains to the minority of patients who have some insight—in other words, those who acknowledge that they really don't look as bad as they think. With these patients, it is helpful to reinforce that this view is correct. In general, it is usually more fruitful to focus on the distress and impairment that the appearance concerns are causing the patient rather than on how they look. Such a focus may facilitate referral to a mental health professional.

It is usually useless, and frustrating for patients, to simply advise them to stop picking their skin. Most patients have tried countless times to stop but are unable to. The picking behavior is a compulsive activity over which patients have little or no control (3,11). Educating them that the picking is a symptom of BDD, and is treatable, can be helpful. It should be kept in mind that although many individuals who pick their skin have BDD, skin picking is a heterogeneous symptom that can present as a symptom of other disorders (50). To determine whether the picking is a symptom of BDD, the dermatologist should determine whether the purpose of the picking is to improve appearance and whether the definitional criteria for BDD are met.

3. *It is probably best to avoid cosmetic procedures.* Although definitive data on the treatment outcome of such treatment for BDD are lacking and no one can predict how a given patient will respond, the data presented above suggest that these treatments are unlikely to be successful and may even make the patient worse. In some cases, such treatment precipitates psychosis, suicidal behavior, or violence. We suggest telling patients that because they have BDD, you are concerned that they will be unhappy with the treatment—that surgery and dermatological treatment are unlikely to be successful for this problem and can even make it worse.

It is probably also best to avoid doing "a little something" to appease the patient, as this approach, too, can be unsuccessful—even disastrous. In one case, for example, a surgeon refused to do the extensive surgery requested by the patient but did give him some facial creams. In the patient's view, the creams created huge, dark spots on his skin. As a result, he went on a rampage with a hammer, destroying his parents' furniture and threatening to harm his family members. However, the treatment outcome of minor procedures, like that of any nonpsychiatric treatment for BDD, requires further research.

4. *Attempt to refer the patient to a psychiatrist for treatment.* Rather than referring the patient to another dermatologist, we recommend attempting to refer the patient to a psychiatrist for treatment with an SRI. This can be facilitated by using the psychoeducational approach discussed above, telling patients that they have a body image problem that is best treated by someone with expertise in the condition. It is of course best to refer to a psychiatrist familiar with BDD and its treatment.

If patients resist referral because they continue to believe the problem is physical, not psychological, focus on the large amount of time they spend obsessing about how they look, the amount of distress it is causing them, and how it is affecting—even ruining—their life (3). Focusing on psychiatric treatment's potential to decrease suffering and improve functioning may facilitate the referral.

If the patient wants to try therapy instead of medication, keep in mind that most mental health professionals are not trained in CBT and even fewer have expertise in treating BDD with CBT. It is important to refer to a therapist (a physician, psychologist, or social worker) who is trained in CBT and familiar with BDD.

If a patient is severely depressed or suicidal, an SRI is needed. In this case, we recommend not referring the patient for CBT alone.

5. For skin pickers, a combination of psychiatric and dermatological treatment may be best. One group of BDD patients who may require dermatological treatment are those who pick their skin. Because they can do considerable damage to their skin, dermatological treatment may be necessary. However, the dermatological treatment will not stop the picking and should be combined with the psychiatric treatment described above.

6. For low-risk patients who refuse referral to a psychiatrist or a mental health professional trained in CBT, consider treating the patient yourself with an SRI. SRIs are relatively straightforward to use, although drug interactions must be considered (this is less of a concern with citalopram, escitalopram, and sertraline). For patients who refuse referral to a mental health professional, it is probably better to treat with an SRI yourself or refer the patient to his or her general practitioner for SRI treatment, rather than forgoing treatment. It is best to do this after consulting with a psychiatrist familiar with BDD, if possible. If this approach is used, the patient's suicidality must be frequently monitored. If patients are or become suicidal or severely depressed, they should be referred to a psychiatrist familiar with BDD.

To determine whether an SRI will work, patients should receive a SRI trial 12–16 weeks in duration. The highest SRI dose recommended by the manufacturer or tolerated by the patient should be used if a lower dose is ineffective (43). If this fails, another SRI should be tried (43). If several SRIs fail, referral to a psychiatrist should again be considered. Many patients who respond to an SRI will require chronic treatment, as the risk of relapse appears high with SRI discontinuation (36,37). More detailed recommendations on the pharmacotherapy of BDD are provided elsewhere (43).

CONCLUSIONS

In recent years BDD has gone from being a neglected psychiatric disorder to one that is becoming better recognized and understood. Nonetheless, research on this disorder is still in its early stages, and much more investigation of BDD is needed, especially in dermatological settings. Available data indicate that the disorder is fairly common, frequently presents to dermatologists, often responds poorly to dermatological treatment, and usually responds well to SRIs and CBT. Treatment recommendations will be modified in the future as more research is done. In the meantime, it is important that dermatologists screen patients for BDD and accurately diagnose this condition, as available psychiatric treatments are often efficacious for patients who suffer from this distressing and sometimes disabling disorder.

REFERENCES

1. Phillips KA. Body dysmorphic disorder: the distress of imagined ugliness. Am J Psychiatry 148:1138–1149, 1991.
2. Phillips KA, McElroy SL, Keck PE Jr, Pope HG Jr, Hudson JI. Body dysmorphic disorder: 30 cases of imagined ugliness. Am J Psychiatry 150:302–308, 1993.
3. Phillips KA. The broken mirror: understanding and treating body dysmorphic disorder. New York: Oxford University Press, 1996.
4. Cotterill JA. Body dysmorphic disorder. Dermatol Clin 14:457–463, 1996.
5. American Psychiatric Association. Diagnostic and Statistical Manual of Mental Disorders. 4th ed. Washington, DC: American Psychiatric Publishing, 1994.
6. Cotterill JA. Dermatological non-disease: a common and potentially fatal disturbance of cutaneous body image. Br J Dermatol 104:611–619, 1981.
7. Bishop ER. Monosymptomatic hypochondriacal syndromes in dermatology. J Am Acad Dermatol 9:152–158, 1983.
8. Koblenzer CS. The dysmorphic syndrome. Arch Dermatol 121:780–784, 1985.
9. Koblenzer CS. The broken mirror: dysmorphic syndrome in the dermatologist's practice. Fitz J Clin Dermatol March/April 1994:14–19.
10. Zaidens SH. Dermatologic hypochondriasis: a form of schizophrenia. Psychosom Med 12:250–253, 1950.
11. Phillips KA, Taub SL. Skin picking as a symptom of body dysmorphic disorder. Psychopharmacol Bull 31:279–288, 1995.
12. Gupta MA, Gupta AK, Haberman HF. Neurotic excoriations: a review and some new perspectives. Compr Psychiatry 27:381–386, 1986.
13. Hanes KR. Body dysmorphic disorder: an underestimated entity? [letter]. Austral J Dermatol 36:227–229, 1995.
14. Phillips KA, Diaz S. Gender differences in body dysmorphic disorder. J Nerv Ment Dis 185:570–577, 1997.
15. Veale D, Boocock A, Gournay K, Dryden W, Shah F, Willson R, Walburn J. Body dysmorphic disorder: a survey of fifty cases. Br J Psychiatry 169:196–201, 1996.
16. Hollander E, Cohen LJ, Simeon D. Body dysmorphic disorder. Psych Ann 23:359–364, 1993.
17. Pope HG, Phillips KA, Olivardia R. The Adonis Complex: The Secret Crisis of Male Body Obsession. New York: The Free Press, 2000.
18. Phillips KA, McElroy SL, Keck PE Jr, Pope HG Jr, Hudson JI. A comparison of delusional and nondelusional body dysmorphic disorder in 100 cases. Psychopharmacol Bull: 179–186, 1994.
19. O'Sullivan RL, Phillips KA, Keuthen NJ, Wilhelm S. Near fatal skin picking from delusional body dysmorphic disorder responsive to fluvoxamine. Psychosom 40:79–81, 1999.
20. Phillips KA. Quality of life for patients with body dysmorphic disorder. J Nerv Ment Dis 188:170–175, 2000.

21. Cotterill JA, Cunliffe WJ. Suicide in dermatological patients. Br J Dermatol 137:246–250, 1997.

22. Rosen JC, Reiter J, Orosan P. Cognitive-behavioral body image therapy for body dysmorphic disorder. J Consult Clin Psychol 63:263–269, 1995.

23. Phillips KA, Dufresne RG Jr, Wilkel C, Vittorio C. Rate of body dysmorphic disorder in dermatology patients. J Am Acad Dermatol 42:436–441, 2000.

24. Albertini RS, Phillips KA. 33 cases of body dysmorphic disorder in children and adolescents. J Am Acad Child Adolesc Psychiatry 38:453–459, 1999.

25. Phillips KA, Grant J, Albertini RS, Stout R, Price LH. Retrospective follow-up study of body dysmorphic disorder. New Research Program and Abstracts, American Psychiatric Association 152nd Annual Meeting. Washington, DC: American Psychiatric Association, 1999:151.

26. Phillips KA, McElroy SL. Personality disorders and traits in patients with body dysmorphic disorder. Compr Psychiatry 41:229–236, 2000.

27. Neziroglu F, McKay D, Todaro J, Yaryura-Tobias J. Effect of cognitive behavior therapy on persons with body dysmorphic disorder and comorbid axis II diagnoses. Behav Ther 27:67–77, 1996.

28. Perugi G, Akiskal HS, Lattanzi L, Cecconi D, Mastrocinque C, Patronelli A, Vignoli S, Berni E. The high prevalence of "soft" bipolar (II) features in atypical depression. Compr Psychiatry 39:63–71, 1998.

29. Phillips KA, Nierenberg AA, Brendel G, Fava M. Prevalence and clinical features of body dysmorphic disorder in atypical major depression. J Nerv Ment Dis 184:125–129, 1996.

30. Sarwer DB, Whitaker LA, Pertschuk MJ, Wadden TA. Body image concerns of reconstructive surgery patients: an underrecognized problem. Ann Plast Surg 40:403–407, 1998.

31. Sarwer DB, Wadden TA, Pertschuk MJ, Whitaker LA. Body image dissatisfaction and body dysmorphic disorder in 100 cosmetic surgery patients. Plast Reconstr Surg 101:1644–1649, 1998.

32. Ishigooka J, Iwao M, Suzuki M, Fukuyama Y, Murasaki M, Miura S. Demographic features of patients seeking cosmetic surgery. Psychiatry Clin Neurosci 52:283–287, 1998.

33. Phillips KA, McElroy SL, Lion JR. Body dysmorphic disorder in cosmetic surgery patients [letter]. Plast Reconst Surgery 90:333–334, 1992.

34. Ladee GA. Hypochondriacal Syndromes. Amsterdam: Elsevier, 1966.

35. Hollander E, Liebowitz MR, Winchel R, Klumker A, Klein DF. Treatment of body dysmorphic disorder with serotonin reuptake blockers. Am J Psychiatry 146:768–770, 1989.

36. Phillips KA, Dwight MM, McElroy SL. Efficacy and safety of fluvoxamine in body dysmorphic disorder. J Clin Psychiatry 59:165–171, 1998.

36a. Phillips KA, Albertini RS, Rasmussen SA. A randomized placebo-controlled trial of fluoxetine in body dysmorphic disorder. Arch Gen Psychiatry 59:381–388, 2002.

37. Phillips KA, Albertini RS, Siniscalchi J, Khan A, Robinson M. Effectiveness of pharmacotherapy for body dysmorphic disorder: a chart-review study. J Clin Psychiatry 62:721–727, 2001.

38. Perugi G, Giannotti D, Di Vaio S, Frare F, Saettoni M, Cassano GB. Fluvoxamine in the treatment of body dysmorphic disorder (dysmorphophobia). Int Clin Psychopharmacol 11:247–254, 1996.

39. Hollander E, Allen A, Kwon J, Kwon J, Mosovich S, Schmeidler J, Wong C. Clomipramine vs desipramine crossover trial in body dysmorphic disorder: selective efficacy of a serotonin reuptake inhibitor in imagined ugliness. Arch Gen Psychiatry 56:1033–1039, 1999.

40. Simeon D, Stein DJ, Gross S, Islam N, Schmeidler J, Hollander E. A double-blind trial of fluoxetine in pathologic skin picking. J Clin Psychiatry 58:341–347, 1997.

41. Kalivas J, Kalivas L, Gilman D, Hayden CT. Sertraline in the treatment of neurotic excoriations and related disorders. Arch Dermatol 132:589–596, 1996.

42. Hollander E, Cohen L, Simeon D, Rosen J, DeCaria C, Stein DJ. Fluvoxamine treatment of body dysmorphic disorder [letter]. J Clin Psychopharmacol 14:75–77, 1994.

43. Phillips KA. Pharmacologic treatment of body dysmorphic disorder: a review of the evidence and a recommended treatment approach. CNS Spectrums 7:453–460, 2002.

44. Neziroglu FA, Yaryura-Tobias JA. Exposure, response prevention, and cognitive therapy in the treatment of body dysmorphic disorder. Behav Ther 24:431–438, 1993.

45. Wilhelm S, Otto MW, Lohr B. Cognitive behavior group therapy for body dysmorphic disorder: a case series. Behav Res Ther 37:71–75, 1999.

46. Veale D, Gournay K, Dryden W, Boocock A, Shah F, Willson R, Walburn J. Body dysmorphic disorder: a cognitive behavioral model and pilot randomized controlled trial. Behav Res Ther 34:717–729, 1996.

47. McKay D. Two-year follow-up of behavioral treatment and maintenance for body dysmorphic disorder. Behav Mod 23:620–629, 1999.

48. Dufresne RG, Phillips KA, Vittorio CC, Wilkel CS. A screening questionnaire for body dysmorphic disorder in a cosmetic dermatologic surgery practice. Dermatol Surg 27:457–462, 2001.

49. Phillips KA, Van Noppen B, Shapiro L. Learning to Live with Body Dysmorphic Disorder. Milford, CT: Obsessive-Compulsive Foundation, 1997.

50. http://www.BodyImageProgram.com

51. Arnold LM, McElroy SL, Mutasim DF, Dwight MM, Lamerson CL, Morris EM. Characteristics of 34 adults with psychogenic excoriation. J Clin Psychiatry 59:509–514, 1998.

52. Phillips KA, Grant J, Siniscalchi J, Albertini RS. Surgical and nonpsychiatric medical treatment of patients with body dysmorphic disorder. Psychosomatics 42:504–510, 2001.

53. Phillips KA, Najar F. An open-label study of citalopram in body dysmorphic disorder. J Clin Psychiatry, in press.

12

The Spectrum of Dermatological Self-Mutilation and Self-Destruction Including Dermatitis Artefacta and Neurotic Excoriations

Myriam Van Moffaert
University Hospital
Ghent, Belgium

THE SPECTRUM OF DERMATOLOGICAL SELF-MUTILATION AND SELF-DESTRUCTION: COMMON ISSUES

The spectrum of self-induced dermatological conditions is very extended. Self-mutilative and self-destructive psychological tendencies tend to express themselves in a continuum of behaviors motivated by a myriad of causes ranging from simple distress to perverse intentions, and the underlying psychiatric disorders are the most complicated. Although the definitions of both dermatitis artefacta and neurotic excoriations suggest specific skin lesions, specific motivations, and specific underlying psychiatric conditions, it must be emphasized that the spectrum of self-indiced dermatological disorder is very extended. Patients with cutaneous artefacts present their double morbidity—dermatological and psychiatric—to the dermatologist, so most of the burden of detecting, diagnosing, and treating these difficult cases falls on that physician (1). The dermatologist will find guidelines in this chapter for the management of a wide range of artificial dermatosis, from lesions inflicted through tics and obsessive-compulsive behavior such as neurotic excoriations, nail biting (onychophagy), and hair pulling (trichotillomania, trichophagy) to the different types of dermatitis artefacta and even cases of clear malingering or pathomimesis (simulating a dermatosis with a motive of definite material gain, such as release from prison or obtaining a sickness allowance) (2,3).

According to the manner of production, self-induced dermatologial lesions may appear as burns, abrasions, erosions, scratches, ulcers, or bullae. Patients with cutaneous factitious disorders are quite ingenious in simulating well-defined dermatoses. They may provoke cutaneous lesions in a unique event or attempt repetitive actions, all resulting in a difficult-to-diagnose skin condition (4). There are types of dermatitis artefacta, such as trichotillomania, which run a completely automatic course. Other types of dermatitis artefacta follow an ingenious procedure: first a concoction is made, which is then injected subcutaneously or intravenously accompanied by an extensive ritual. There is a marked variation in the degree of consciousness and free will involved in the different types of dermatitis artefacta.

The act of provoking the cutaneous lesions frequently has a relaxing effect (4). Particularly in the case of bleeding lesions, the moment they see the blood flowing, patients experience a very pleasant sensation, which is sometimes compared to an orgasm or the high after drug-taking. Pain perception is often altered during self-mutilation: instead of pain, many patients experience delight. Remarkably enough, when the self-mutilation lesions are being treated, for example, when a cut is being sutured, some patients also show reduced sensitivity to pain. The relaxing effect and the experience of lust connected with self-mutilation can become addictive, and the patient becomes dependent on self-mutilation. Individuals who suffer from unpleasant states of depersonalization and derealization (the pathological sensation of alienation and the loss of the sense of reality towards oneself or the familiar environment, respectively) have a marked compulsion to provoke painful physical sensations and self-mutilation in order to arrest the depersonalization or derealization (5).

Physicians generally believe self-destruction and self-mutilation in a patient equates with a severe psychopathology, and the very act of cutaneous self-mutilation involved in dermatitis artefacta is generally regarded as a severe behavioral disorder. It is not sufficiently recognized that there is an element of self-destruction in many everyday behavioral patterns such as smoking, excessive alcohol intake, speeding, frequent changing of sexual partner without adequate protection, and high-risk sports.

Self-destructive behavior is in fact situated in a continuum, and the skin is of all organs and organic systems the organ most often chosen in cases of self-mutilation and factitious skin disorder. Several reasons are at hand—first and most obvious the skin's easy accessibility. The skin literally needs much "handling" due to normal daily hygiene, so "manipulations" may be a mere exaggeration of nonpathological interaction with the skin. The skin is also a favorite area for the discharge of all kinds of tension: in situations of tension and frustration there is an increase in the number and intensity of "displacement" motions, i.e., all kinds of rubbing, scratching, and picking imitating normal cleansing movements (6,7).

Apart from accessibility, the visibility of a skin injury and the fact that the skin is an organ of communication and expression are also important. Furthermore, the skin forms a protective layer between the individual and the outside world and plays an important part in one's concept of oneself (Didier Anzieu's term *le Moi-Peau*—the concept of the self, relating to the boundary between the individual and the environment, i.e., the cutaneous envelope) (8). Finally, the skin is essential for the exchange of experience between the individual and his immediate environment and has a specific role in interhuman contact. Next, a cultural dimension may be at play in dermatitis artefacta (9). The line between acts that are accepted as normal interference with one's own body (depilation, tattooing) and self-inflicted physical changes regarded as self-mutilation behavior varies from culture to culture and also within a particular culture according to factors such as age and sex. Shaving of hair is part of some religious rites (e.g., the tonsure several years before a priest is ordained in the Roman Catholic church). In some primitive African and south American populations cutaneous mutilations (mainly epidermal scarification) and the resulting scars have been accepted as an aesthetic procedure and as part of the strutting behavior of warriors. Another example is the former custom of inflicting a *Schnitze* (cut) on members of certain German student associations.

Aggravation of a preexisting genuine dermatosis by stress and anxiety is part of the self-mutilative spectrum in dermatological practice. The occurrence as well as the severity of many genuine dermatological disorders is influenced by emotional factors and, thus, through involuntary behavioral factors such as rubbing, skin-picking and scratching, and dermatoses (e.g. eczema, alopecia, psoriasis, and urticaria) may be aggravated and thus strongly affected by nonspecific emotional stress factors and specific life events (10). Stress, anxiety, and the resulting scratching may affect the onset and duration of the disorder or trigger a relapse and thus influence patient compliance with medications (11). Although the primary cause of atopic dermatitis is immunological, psychological factors play a part in precipitating and maintaining the lesions, while emotional elements also have a strong effect on the itch-scratch cycle (12). In infantile eczema the role of emotional factors is beyond question. Maternal or parental rejection of atopic children is crucial to the development of the disorder (13). Consequently, a psychosomatic treatment principle has been suggested in which the concentration of active substances in ointments for treating the disorder is reduced, which necessitates more frequent applications (13). This may result in an increase in skin contact and cuddling, which has a beneficial effect on the disease. Attacks or relapses of alopecia areata are induced by stress factors and neurotic personality features (14). Neuroendocrinological investigations support the hypothesis that patients with psoriasis have personality features that result in the interpretation of challenging situations as more stressful than they would be interpreted by individuals without psoriasis (14). Patients with psychogenic pruritus (pruritus anogenitalis and pruritus vulvae, in particular) have distinguishing character features such as semi-permeability (extreme vulnerability to the feelings of others), the inability to manage aggressive tendencies, character armoring (resistance to others' perceptions of self), exaggerated cleanliness, and fear of disorder: all these particularities may engender excessive washing or other rituals, which can aggravate the authentic dermatosis. Of course one may argue that the use of the term "dermatitis artefacta" should be reserved for lesions totally made by the patient de novo, but as neurotic excoriations are part of this discussion it seems illogical not to include aggravation of authentic dermatosis by stress-related conditions.

NEUROTIC EXCORIATIONS AND DERMATITIS ARTEFACTA: DIFFERENCES AND SIMILITUDES

Dermatitis artefacta, or factitial dermatitis, is diagnosed when the patient uses a more elaborate method than simple excoriation to self-induce skin lesions. Skin lesions are provoked by numerous mechanical means or by the application of chemical irritants and caustics. The act of creating lesions may be conscious (e.g., secondary gain) or unconscious, but the patient almost always denies doing so (15). The pseudo-patient may mimic an existing dermatological condition or create a "mysterious dermatosis," thus posing for the dermatologist a diagnostic enigma not conforming to the dermatological textbooks. The. aim to become a patient is guided by different, often co-existing motivations: the passive role of the patient in itself, as the center of medical attention, sometimes aggravated by the aim of becoming a difficult case in terms of diagnosis and treatment, or the pursuit of sickness leave or benefit. Sometimes a main or side goal is challenging physicians or duping them as a revenge on the medical profession (15).

Neurotic excoriations are more the result of unconsciously motivated repetitive behavior, skin picking, and scratching caused by different motivations ranging from simple stress- and tension-reducing scratching to outright obsessive-compulsive disorder. Patients usually acknowledge, in contrast to the outraged denial of dermatitis artefacta patients, that they feel an uncontrollable urge to gouge and pick at their skin and are obsessively involved in a vicious circle. Repeated picking and digging and scraping produces the characteristic excoriations, usually on parts readily accessible to the hands.

The main difference between neurotic excoriations and dermatitis artefacta lies in the underlying psychopathology and the fact that the fingers and fingernails are used to create lesions, in contrast to the more elaborate measures (sharp objects, chemicals, cigarette butts, etc.) used to create dermatitis artefacta (6).

Some types of self-induced dermatological lesions are more the result of minor tics. The essential feature of trichotillomania is the recurrent pulling out of one's hair, resulting in noticeable hair loss (16). Together with nail-biting, lip-biting (factitious cheilitis is a persistent crusting and scaling of the lips, through continued biting), and excoriations, trichotillomania is one of the several behaviors that are part of normal human self-grooming but that may escalate to an obsessive-compulsive syndrome. The patient with trichotillomania selects a part of the scalp to be pulled and ritualistically twists, scrutinizes, and may even eat (trichophagy) the hair after it has been extracted. Other cases involve the deliberate infliction of bruises or edema caused by elastic bands.

Dermatitis artefacta and neurotic excoriations are both gender-specific. Both are far more present in female patients. In dermatitis artefacta, estimates of female-to-male ratios vary from 3:1 to 8:1, depending on the source. It can present at any age, but is most common in adolescents and young adults. It is very common for the patient to have some affiliation with the health care field, either through employment or a family member. Women with personality traits such as emotional immaturity and relational difficulties are most at risk when conflictual events and stresses precipitate the onset of factitious lesions (17). These patients often have a history of psychosomatic illnesses. In children there may be evidence of an underlying anxiety or adjustment disorder or a dysfunctional mother-child relationship, including physical or emotional abuse. Adult patients often display borderline personality traits, characterized by infantile, dependent, manipulative behavior and poor impulse control. A thorough history may reveal a psychosocial stressor that occurred just before the condition appeared. While "secondary gain" may motivate the activity, the patient may (in the case of malingering) or may not (in the case of unconsciously wanting to assume the invalid role) be aware of it. Neurotic excoriations are also more common in women and can occur at any age, although the most severe and recalcitrant cases usually appear between the third and fifth decades.

A diagnosis of self-induced skin lesions should not be made simply by exclusion. It should be suspected, however, in a patient with bizarre skin lesions and a "hollow history"—a history of psychosomatic/emotional illness, recent psychosocial stressors, and typical affect of patient and family. Other supporting evidence includes a multiplicity of prior consultations with other phycisians, extensive studies with negative results, long lists of ineffective treatments, and the patient's past or present association, direct or indirect, with the health care field.

Lastly, the prognosis of dermatitis artefacta and neuroric excoriation differs in the psychiatric sense. Neurotic excoriations tend, untreated, to become a chronic condition, without an aggravation to more severe self-destructive behavior, and complicated with social phobia only (i.e., the fear of being seen by others, mainly strangers; this results in a "housebound" syndrome). Dermatitis artefacta has a more escalating evolution profile. Dermatitis artefacta may become part of a self-mutilation career, which typically starts in adolescence with direct low-lethal self-mutilation (cigarette burns or slight epidermal scratches). After adolescence this occasional self-mutilation develops into a chronic condition with considerable psychiatric morbidity such as pronounced social withdrawal or drug overdose. The typical career of a self-mutilator continues with repetitive psychiatric and medical hospitalization. The hospitalization period is strikingly long on average, which indicates that the majority of patients are resistant to therapy, or at least that the treatment seems to have little effect. This observation has significant implications for public health care.

NEUROTIC EXCORIATIONS

Neurotic excoriations were described by Brocq in 1889 (see Ref. 11) as *acné excoriée des jeunes filles*, the name given to self-inflicted lesions on a preexisting acne condition in young neurotic women.

Neurotic excoriations on healthy or previously diseased (mostly juvenile acne) skin is a frequent problem encountered in liaison-psychiatry. Patients suffer from an irresistible urge to excoriate the skin. Excoriations usually start during adolescence, as an extension of cleaning procedures for removing comedos. The compulsion becomes uncontrollable and leads to an imperative urge to dig into the skin in order to remove imaginary foreign substances (18). Because patients, by definition, can inflict lesions only to those areas of the body that are reachable, and because they tend to excoriate areas that are readily accessible, the distribution of the lesions can give the clinician a valuable clue. More specifically, patients with neurotic excoriations usually show a striking sparing of the upper lateral back area bilaterally, referred to as the "butterfly sign." There is also a preponderance of involvement on the extensor arm as compared to the medial arm, and on the anterior thigh as opposed to the posterior thigh. Even though this distribution of self-induced, excoriated lesions is highly suggestive of a psychogenic condition, it is not diagnostic because any condition that has pruritus as the primary symptom (uremic pruritus, scabies, idiopathic pruritus, etc.) can result in a similar distribution. Therefore, clinicians must be careful not to make the diagnosis on the basis of the morphology and the distribution of the lesions alone. One still needs to investigate other causes and search for psychopathology through either direct questioning or clinical observation.

Once the process of self-picking has begun, a focal itch or other sensation in uninvolved skin may initiate scratching, or tissue damage from scratching may trigger itching in either case. The itch-scratch cycle becomes a part of the clinical picture and may take on a life of its own. The underlying psychopathology can vary, but the most common findings are obsessive-compulsive disorder, anxiety, and depression. In mild or transient cases, especially in childhood, it may simply be a response to stress in a patient with obsessive-compulsive tendencies. In many persistent and recurrent cases, however, psychiatric evaluation will reveal a true obsessive-compulsive disorder. Classified as a type of anxiety disorder, this is defined as recurrent, uncontrollable thoughts that the patient finds senseless and intrusive (obsessions), causing increasing anxiety which can only be relieved by performing certain repetitive acts (compulsions, in this case, picking at the skin). Depressed patients, especially of the agitated rather than the retarded subtype, can also present with excoriations. A careful history may elicit symptoms of depression such as poor appetite, disturbed sleep, low energy, depressed mood, and crying episodes. Patients with generalized anxiety disorder may also present with excoriations. When tension mounts for these patients, they may focus on any blemish on the skin and channel their anxious energy to it. The neurotic excoriations sometimes occur in association with a psychiatric body image disturbance called body dysmorphic disorder.

DERMATITIS ARTEFACTA

Dermatitis artefacta are self-indiced cutaneous artefacts, which are not merely the result of a tic or an obsessive severe scratching, but the result of a more purposeful, sometimes quite ingenious, action to provoke skin lesions. Dermatitis artefacta includes a spectrum of lesions ranging from minimal aggravations of a previous genuine dermatosis to intentional cutaneous self-injury, which may be life-threatening because of gangrene or generalized infection. Artificial skin lesions are usually located in areas easily reached by the dominant hand. The morphology of dermatitis artefacta lesions is often bizarre, linear instead of round or oval-shaped, with clear-cut, angulated or geometric edges and differences in the course of lesion formation, which differentiate them from a natural dermatosis in which the lesions evolve more or less in the same pattern. An important clue to the diagnosis is the presence of completely normal, unaffected skin immediately adjacent to the often horrific-appearing lesions.

The "hollow history" is a very consistent finding in cases of factitial dermatitis. This term refers to an astonishing vagueness and inability of the patient to give any details about the appearance and evolution of skin lesions. The only information obtainable is that the lesions appeared "suddenly", without any preceding signs or symptoms. While the patient is seemingly unmoved by these puzzling and disfiguring lesions, which often appear painful, the family is frequently angry and accusatory of what they perceive as medical incompetence.

Dermatitis artefacta occurs in several psychiatric syndromes such as schizo-affective psychosis, monosymptomatic hypochondriacal psychosis (in psychodermatology the most common clinical type is the delusion of parasitosis or dermatozoal delusion), mental deficiency, melancholia, epileptic twilight states, during pathological alcohol intoxication, or in cocaine or LSD abuse. In addition, dermatitis artefacta sometimes appears to be the result of psychiatric conditions such as severe obsessive syndromes or anxiety paroxysms. However, dermatitis artefacta within the framework of major psychiatric pathology is relatively rare; e.g., the incidence of self-mutilation in hospitalized schizophrenics is 6% (11). Repetitive dermatitis artefacta, especially with the purpose of becoming a "false patient" is most frequent in borderline individuals, who exhibit typical personality disorders with emotional and relational instability, impulsiveness, mood dysregula-tion, and inadequate aggression (19). In borderline problems the act of cutaneous self-mutilation signifies the acting out of separation problems, i.e., the adult relives the intense feelings of desolation and rage that normally occur in the young child who is left on his own.

Recently the connection between dermatitis artefacta and a type of body image disturbance has been emphasized. Body dysmorphic disorder (BDD) has many dermatological subtypes. BDD is characterized by a sense of personal ugliness, cosmetic defect, or deformity. The impetus for these thoughts can be a nonexistent skin defect or minor skin defects such as blemishes and red spots, or wrinkling and changing of the skin with aging (20,21). The imagined or exaggerated defects (BDD comes in a continuum from overvalued ideas to frank psychosis) become the focus of obsessive thought or phobic avoidance. BDD on the skin leads to urgent requests for incisive dermatological treatment (laser therapy or transplant) and/or cosmetic surgery. BDD patients who are denied access to medical treatment may take the initiative to self-treatment. Paradoxically, in this self-treatment they may aggravate a minor skin condition or even provoke lesions on an unblemished skin. Physicians may find it difficult to understand that a patient aggravates a skin problem while his obvious wish seems to be freed of it, but the ambivalence between wishes and behavior is very common in BDD patients and is in fact typical for their psychodynamics.

Another psychiatric disorder sometimes overlapping with dermatitis artefacta is monosymptomatic hypochondriacal psychosis (MHP), a delusional belief of being diseased, despite the absence of factual evidence (18) sometimes accompanied by hallucinatory symptoms (22,23) which can include cancerophobia, parasitosis, or bromosidrosis. In parasitosis or Ekbom's syndrome there are frank delusions of infestation in which the patient believes herself to be infested with parasites or insects, sometimes accompanied by tactile hallucinations of insects crawling over the skin (formication), even psychotic beliefs of a life cycle of various "subcutaneous insects." The specific artificial lesions are digging lesions made in an attempt to remove the parasites. Another analogous particular type of MHP is a variety of delusional syndromes where the patient feel a foreign body (glass particles, sugar crystals, hair from a pet, etc.) under the skin. Some patients suffer from the delusion of emitting an offensive body odor (bromosidosis) (24). This "olfactory reference syndrome" is a psychiatric disorder that is difficult to categorize and treat. In the literature and in our personal practice, cases of suicide are reported. The treatment is combined cognitive-behavioral therapy with antipsychotic medication, nonacceptance of which by the patient is the main obstructive factor in the management. Lastly, patients may interpret benign skin lesions as skin cancer, interpret wrinkles resulting from normal aging as pathological, or be convinced that they suffer from a venereal disease (e.g., simple skin blemishes are taken for Kaposi lesions in insecure individuals with sexual experiences that for them were anxiety provoking).

Psychiatric disorders (anxiety, depression, BDD, MHP) may be the underlying cause of dermatitis artefacta, but the lesions, even if self-provoked, hurt and diminish the patient's self-esteem and ego and may in turn become the cause of anxiety, social phobia, and depression (15). Often the impact of psychiatric illness is blurred and bidirectional—it becomes a question of which came first—"the chicken or the egg"? Indeed, psychiatric disorder is both cause and consequence of self-provoked skin lesions. Skin disease frequently leads to reactive psychological problems because the direct visibility of skin lesions leads to undeserved professional or social stigmatization. But patients with dermatitis artefacta also tend to experience a "leper complex," with their appearance lowering their self-esteem. In addition, they have to cope with the inconvenience caused by the dermatosis and by its treatment, which often includes occlusive dressings and the need to wear a cap or to apply smelly ointments (25).

Psychiatric disorders are often at the cause of self-mutilation in dermatology and may also be the consequence of the visible, often horrific, lesions of dermatitis artefacta. But there is a third psychiatric complication, comorbidity. Indeed, comorbid depression is very common in patients with psychocutaneous disorders, dermatitis artefacta in particular. Stress-inducing life events, including loss of a loved one (through death or separation) and subsequent reactive depression, are associated with alopecia areata (26) and psoriasis (27). The depression is a response to, rather than a cause of, the illness. Anxiety is both causative and reactive in general tension-provoking itch, a condition that leads to scratching partially as a tension-reducing habit (28). Many skin disorders, acne and alopecia in particular, are complicated by social phobia (29). Dermatitis artefacta in the genital area generally cause deterioration of the patient's sex life (25) This effect is often overlooked, and we strongly recommend that physicians inquire explicitly about the patient's sexual activity and feelings of sexual (un)attractiveness.

RELATED ENTITIES: WRIST SLASHING, MUNCHAUSEN SYNDROME, POLLE SYNDROME

In addition to typical dermatitis artefacta, other types of self-mutilation involve some cutaneous lesions, e.g., wrist slashing. Indeed, wrist cutting or wrist slashing is not always intended as a suicidal act. In extreme stress situations, some self-mutilators inflict superficial cuts on the wrist or the inner side of the arm without specifically aiming at the radial arteries. In these cases the diagnosis is obvious (30).

Another related type of cutaneous self-mutilation, related to wrist cutting, is the syndrome of "delicate self-cutting," in which the self-mutilator induces superficial cuts as a reaction to conflicts and tension (30). The self-mutilator (usually a woman) generally uses a razor blade or another object that can cause superficial cutaneous scratches. The cuts are mainly located on the flexor surface of the wrist and arms, but the scars can also be found on the legs, chest, and abdomen. In delicate self-cutting the scars are generally parallel, but scratchers who are less careful in their self-mutilation exhibit indiscriminate scars.

A separate group of self-mutilation patients practice the subcutaneous insertion of needles or other pointed objects, and by continuous pressure they manage to push the needles deep into the tissues. The ingestion of various objects as well as the insertion of all kinds of needles or other objects into the orifices of the body is relatively frequent among sexual deviants. Superficial injury of genital mucosa and the insertion of objects (hairpins, needles) into the vagina and the urethra are not generally intended as self-mutilation, but are rather part of perverted sexual acts whereby pain and mutilation are essential ingredients of the masochistic and sadistic sexual experience (15).

Some of the self-inflicted dermatological lesions contain next to a component of self-mutilation a second aim: to feign a genuine dermatological illness. These "factitious disorders"—a diagnostic category coined in the DSM-IV—consist of physical symptoms that are intentionally produced or feigned, and may be classified according to the organ of choice; in the abdominal type patients complain of acute abdominal pain in the absence of any reason; in the hemorragic type hematuria may be produced by the ingestion of anticoagulants or anemia may be provoked by repetitive self-provoked genital or rectal wounds. A particular type of factitious illness with dramatic symptom presentation is the Munchausen syndrome. This refers to patients who fabricate a plausible history of illness by simulating impressive syndromes. Asher (3) coined the phrase in analogy with the adventurous but fictitious stories about a German baron, Karl Friedrich Hieronymus von Münchhausen (1720–1797), as told by Rudolf Erich Raspe in his "Baron Munchausen's Narrative of his Marvellous Travels and Campaigns in Russia" (1785). Munchausen patients force hospitals to admit them on the grounds of alarming complaints. It is striking that these "hospital hobos" in their pursuit of hospitalization do not shrink from painful and complicated diagnostic examinations. Many undergo more than one laparotomy, and even trepanations (perforation of the skull) have been reported. In this respect their problems are also related to self-mutilation, although the Munchausen patient does not personally perform self-mutilation but compels doctors to perform useless surgery—hence the terms "laparatomia migrans," "scalpellophilia," and "surgicomania." The typical Munchausen patient presents as an emergency case at night or on the weekend, when the least experienced doctors are on duty. The Munchausen syndrome also includes psychiatric symptoms such as pathological lying (pseudologia fantastica). Most patients suffer from a psychopathic personality disorder. Since they come to the doctor with a false cry for help, a therapeutic relationship based on trust is generally impossible.

Effective therapy has not yet been described, though some patients have been stabilized with supportive psychotherapy (31).

A complex of symptoms in children artificially induced by their parents, a sort of Munchausen syndrome by proxy, has been termed Polle syndrome, after Baron von Münchhausen's son, who was supposed to have died under mysterious circumstances. There are reports of parents who insist on medical examination of their children because of symptoms, e.g., ecchymoses, caused by the parents themselves. This pathology has not been extensively investigated, but is probably connected with child abuse (battered children). In contrast, the parents are often very worried about the child's health in these "factitious disorders by proxy." It is not yet clear whether the extreme concern for the child is a reason for the repeated medical examination of the child whereby the provoked symptoms serve to alarm the doctor or whether the parents' preoccupation is feigned and masks child abuse.

TREATMENT OF THE SELF-DESTRUCTIVE DERMATOLOGICAL SPECTRUM DISEASES

Medical-Psychiatric Aid for Self-Mutilators

General practitioners and somatic specialists will prefer to refer self-mutilators to a psychiatrist because of the psychiatric basis of self-destructive behavior. However, experience has shown that the majority of self-mutilators respond negatively to such a referral. Immediate referral to a psychiatrist usually results in the patient dropping out or embarking on "doctor shopping."

It is strategically preferable not to suggest direct psychiatric referral initially, but to play along with the self-mutilator's somatic presentation. Attempts can be made to come to an agreement about the frequency and type of examinations. Sometimes this offer of medical attention and acceptance is enough to prevent the self-mutilation from getting worse.

While some aspects of self-destruction are still untreatable, underlying problems such as depression, psychosis, conversion symptoms, toxicomania, or organic-cerebral pathology are amenable to treatment. Supportive psychosocial therapy can in any case have a positive influence on the precipitating situational tension. A simultaneous or consecutive combination of biological, psychotherapeutic and behavior-therapeutic techniques is often required. The purely somatic approach to the problem (e.g., local antibiotic cream for infected lesions, blood transfusion in iron deficiency anemia caused by repeated wrist cutting) may seem pointless but often has a therapeutic effect in itself. However, it is obvious that a placebo, a simple cream, physiotherapy, or massage cannot deal directly with the complex underlying psychiatric problems.

Management by the Dermatologist: General Guidelines

Patients with dermatitis artefacta (pure self-mutilation and/or factitious disorders) are often referred by the dermatologist or plastic surgeon to the psychiatrist because of the psychiatric basis of self-destructive behavior. However, it appears from case studies that most dermatitis artefacta patients react negatively if they are referred at once and will either abandon the treatment or try "doctor shopping" (31). In combined dermatological-psychiatric disorders, referral for psychological counseling and even vigorous psychiatric treatment may be necessary, but many patients with psychodermatological disorders will resent or even refuse referral. Therefore, it is mandatory for all physicians confronted with psychocutaneous problems to have some knowledge about the treatment possibilities and to be willing to treat both the dermatological and the psychiatric components of the disorders.

It is strategically preferable not to suggest direct psychiatric referral to dermatitis artefacta patients initially, but to play along with the somatic presentation. Usually patients deny that they are producing the lesions. Brusque confrontation with the self-inflicted cause of dermatitis artefacta should be avoided. Generally well accepted is the interpretation of the lesions in a more indirect psychosomatic way, inferring that the persistent lesions cause stress and that their course may be aggravated by frustrations. Attempts can be made to come to an agreement about the frequency and type of examinations. Sometimes this offer of medical attention and acceptance is enough to stop the dermatitis artefacta from becoming worse (1).

The psychotherapeutic effect of treating symptoms may be beneficial because it manifests medical concern for the patient with a factitious disorder. The caring environment offered by hospitalization may also have a positive effect. However, the nursing staff need to be carefully briefed so that they react supportively to the patient and do not say or do anything to imply that the condition is self-inflicted.

The choice of psychotropic agent in dermatitis artefacta is usually based on treatment of symptoms or of presumed underlying psychiatric pathology. In pharmaceutical treatment of a depression pathology, it should not be forgotten that these self-destructive patients also have a distinct tendency to be suicidal, so treatment needs to be "suicide-safe" as well as effective, making one of the newer antidepressants a safer choice. Furthermore, some of the selective serotonin-reuptake inhibitors (SSRIs) have an anticompulsive effect and may thus reduce the obsessive-compulsive part of some types of self-mutilation, e.g., acne excoriée, trichotillomania, and delicate self-cutting. Anxiolytics are indicated in self-mutilation conditioned by tension and anxiety. Antiepileptics can be used in the presence of epileptic fits or the equivalent. In borderline patients, low doses of neuroleptics have some effect in prevention of repetitive self-aggressive behavior (deliberate suicidal acts).

A behavioral dimension in the treatment is particularly indicated for lesions caused by compulsive behavior such as tics, excessive scratching, or aggravation of existing lesions. A second indication for behavioral therapy is self-mutilation that persists in the form of a tic after psychotherapeutic resolution of the underlying psychodynamic conflicts.

Aversion therapy in which self-mutilation behavior is linked with an aversive stimulus is useful. This treatment consists of applying a negative stimulus (a weak electric impulse) following unwanted behavior, e.g., scratching or excoriating. The aversion treatment tries to alleviate the self-mutilating behaviors by applying the negative stimulus with gradually increasing discomfort. However, this aversion treatment encounters understandably ethical criticism. We believe the treatment to be obsolete. An alternative and more accepted treatment is systematic desensitization, which progressively increases mental resistance against the specific tensions preceding self-mutilation by exercises confronting the patient—first imaginary, then real—with tense situations increasing in intensity (1).

Behavior-corrective techniques are particularly useful in the case of skin artefacts. Substitute "grooming sessions," in which a nurse teaches less aggressive skin-care techniques, are recommended for patients with dermatitis artefacta due to compulsive-aggressive skin "care." Relaxation techniques may contribute to improving tension-related types of dermatological self-destructive actions: sessions of relaxed breathing and muscle-relaxing exercises (e.g., the Jacobson method) (32) consist of alternatively tensing a muscle group and then relaxing the same muscles. The patient learns to focus on specific parts of the body with tension, and then learns to diminish the tension. Relaxation techniques are not very specific, and their effectiveness is not (yet) confirmed in evidence-based trials, but the technique is therapeutic because of the general tension-reducing effect and the positive physical awareness achieved during the sessions. Most self-mutilators are not very motivated for psychotherapy: they are unaware or in denial of their psychological difficulties, and they have a tendency to somatize. Therefore, attempts should be made to integrate the psychotherapy in the somatic treatment. By integrating psychological relaxation in sessions of bodily relaxation, the psychological part of the treatment becomes more readily accepted.

It is useful, as a beginning point of some form of psychotherapy, to extend the somatic approach to a wider psychosocial context in which the dermatitis artefacta patient can discuss his individual living circumstances and tensions. This simple technique appears to have a favorable therapeutic effect. Venting rancor and aggression on the consulting physician in particular and the medical profession in general is a form of catharsis. A nonjudgmental attitude on the part of the doctor in particular is a corrective emotional experience for the self-mutilation patient and a counterweight to his own hostility and aggressiveness.

Psychotropic Drug Treatment of Dermatitis Artefacta

Psychopharmacological treatment should always be part of an approach that combines medical and psychobiobehavioral management. Clinical experience shows that psychotropic drugs can radically change the course of a psychodermatological condition such as dermatitis artefacta. Although empirically the use of antidepressants and anxiolytics is known to be useful in a variety of dermatitis artefacta, these findings still require confirmation in controlled trials. However, the use of antipsychotic drugs in delusional skin disorders complicated with cutaneous self-mutilation is well documented.
Objective assessment of the efficacy of psychotropic drugs in dermatitis artefacta is difficult. On the one hand, psychotropic agents often improve the psychiatric symptoms initially and subsequently (and often only indirectly) have an effect on the somatic symptoms. On the other hand, there is a considerable placebo response in this patient population.

Antipsychotic Drugs

Antipsychotic drugs are useful treatments for dermatological syndromes that are the "cutaneous" expression of psychotic conditions. Antipsychotics are used in moderate to high dosages in dermatitis artefacta within the frame of monosymptomatic hypochondriacal psychoses. Pimozide seems efficaceous in patients with a combination of pain and a creeping type of paraesthesia, leading to digging lesions (33). Pimozide (Orap R) 2–12 mg/day is the drug of choice in delusions of parasitosis (23). Other antipsychotic drugs are effective if prescribed in equivalent doses to pimozide, e.g., chlorpromazine (Thorazine R) 100–400 mg/day or trifluoroperazine 10–15 mg/day. If parasitosis delusions with dermatitis artefacta respond to pimozide, after a treatment of several weeks gradual tapering of dosage to as low as 1 mg/day may be attempted.

Treatment failures with antipsychotic drugs are mostly due to compliance problems in uncooperative patients. Approximately 10% of patients receiving long-term antipsychotic treatment experience iatrogenic parkinsonism, characterized by extrapyramidal rigidity, cogwheel phenomenon, and tardive dyskinesia. Tardive dyskinesia is an infrequent but difficult late side effect of antipsychotic drug treatment. Fortunately, this adverse effect is extremely rare during use of pimozide, particularly if used at moderate doses of 4–8 mg/day. Adverse effects such as sedation, apathy, or a generalized neuroleptized syndrome (a general mental retardation combined with muscular stiffness, also called "camisole chimique") are dosage-dependent. Other adverse effects, such as dryness of the mouth, constipation, and blurred vision, are accepted by most dermatitis artefacta patients if they have been informed of the possibility of their occurrence beforehand and if treatment brings some relief from their delusions or pain.

Antipsychotics are also associated with anticholinergic adverse effects. Narrow angled glaucoma, prostatic enlargement, and arrhythmia are contraindications. It remains to be confirmed whether the older (sulpiride, amisulpiride) and newer atypical neuroleptics (risperidone, olanzapine) (34) improve results in psychodermatological drug management with fewer side effects.

Antidepressant Drugs

In dermatitis artefacta depression is often part of the etiology (self-hate resulting in self-provoked facial lesions) but more often is a reaction to the disfigurement of a skin disease. Clinical experience indicates that antidepressants alleviate the psychological stress of chronic dermatitis artefacta and help to relieve reactive depression following aesthetically handicapping skin lesions.

Several trials involving patients with psychosomatic skin disorders comparing tricyclics and monoamine oxidase inhibitors (MAOIs) were indicative of some relief of depressive symptoms concomitant with an improvement of the skin disorder.

Antidepressants with a selective antiobsessional effect, such as clomipramine and fluvoxamine, have been shown to be useful in the treatment of trichotillomania (35). Doxepin, which combines antidepressant efficacy with antianxiety and antihistaminergic properties, breaks the itch-scratch cycle that may be part of the cause of chronic dermatitis artefacta.

The use of tricyclics and MAOIs by nonpsychiatrist physicians has always been limited because these physicians are fearful of their potentially serious adverse effects: autonomic adverse effects such as dry mouth, micturition difficulties, postural hypotension, and cardiovascular effects (tachycardia, electrocardiogram changes with a risk of ventricular arrhythmia) and potential lethality in overdose. Notably, the older nonselective and irreversible MAOIs induce dangerous hypertensive crises if they are combined with sympathomimetic agents, tricyclic antidepressants, or tyramine-containing food, such as cheese (36). Therefore, their use in general psychodermatological practice has always been limited.

Second-generation antidepressants having fewer side effects, such as fluvoxamine, fluoxetine, paroxetine, sertraline, mianserin, trazodone, and viloxazine, have been tried, both in open studies and in double-blind trials in psychodermatological conditions. For example, the efficacy of fluvoxamine was demonstrated in a double-blind, placebo-controlled trial involving 70 patients with psychodermatological disorders (37). Patients presented with a variety of symptoms, including pruritus anogenitalis, dermatitis artefacta, generalized psychogenic pruritus, chronic urticaria, alopecia areata, acne excoriée, trichotillomania, glossopyrosis, chronic facial pain, and monosymptomatic skin hypochondriasis. The best treatment outcome was obtained in patients with syndromes with self-destructive and compulsive features, such as excoriated acne, trichotillomania, and dermatitis artefacta.

From a clinical point of view, the fact that SSRIs are better tolerated than tricyclic antidepressants is very important, as patients with somatic discomfort will become noncompliant if their drug treatment has noticeable physical adverse effects (38).

Anxiolytic Drugs

Anxiety states may be contributive, concomitant, or secondary to dermatitis artefacta. Anxiety is sometimes relieved by scratching (without itching as trigger) as a kind of "displacement" behavior (i.e., gestures that mimic washing or grooming rituals and are performed by primates and humans in stressful situations) (39). The temporary use of an anxiolytic is appropriate if psychological stress, tension, anxiety, hostility, or irritation are important factors in dermatitis artefacta (39).

The correct use of benzodiazepines may reduce the underlying tension and hostility that often constitute an important factor in self-provoked lesions, because they may help the skin to heal by lowering the intensity of scratching. Chronic psychosomatic skin complaints respond well to benzodiazepines with a long half-life, such as diazepam (39). Alprazolam, which is metabolized much more quickly than diazepam, has an interesting profile because it seems to have antidepressant as well as anxiolytic properties (39). Alprazolam is recommended in particular in the treatment of depressed patients with psychocutaneous disorders who also have underlying cardiac disorders that may be exacerbated by tricyclic antidepressants.

However, in view of the risks of dependency and the possibility of withdrawal effects such as rebound anxiety on discontinuation of the treatment, the prescription of an anxiolytic, in particular a benzodiazepine, must be closely monitored. If treatment with a benzodiazepine is instituted, therapy should be limited to a few weeks, covering only the acute anxiety situation.

Other Agents

Hydroxyzine is an antihistaminic that has been used successfully as a tranquilizer in patients with urticaria (40). Cerebral endorphins have a possible role in itch and pain, and morphine can cause pruritus. The role of endogenous opioid compounds (endorphins) and of antiopiate agents has been investigated in self-mutilative behavior (41). Antiopiate (naloxone) agents blocked, at least temporarily, the self-mutilation. However, it is still speculative whether opioid antagonists or other agents such as gamma-aminobutyric acid (GABA) analogs (42) are useful in dermatitis artefacta (43).

CONCLUSIONS

Symptomatic treatment can still have a beneficial psychotherapeutic effect since it is a symbol of medical concern for the self-mutilator (44). Hospitalization in itself and the inherent caring atmosphere will also have a favorable effect. It is important that the hospital nursing staff be properly briefed so that they can be supportive in their dealings with the patient and will not reproach the patient verbally or nonverbally for being the cause of the medical problem.

The indication for a certain type of psychotropic agent in self-mutilation syndromes is still based (for the time being) on rather symptomatic criteria according to the concomitant psychiatric symptoms or to the presumed causative psychiatric pathology. Antidepressants have proved their effect in self-mutilation based on depression pathology. When a depression pathology is treated with pharmaceutical agents, it should be borne in mind that these self-destructive patients also have a marked tendency towards suicide. Therefore, treatment that is both effective and "suicide-safe" should be chosen, tricyclics and MAOIs best avoided, and SSRIs recommended.

Anxiolytics are indicated in self-mutilation conditioned by tension and anxiety. Antiepileptics may be used in self-mutilation in the presence of epileptic fits or the equivalent. In borderline patients, low doses of neuroleptics prevent repetitive self-aggressive behavior (deliberate suicidal acts) to a certain extent.

Treatment focused on the self-mutilation act is particularly indicated for lesions caused by compulsive behavior such as tics, excessive scratching, aggravation of existing lesions, e.g., in acne excoriée. A second indication for behavioral therapy is self-mutilation that persists in the form of a tic after psychotherapeutic resolution of the underlying psychodynamic conflicts.

REFERENCES

1. Van Moffaert M. Integration of medical and psychiatric management in self-mutilation. Gen Hosp Psychiatry 1990; 13:1–9.
2. Thretowan D, Enoch WH. The Münchhausen syndrome. In: Uncommon Psychiatric Syndromes. Bristol, England: John Wright & Sons, 1979.
3. Asher R. Munchausen's syndrome. Lancet i(260):339–341, 1951.
4. Van Moffaert M. Training future dermatologists in psychodermatology. Gen Hosp Psychiatry 1986; 8:115–118.
5. Ford CV. The Somatizing Disorders: Illness as a Way of Life. New York: Elsevier, 1983.
6. Medansky RS, Handler RM. Dermatopsychosomatics: classification, physiology, and therapeutic approaches. J Am Acad Dermatol 1981; 5:125–135.
7. Keehn JD. Animal Models for Psychiatry. London: Routledge and Kegan Paul, 1986.
8. Anzieu D. Le Moi-Peau. Paris: Bordas, 1985.
9. Meninnger K. Man Against Himself. New York: Harcourt, Brace & World, 1938.
10. Wittkower ED, Lester E. Hautkrankheiten in psychosomatischer Sicht. Acta Psychosom Documenta Geigy 1960; 6:1–39.
11. Whitlock FA. Psychophysiological Aspects of Skin Diseases. London: Saunders, 1970.
12. Panconesi E. The future is here: cutaneous psychoneuroimmunology as a premise. In: Panconesi E, ed. Stress and Skin Diseases: Psychosomatic Dermatology. Philadelphia: Lippincott, 1984; 78–93.
13. Beveridge GW. Diseases of the skin: infantile eczema. Br Med J 1974; 1:154–155.
14. Fava GA, Perini GI, P Santonastaso P. Life events and psychological distress in dermatologic disorders; psoriasis, chronic urticaria and fungal infections. Br J Med Psychol 1980; 53:277–282.

15. Van Moffaert M. Psychosomatics for the practising dermatologist. Dermatologica 1982; 165:73–84.

16. Panconesi E, ed. Stress and Skin Diseases: Psychosomatic Dermatology. Philadelphia: JB Lippincott, 1984.

17. Brenner S, Politi Y. Dermatologic diseases and problems of women throughout the life cycle. Int J Dermatol 1995; 34(6):369–379.

18. Cotterill JA. Dermatological non-disease: a common and potentially fatal disturbance of cutaneous body image. Br J Dermatol 1981; 104:611–619.

19. Nadelson T. False patients, real patients: a spectrum of disease presentation. Psychother Psychosom 1985; 44.

20. Hay GG. Dysmorphophobia. Br J Psychiatry 1970; 116:399–406.

21. Philips KA. The Broken Mirror: Understanding and Treating Body Dysmorphic Disorder. New York: Oxford University Press, 1996.

22. Munro A. Monosymptomatic hypochondriacal psychosis manifesting as delusions of parasitosis. Arch Dermatol 1978; 114:940–943.

23. Lyell A. Delusions of parasitosis. Br J Dermatol 1983; 108:485–499.

24. Bishop EM. Monosymptomatic hypochondriacal syndromes in dermatology. J Am Acad Dermatol 1983; 9:152–158.

25. Renshaw D. Sex and the dermatologist. Int J Dermatol 1980; 19:469–471.

26. Macalpine I. Is alopecia areata psychosomatic? Br J Dermatol 1958; 70:147–158.

27. Arnetz BB, Fjellner B, Eneroth P. Stress and psoriasis: psychoendocrine and metabolic reactions in psoriatic patients during standardized stress or exposure. Psychosom Med 1985; 47:528–541.

28. Fjellner B, Arnetz B, Eneroth P. Pruritus during standardized mental stress. Acta Derm Venereol 1985; 65:199–205.

29. Musaph H. Psychodermatology. In: Hill OW, ed. Modern Trends in Psychosomatic Medicine. Vol 3. London: Butterworths, 1976:320.

30. Pao PE. The syndrome of delicate self-cutting. Br J Med Psychol 1969; 42:195–205.

31. Axen DM. Chronic factitious disorders: helping those who hurt themselves. J Psychosoc Nurs 1986; 3:19–27.

32. Jacobson E. Progressive Relaxation. Chicago: University of Chicago Press, 1938.

33. Frithz A. Delusions of infestation: treatment by depot injections of antipsychotic drugs. Clin Exp Dermatol 1979; 4:485–488.

34. Koblenzer CS. Dermatitis artefacta: clinacal features and approach to treatment. Am J Clin Dermatol 2000; 1:47–55.

35. Swedo SE, Henrietta LL, Rappoport JL. A double-blind comparison of clomipramine and desipramine in the treatment of trichotillomania (hair pulling). N Engl J Med 1989; 321:497–501.

36. Friedman S, Kantor I, Sobel S. On the treatment of neurodermatitis with a monoamine oxidase inhibitor: the chemotherapy of psychosomatic illness through a REM suppression. J Nerv Ment Dis 1978; 166:117–125.

37. Hendryckx B, Van Moffaert M, Spiers R. The treatment of psychocutaneous disorders: a new approach. Curr Ther Res 1991; 49:111–119.
38. Sarti MG, Cossidenti A. Therapy in psychosomatic dermatology. In: Panconesi E, ed. Stress and Skin Diseases: Psychosomatic Dermatology. Philadelphia: Lippincott, 1984.
39. Koo JM, Strauss GD. Psychopharmacologic treatment of psychocutaneous disorders: a practical guide. Semin Dermatol 1987; 6:83–93.
40. Van Moffaert M. Hydroxyzine in the treatment of anxiety states. In: Nutt D, Ballenger J, eds. Anxiety Disorders. Oxford, England: Blackwell Science, 2002.
41. Richardson JS, Zaleski WA. Naloxone and self-mutilation. Biol Psychiatry 1983; 18:99–101.
42. Primrose DA. Treatment of self-injurious behaviour with a GABA (gamma-aminobutyric acid) analogue. J Ment Defic Res 1979; 23:163–174.
43. Bernstein JE, Swift RM, Soltani K. Antipruritic effect of an opiate antagonist, naloxone hydrochloride. J Invest Dermatol 1982; 78:82–83.
44. Koblenzer CS. Psychocutaneous Disease. Orlando, FL: Grune & Stratton, 1987.

13

Obsessive-Compulsive Disorders in Dermatology Patients

Julia K. Warnock
University of Oklahoma Health Sciences Center
Tulsa, Oklahoma, U.S.A.

Thelda Kestenbaum
University of Kansas Medical Center
Kansas City, Kansas, U.S.A.

INTRODUCTION

Obsessive-compulsive disorder (OCD) is a disabling anxiety disorder that is estimated to affect 2–3% of the general population of the United States. Until fairly recently OCD was considered a rare disorder with a poor prognosis. Advancements in the diagnosis, biology, and treatment have altered the prognosis favorably. OCD is estimated to be the fourth most common psychiatric disorder following phobias, substance abuse disorders, and the major depressive disorders (1). New treatment approaches, particularly pharmacotherapy and cognitive behavioral therapy, have significantly improved the clinical outcome for the majority of patients. A significant proportion of individuals suffering from OCD or an obsessive-compulsive spectrum disorder will have cutaneous lesions as part of their pathology, thus are likely to consult with a dermatologist. A patient with OCD may present to a dermatologist with common symptoms or signs such as compulsive hand and/or body washing, neurotic excoriations, compulsive hair pulling (trichotillomania), acne excoriée or compulsive skin picking, onychotillomania, fears of contamination or infestation, or a debilitating preoccupation or concern with an imagined or minor defect in appearance. The dermatologist familiar with the diagnosis and treatment of OCD in clinical practice can help reduce the significant morbidity associated with this common disorder.

DIAGNOSIS

OCD is characterized by recurrent and persistent obsessions or compulsions that are severe enough to be time consuming or cause impairment in relationships, employment, school, or social activities (2). Obsessions are recurrent and persistent ideas, impulses, images, or thoughts that cause distress and anxiety. The patient usually realizes that the obsessions are irrational, disturbing, and inappropriate but is unable to ignore or suppress them. Obsessions may involve themes of contamination (dirt, germs), somatic concerns (infestations, body odor, infection), sexual content (forbidden thoughts or imagery), religion (concern with blasphemy or sacrilege), aggressive impulses, repeated doubts (doors locked, appliances turned off), or symmetry. The individual with obsessions frequently has compulsive symptoms, as well. Compulsions are repetitive motor acts often performed in a stereotypical manner. The patient feels compelled to perform the actions in order to reduce a feeling of mounting tension. The performance of the irrational act relieves the patient of an uneasy feeling of distress. Compulsive behaviors may present in a wide variety of symptoms and signs to the dermatologist. They may range from simple actions, such as touching, lip licking, tapping, or rubbing, to more complex actions, such as cutaneous self-injurious behaviors (neurotic excoriations, nail biting, skin picking, hair pulling) or cleaning, washing, and grooming rituals. Thus, a diverse array of lesions on the skin may be present in patients with OCD or OCD spectrum disorders.

NEUROBIOLOGY OF OCD

Specific neuroanatomic regions and neurotransmitter systems have been implicated in the pathophysiology of OCD. Neurochemical mechanisms important in this disorder have been implicated by the response of OCD patients to serotonergic agents that block the presynaptic uptake of serotonin. Serotonin dysfunction is suggested when agents such as clomipramine (Anafranil), fluoxetine (Prozac), sertraline (Zoloft), fluvoxamine (Luvox), or paroxetine (Paxil) are effective in the treatment of OCD. Further evidence indicates that *m*-chlorphenylpiperazine (m-cpp), a mixed serotonin receptor agonist, can induce obsessional symptoms in OCD patients, but not in healthy controls (3). Robust findings from neuroimaging studies indicate that a prefrontal cortex–basal ganglia–thalamic circuit may be the pathway involved in the expression of obsessions and compulsions (4). Neurological disorders associated with OCD such as Tourette's syndrome, Huntington's disease, Sydenham's chorea, and Parkinson's disease, which are associated with basal ganglia disease, also implicate the basal ganglia in OCD pathology. Children who develop OCD and/or tic disorders following streptococcal infections are described as having PANDAS (Pediatric Autoimmune Neuropsychiatric Disorders Associated with Streptococcal Infections). It is believed that, in PANDAS, the antibodies produced against the invading bacteria interact with the basal ganglia to cause tics and/or OCD.

EPIDEMIOLOGY

OCD affects approximately 2–3% of the U.S. population (5), making it the fourth most common mental disorder (1). Approximately one half to one third of adult patients with OCD developed symptoms during the childhood years. One investigation (6) reported that the mean age of onset of OCD symptoms was 14.5 years. Further, the investigators noted that the typical patient does not reveal his symptoms to a family member or friend until 8 years later, at age 22. The patient finally presents to a health care professional, typically, at a mean age of 25. However, the correct diagnosis is not made, on average, until the age of 30.4 ± 13 years. In addition, patients typically do not obtain appropriate treatment until a mean age of 31.7 ± 12.9 years. Note the substantial gap of 10.2 years between the onset of OCD symptoms (14.5 years) and the first attempt to seek professional help. A significant gap of 17.2 years also exists between the onset of symptoms and receipt of appropriate treatment (31.7 years) (6). The estimated prevalence of OCD in children and adolescents is about 1% (7), with the most likely cutaneous presentation being trichotillomania (hair pulling), onychotillomania, onychophagia (nail biting), and acne excoriée (8). The prevalence of OCD among patients presenting to a dermatologist with chronic pruritic conditions may be as high as 14% (9).

CORMORBIDITY

Patients presenting with OCD are at substantial risk of having an additional psychiatric disorder such as major depression (38.9%), panic disorder (15.5%) or social phobia (10.1%) (6). Hollander and colleagues (6) also reported high rates of OCD spectrum–related disorder in patients with OCD, including body dysmorphic disorder (current = 15%; past = 23%), skin picking (current = 11%; past = 15%), and nail biting (current = 10%; past = 13%).

OBSESSIVE-COMPULSIVE SPECTRUM–RELATED DISORDERS

Recent psychiatric literature suggests that some disorders may overlap with OCD and from both a diagnostic and treatment perspective may be usefully thought of as obsessive-compulsive spectrum disorders. The dermatologist should note, in particular, two obsessive-compulsive spectrum disorders that deserve special consideration: 1) cutaneous self-injurious behaviors, (e.g., skin picking as in acne excoriée, repetitive scratching or rubbing of the skin as in neurotic excoriations, trichotillomanis, and nail biting) and 2) body dysmorphic disorders.

Cutaneous Self-Injurious Behaviors

Self-injurious behavior (SIB) is the infliction of direct physical injury to one's own body without lethal intent (10). Skin lesions that result from self-injurious behaviors may indicate the dermatological expression of one of a number of different psychiatric disorders (11). When examining a patient with suspected SIB, the dermatologist must consider not only the cutaneous pathology, but the psychiatric diagnosis as well. The dermatologist must determine the "psychiatric context" of the SIB. If the patient is delusional (e.g., delusions of parasitosis) or has a severe manipulative, demanding personality disorder (e.g., dermatitis artefacta in a borderline personality disorder), then the patient is not likely to have OCD or a related spectrum disorder. Treatment options are different for various psychiatric disorders. The focus of this discussion is the forms of SIB that have a compulsive quality to the self-injury. Both SIB and OCD have in common intrusive urges to commit an act that is perceived as senseless. There may also be a sense of mounting tension with attempts to resists the impulse and relief of anxiety upon completion of the act. The more common manifestations of OCD spectrum–related disorders that involve self-injury in dermatology include trichotillomania, onychotillomania, onychophagia, acne excoriée, and neurotic excoriations (12). Lipinski (13) suggests that patients with a variety of SIB should be carefully evaluated for the presence of other signs and symptoms of OCD. He discusses a patient with both OCD and self-inflicted lesions caused by biting, cutting, and burning the skin who responded to a trial of clomipramine (Anfranil) at 250 mg for 6 weeks. Simeon and colleagues (10) note that the skin picking involved in neurotic excoriations may be repetitive and ritualistic and frequently leads to a reduction in tension. These types of patients with SIB have significant comorbidity with OCD, and both appear to have good response to the serotonergic reuptake agents.

Trichotillomania is another disorder that may be conceptualized as an OCD spectrum disorder. In some cases, the repetitive hair pulling is performed in a ritualized fashion simulating some aspects of OCD. In addition, both OCD and trichotillomania show a selective response to the serotonergic reuptake inhibitors. Swedo et al. (14), in a double-blind crossover comparison trial, demonstrated that clomipramine (Anfranil), but not desipramine (Norpramin and other generics), to be effective in the short-term treatment of trichotillomania. Other investigators (15) suggest that this finding provides support for a neurobiological overlap between OCD and trichotillomania.

Body Dysmorphic Disorder

The essential feature of body dysmorphic disorder (BDD) as defined in DSM-IV (2) is a preoccupation with an imagined defect in appearance. If a slight anomaly is present, the concern of the patient is excessive. Examples seen by the dermatologist may include worrying about body odor, "thinning" hair, or overconcern about nose size, facial blemishes, or scars. These patients may spend hours each day thinking about and frequently scrutinizing and checking their "defect." While BDD is classified in the DSM-IV as a somatoform disorder (2), Phillips and colleagues (16) discuss the evidence supporting the concept that BDD may be related to OCD.

BRIEF PSYCHIATRIC INTERVIEW: DESIGNED FOR THE DERMATOLOGIST EXAMINING A PATIENT SUSPECTED OF OCD OR RELATED SPECTRUM DISORDER

Patients with OCD or related spectrum disorder presenting to the dermatologist are likely to be willing to discuss their symptoms if a warm, nonjudgmental environment is provided. As alluded to earlier, health care professionals often fail to provide their patients with a timely diagnosis of

OCD. The patient may feel embarrassed or shameful that they induced the lesion on his or her skin. After careful examination of the skin, useful questions may include: How much time do you spend examining your skin? washing? cleaning? How much time do you spend worrying about germs? contamination? checking yourself in the mirror? Do you notice that you have certain thoughts or habits that take up a significant amount of your time, such as counting or rearranging things? If the total amount of time that the patient reports engaging in obsessive thinking or performing compulsions is more that 1 hour per day, then the diagnosis of OCD or an OCD spectrum–related disorder is likely. The Yale-Brown Obsessive-Compulsive Scale (Y-BOCS) (17) may be incorporated into the dermatologist's practice to rate the severity of symptoms at the initial interview. The Y-BOCS symptom checklist consists of important items that help confirm the diagnosis of OCD and measures the severity of both obsessions and compulsions. The total Y-BOCS score can range from subclinical to extreme. In addition, the Y-BOCS can be easily readministered during follow-up appointments to assess improvements in symptoms with the selected treatment. A decrease in that time that the patient spends on OCD-related activities is a good marker over time to determine improvement.

The family history is often helpful for the dermatologist who is examining the patient for OCD or a related disorder. Ask the patient if any family member has a similar or related problem. Try to determine if that relative had a successful treatment. If the relative did have a successful treatment, attempt to identify the psychotropic medication and the dose at which remission was achieved. Information of this type may be very helpful in initiating a treatment plan for that particular patient.

TREATMENT STRATEGIES FOR OBSESSIVE-COMPULSIVE DISORDERS AND RELATED SPECTRUM DISORDERS

Pharmacological Treatment

Clomipramine (Anfranil) was the first psychotropic medication approved by the U.S. Food and Drug Administration (FDA) for the treatment of OCD in 1989. Since then, four other pharmacological agents, all selective serotonin reuptake inhibitors (SSRIs)—fluvoxamine (Luvox), fluoxetine (Prozac), sertraline (Zoloft), and paroxetine (Paxil)—have received approval from FDA for the treatment of adults with OCD. Three of these medications are approved by FDA for use in children: clomipramine (Anfranil), fluoxetine (Prozac), and sertraline (Zoloft). Citalopram (Celexa), the fifth SSRI introduced in the United States, has been used for the treatment of depression and OCD in Europe. Escitalopram (Lexapro), the most recent SSRI introduced in the United States, is the isomer of citalopram and is likely to be as effective in the treatment of OCD as the other SSRIs.

Clomipramine (Anafranil) has been shown in numerous placebo-controlled trials to be effective in reducing OCD symptoms (18). The mechanism of action of clomipramine and the SSRIs in reducing symptoms is unclear at this time. However, the serotonergic hypothesis for OCD gained credibility from controlled trials in which the antidepressants that block serotonin reuptake are effective, whereas antidepressants that involve other neurotransmitter systems are ineffective (19,20). The usual starting dose of clomipramine is 50 mg, with increase of 50 mg every 4–5 days. The target dose is around 250 mg; less than 200 mg is usually inadequate. One advantage of clomipramine is that the plasma level can be monitored. However, clomipramine is a tricyclic, which is associated with anti-cholinergic and antiadrenergic side effects. These side effects may include dry mouth, sedation, orthostasis, weight gain, urinary retention, and blurry vision. This medication may be lethal in overdose. An electrocardiogram (ECG) is required to monitor pediatric patients.

The SSRIs (fluoxetine, paroxetine, sertraline, and fluvoxamine) have been demonstrated to be effective in the treatment of OCD in separate multicenter, placebo-controlled trials (21). The SSRIs are generally better tolerated than clomipramine, and at this point in time there is little doubt that the serotonin reuptake inhibitors are the first-line pharmacotherapy for treatment of OCD (22), especially for dermatologists (23). In terms of the typical dosing strategy, it is suggested that the clinician begin at the typical starting dose for the treatment of depression. However, the SSRI will need to titrated to the maximum tolerated dose at which the most improvement in OCD symptoms are noted. For example, sertraline (Zoloft) may be initiated at 50 mg/day and may be increased in increments of 25 mg each 4–6 weeks until complete remission of the OCD symptoms is obtained, up to a maximum of 200 mg/day.

The dermatologist using an SSRI in the treatment of patients must be aware that the duration of treatment is extremely important. Psychiatric clinical and research experience indicates that improvement in OCD symptoms continues to occur when the medications are taken beyond 8- or 12-week trials. A patient demonstrating partial improvement in hand-washing rituals after 4–5 weeks of pharmacotherapy may be expected to continue to improve over the next several weeks or even months. In addition, the practitioner should note that generally higher doses of the SSRI may be required for the patient with OCD to obtain maximum response (24) as compared to the treatment of depression. The typical side effects of the SSRIs, such as nausea, diarrhea, agitation, headaches, and sexual dysfunction, may increase at the higher doses. The clinician may minimize side effects by increasing the dose slowly. It is also important to note that the cessation of pharmacotherapy results in a return of OCD symptoms in most patients. With discontinuation of clomipramine, for example, 89% of the patients had a significant relapse of their OCD symptoms by the end of a 7-week placebo trial period (25). Thus, for patients with OCD considering discontinuation of their medication, the dermatologist should inform them of their high chance of relapse with discontinuation (23). It is often helpful for the dermatologist to remind the patient that the normal course of the illness is to wax and wane. Good treatment will require vigilant attention to long-term management. If available, referral to a clinician experienced in cognitive-behavioral therapy (CBT) may be helpful in prevention of relapse.

Cognitive-Behavioral Therapy

While there are numerous psychotherapeutic approaches touted in the treatment of patients with OCD, only CBT has been demonstrated in randomized, controlled trials to be effective (26). CBT, especially in combination with pharmacotherapy, has improved the prognosis in the treatment of OCD. The techniques used in CBT to reduce compulsive rituals include three components: 1) actual exposure to the feared situations, 2) imaginal exposure to feared consequences, and 3) response prevention, in which support is given to the patient to resist the urge to engage in the compulsive ritual (27). Exposure involves gradually and repeatedly bringing the patient into contact with the feared object for as long as possible. Following exposure, the patient must refrain from performing the ritual (e.g., handwashing, face picking) after the exposure (response prevention). The exposure/response-prevention principles are based on the behavioral therapy concept that anxiety diminishes over time when the performance of the ritual is blocked. When anxiety reduction is no longer dependent on the rituals, then the ritual compulsion will be extinguished. CBT requires approximately 15–25 individual sessions, daily homework assignments, exposure sessions, and home visits. Foa and colleagues (28) found in their review of the literature that 51% of patients had reductions of at least 70% of their obsessions and rituals; 39% of the patients had a reduction of between 31% and 69%. For patients with OCD or OCD spectrum disorders who present to the dermatologist, CBT may be combined with medications or may be used alone in patients who refuse to consider psychotropic medication.

Augmentation Strategies in OCD Treatment–Resistant Patients

If a patient does not respond to the first-line medication (usually an SSRI), then the dermatologist may switch to another SSRI or may carefully augment the SSRI with clomipramine (Anfranil). An adequate trial is defined as the maximum tolerated dose for at least 12 weeks. CBT may be used to augment pharmacotherapy, if available. A recent case series reported positive results using trazodone (Desyrel and generics) augmentation (doses—150–600 mg/day) of SSRI therapy in five cases of OCD (29). If the patient has comorbid tics, a trial of adjunctive haloperidol (Haldol and other generics), pimozide (Orap), or risperidone (Risperdal) at low doses could be attempted for a few weeks. The newer atypical antipsychotic agents such as olanzapine (Zyprexa), quetiapine (seroquel), ziprasidone (Geodon) or aripiprazole (Abilify), while not approved by the FDA, may offer safer alternatives than the older antipsychotics. If no improvement occurs, discontinuation of the antipsychotic is recommended (24). The dermatologist should refer the patient to a psychiatrist if, after three adequate trials of medication or combination of medication, limited improvement of the patient is observed.

SUMMARY

The evidence suggests that the prevalence of OCD in a dermatology practice may be much higher than in the general population. The dermatologist will observe an interesting array of signs and symptoms in patients that suggests OCD or an OCD spectrum–related disorder. Psychopharmacological agents, such as clomipramine or the SSRIs, either alone or in combination with cognitive behavioral therapy, help a significant majority of patients suffering from this disorder. Exciting new developments and treatment are on the horizon for children who meet PANDAS criteria and have OCD symptoms (30). An increased awareness of the signs and symptoms of OCD and related disorders will enable the dermatologist to appropriately identify and treat patients, thereby reducing the significant morbidity associated with this common disorder.

REFERENCES

1. Rasmussen SA, Eisen JL. Epidemiology of obsessive compulsive disorder. J Clin Psychiatry 51 (suppl): 10–13, 1990.

2. American Psychiatry Association. Diagnostic and Statistical Manual of Mental Disorders. 4th ed. Washington, DC: American Psychiatry Publishing, 1994.

3. Zohar J, Mueller EA, Insel TR, Zohar-Zadouch RC, Murphy DI. Serotonergic responsivity in obsessive-compulsive disorder: comparison of patients and healthy controls. Arch Gen Psychiatry 44:946–951, 1987.

4. Baxter LR Jr. Positron emission tomography studies of cerebral glucose metabolism in obsessive compulsive disorder. J Clin Psychiatry 55(suppl):54–59, 1994.

5. Karno M, Golding JM, Sorenson SB, Burman MA. The epidemiology of obsessive-compulsive disorder in five U.S. communities. Arch Gen Psychiatry 45:1094–1099, 1988.

6. Hollander E, Stein DJ, Kwon JH, Rowland C, Wong, Broatch J, Himelein C. Psychosocial function and economic costs of obsessive-compulsive disorder. CNS Spectrums 2:16–25, 1997.

7. Leonard HL, Rapoport JL. Pharmacotherapy of childhood obsessive-compulsive disorder. Psychiatr Clin North Am 12:963–970, 1989.

8. Koo JY, Smith LL. Obsessive-compulsive disorders in the pediatric dermatology practice. Pediatr Dermatol 8:107–113, 1991.

9. Hatch ML, Paradis C, Friedman S, Popkin M, AR Shalita. Obsessive-compulsive disorder in patients with chronic pruritic conditions: case studies and discussion. J Am Acad Dermatol 26:549–551, 1992.

10. Simeon D, Stein DJ, Hollander E. Depersonalization disorder and self-injurious behavior. J Clin Psychiatry 56(suppl 4):36–39, 1995.

11. Koblenzer CS. Treatment of "cutaneous self-injurious behavior" (CSIB). Int J Dermatol 37:633–634, 1998.

12. Koo J, Gamble C. Pyschopharmacology for dermatology patients. In: Koo J, ed. Psychodermatology. Dermatologic Clinics. Philadelphia: WB Saunders Company, 1996:509–523.

13. Lipinski JF. Clomipramine in the treatment of self-mutilating behaviors (letter). N Engl J Med 324:1441, 1991.

14. Swedo SE, Leonard HL, Rapoport JL, Lenane MC, Goldberger EL, Cheslow DL. A double-blind comparison of clomipramine and desipramine in the treatment of trichotillomania (hair pulling). N Engl J Med 321:497–501, 1989.

15. Stein DJ, Simeon D, Cohen LJ, Hollander E, Trichotillomania and obsessive-compulsive disorder. J Clin Psychiatry 56(suppl 4):28–34, 1995.

16. Phillips KA, McElroy SL, Hudson JI, Pope HG. Body dysmorphic disorder: an obsessive-compulsive spectrum disorder, a form of affective spectrum disorder, or both? J Clin Psychiatry 56(suppl 4):41–51, 1995.

17. Goodman WK, Price LH, Rasmussen SA, Mazure C, Fleischmann RL, Hill CL, Heninger GR, Charney DS. The Yale-Brown Obsessive Compulsive Scale. I. Development, use and reliability. Arch Gen Psychiatry 46:1006–1011, 1989.

18. The Clomipramine Collaborative Study Group. Clomipramine in the treatment of patients with obsessive-compulsive disorder. Arch Gen Psychiatry 48:730–738, 1991.

19. Goodman WK, Price LH, Delgado PL, Palumbo J, Krystal JH, Nagy LM, Rasmussen SA, Heninger GR, Charney DS. Specificity of serotonin reuptake inhibitors in the treatment of obsessive compulsive disorder: comparison of fluvoxamine and desipramine. Arch Gen Psychiatry 47:577–585, 1990.

20. Leonard HL, Swedo SE, Rapoport JL, Koby EV, Lenane MC, Cheslow DL, Hamburger SD. Treatment of obsessive-compulsive disorder with clomipramine and desipramine in children and adolescents. A double-blind crossover comparison. Arch Gen Psychiatry 46:1088–1092, 1989.

21. Pigott TA, Seay SM. A review of the efficiency of selective serotonin reuptake inhibitors in obsessive-compulsive disorder. J Clin Psychiatry 60:101–106, 1999.

22. Rasmussen SA, Eisen JL, Pato MT. Current issues in the pharmacologic management of obsessive compulsive disorder. J Clin Psychiatry 54(suppl 6):4–9, 1993.

23. Warnock JK, Kestenbaum T. Obsessive-compulsive disorder. In: Koo J, ed. Psychodermatology. Dermatologic Clinics. Philadelphia: WB Saunders Company 1996:465–472.

24. Mathew SJ, Simpson B, Fallon BA. Treatment strategies for obsessive-compulsive disorder. Psychiatr Ann 699–708, 2000.

25. Pato MT, Zohar-Kadouch R, Zohar J, Murphy DL. Return of symptoms after discontinuation of clomipramine in patients with obsessive-compulsive disorder. Am J Psychiatry 145:1521–1525, 1988.

26. Foa EB, Kozak MJ. Obsessive-compulsive disorder: long term outcome of psychological treatment. In: Mavissakalian MR, Prien RF, eds. Long Term Treatments of Anxiety Disorders. Washington, DC: American Psychiatric Press, 1996:285–309.

27. Jenike MA. Obsessive-compulsive disorder: efficacy of specific treatments as assessed by controlled trials. Psychopharmacol Bull 29:487–499, 1993.

28. Foa EB, Steketee, Ozarow BJ. Behavior therapy with obsessive-compulsives: from theory to treatment. In: Mavissakalian M, Turner SM, Michelson L, eds. Obsessive-Compulsive Disorder: Psychological and Pharmacological Treatment. New York: Plenum Press, 1985.

29. Marazzitti D, Gemignani A, Dell'Osso L. Trazodone augmentation in OCD: a case series report. CNS Spectrum 4(12):48–49, 1999.

30. NIMH. Welcome to the Official P.A.N.D.A.S. Web Page. HTTP://intramural.nimh.nih.gov/research/pnd. March 2003.

14

Trichotillomania

Dan J. Stein
University of Stellenbosch
Cape Town, South Africa
and University of Florida
Gainesville, Florida, U.S.A.

Bavanisha Vythilingum and Soraya Seedat
University of Stellenbosch
Cape Town, South Africa

Brian H. Harvey
Potchefstroom University for Christian Higher Education
Potchefstroom, South Africa

INTRODUCTION

Hair-pulling is a behavior that has been described since antiquity. The Bible includes a passage in which the prophet Ezra pulls out his hair, and Homer, Shakespeare, and many others have written about hair-pulling in the context of frustration or grief (1). Such depictions are arguably consistent with the symbolic value of hair; hair classically denotes beauty and power, so that loss of hair correspondingly signifies a range of themes involving aggression and sexuality (2).

Clinical descriptions of hair-pulling have an equally venerable history. Hippocrates advised physicians to assess hair-pulling as part of a routine mental status examination and described a case of hair-pulling in the apparent context of depression (1). Cases of trichobezoar were first described in the eighteenth-century medical literature, and hundreds of cases were subsequently published (2). Hallopeau coined the term trichotillomania (TTM) in 1889, from the Greek words *tricho* (hair) and *tillo* (pull) (3).

Over the next several decades, many anecdotal reports of the treatment of TTM appeared, typically written from a psychodynamic (2) or behavioral (4) perspective. Particular impetus to systematic research was given when the diagnosis was included in the official psychiatric nomenclature in 1987 (5) and when researchers at the National Institutes of Health (NIH) reported that, like obsessive-compulsive disorder (OCD), TTM appeared to have a better response to the serotonin reuptake inhibitor clomipramine than to the noradrenaline reuptake inhibitor desipramine (6). This latter work not only suggested a particular mediating psychobiology, but also emphasized the potential therapeutic value of specific interventions.

In this chapter we consider the phenomenology, psychobiology, pharmacotherapy, and psychotherapy of TTM in turn.

PHENOMENOLOGY

Classification

Trichotillomania is classified as a disorder of impulse control in the fourth edition of the Diagnostic and Statistical Manual of Mental Disorders (DSM-TR) (7). Several of the diagnostic criteria (Table 1) are based on such

TABLE 1 Diagnostic Criteria for Trichotillomania

A. Recurrent pulling out of one's hair resulting in noticeable hair loss.
B. An increasing sense of tension immediately before pulling out the hair or when attempting to resist the behavior.
C. Pleasure, gratification, or relief when pulling out the hair.
D. The disturbance is not better accounted for by another mental disorder and is not due to a general medical condition (e.g., a dermatological condition).
E. The disturbance causes clinically significant distress or impairment in social, occupational, or other important areas of functioning.

Source: Ref. 7.

a view; as in other impulse control disorders, it is noted that there is an increase in tension prior to the behavior, and there is subsequently relief, pleasure, or gratification during completion of the behavior.

Nevertheless, the criteria for TTM have been criticized on a number of grounds. In particular, many patients with chronic hair-pulling do not meet diagnostic criterion B or C for TTM (8,9). It is certainly possible that this will result in changes to the diagnostic criteria for TTM in future editions. Although TTM will likely remain in the section on impulse control disorders, it could also be argued that it should be reclassified.

One possibility, for example, would be to classify TTM as a stereotypic movement disorder. This condition is characterized by nonfunctional motoric movements, which can be self-injurious in nature. The diagnosis is typically given to patients with mental retardation, but there is increased awareness that adults of normal intelligence also can demonstrate sterotypic symptoms (10), one of which may be hair-pulling (11). Other common, repetitive, self-injurious behaviors that may have much in common with hair-pulling include skin-picking (12).

A second possibility is that TTM should be classified as an OCD spectrum disorder together with conditions thought to have phenomenological and psychobiological overlaps with OCD (13). On the one hand, TTM differs from OCD in several ways; for example, the two conditions have a significantly different sex ratio (at least in clinical settings), and hair-pulling does not typically follow a preceding obsession (14,15). Nevertheless, there is some heuristic value to considering the nature of the relationship of the two conditions from both a clinical and a research perspective (14,15).

Epidemiology

The prevalence of trichotillomania has not been studied in systematic epidemiological surveys. Nevertheless, studies in college students have suggested that clinically significant hair-pulling is seen in 1–4% of subjects, with an even greater prevalence of nonclinical hair-pulling (1). Similarly, TTM is not an uncommon presentation in dermatology clinics (16).

Females with TTM are far more commonly seen in clinical settings than males ($\sim$10:1 ratio). Nevertheless, studies of childhood TTM and of hair-pulling in college have documented a much more even gender ratio. Perhaps male pattern baldness is sufficiently acceptable to society that males with hair-pulling are less likely to present for treatment. Alternatively, men may initially target mustache and beard and may be able to prevent TTM by shaving these areas (1).

Onset of TTM is typically around the time of puberty, and the course may be chronic (1). Another group of hair-pulling patients has onset during infancy or childhood, but typically this behavior resolves rapidly (17). A range of stressors has been reported anecdotally to precipitate hair-pulling, but apart from female gender and pubertal age, few risk factors have been systematically defined. Some cases of TTM do appear to involve modeling of someone else with hair-pulling or onset in the context of abuse.

There is increasing recognition of the morbidity of trichotillomania. Hair-pulling itself may consume several hours a day. Careful attention to wigs, hats, specific hairstyle, and other forms of disguise may be needed. Patients may expend significant energy in resisting pulling but be unable to do so, sometimes even pulling in public. Consequences include avoiding various social situations, intimate relationships, and medical examinations. Shame and decreased self-esteem are common and crucial to understanding the disorder.

Less common, but potentially dire, are medical complications; the literature notes carpal tunnel syndrome (after repetitive manipulation of hair), corneal scarring (after pulling from eyelashes), dental erosion (after biting and chewing of hair), and a range of gastrointestinal symptoms including intestinal obstruction (after hair-swallowing) (18).

Symptomatology

Hair-pulling is typically from the scalp, although other common sites include the eyebrows and eyelashes, and any area of the body can be involved (1,8). A variety of patterns of alopecia can be seen, and over time changes in the color and texture of hair may emerge. Patients often describe pulling out particular kinds of hair (e.g., coarse hairs), and they may use their hands or an implement (e.g., tweezers). Occasionally patients do not so much pull as break their hair. A minority of patients pull out hair from significant others, from pets, or from dolls. In addition, some patients pull out other kinds of materials, such as carpet strands.

Hair-pulling may be associated with a range of habits, either involving hair (e.g., touching hair, mirror-checking, playing with hair prior to or after pulling) or habits performed together with or in place of hair-pulling (skin-picking, lip-biting, body-rocking). In view of their associated medical complications, oral habits (running hair against lips, biting hair into bits, swallowing of hair or root) are particularly important to inquire about (18).

Patients may pull in response to negative affective cues (e.g., anxiety) or during sedentary contemplatory activities (e.g., reading) (19). At times it may occur in an "automatic" way (with less awareness) rather than a focused way (to decrease tension). In some cases patients describe pruritis as a cue to hair-pulling. Hair-pulling is often worse in the evenings and is sometimes worse premenstrually. A number of user-friendly scales are now available for measuring the severity of hair-pulling, and may form a useful part of the initial clinical evaluation.

Given the increasing awareness of obsessive-compulsive disorder and OCD spectrum disorders in the media, patients increasingly present to mental health professionals for help. Nevertheless, in younger patients and in patients presenting to dermatologists, denial of hair-pulling may occur. Covering the hair with a bandage in order to observe whether regrowth takes place may be useful in younger patients (19). More rarely, scalp biopsy may be done (21); this reveals characteristic findings in trichotillomania, including catagen hairs, pigment casts, traumatized hair bulbs, and trichomalacia.

Comorbidity

Patients with trichotillomania commonly have comorbid mood and anxiety disorders, including OCD (1). Major depression was the most commonly associated mood disorder and generalized anxiety disorder the most commonly associated anxiety disorder in a large series of TTM patients. A range of other comorbid psychiatric disorders can also be seen, including both axis I and II disorders. Notably, however, some work has found that no particular personality disorder or trait appears characteristic of patients with TTM (1). Conversely, hair-pulling may be seen in a number of disorders, including Tourette's syndrome.

PSYCHOBIOLOGY

Neurochemistry

The finding that clomipramine was more effective than desipramine in obsessive-compulsive disorder has also been found in a number of other disorders with repetitive behaviors, suggesting that serotonin is particularly important in these putative OCD spectrum disorders (13). Indeed, TTM was one of the first disorders for which this response pattern was demonstrated (6). Nevertheless, subsequent trials of selective serotonin reuptake inhibitors (SSRIs) in hair-pulling have not been uniformly positive (22).

A range of studies have assessed serotonin function in TTM, assessing static measures such as cerebrospinal fluid concentrations of the serotonin metabolite 5-hydroxyindoleacetic acid (CSF 5-HIAA), or dynamic measures such as the behavioral or endocrine response to administration of serotonin agonists (23). In a number of such studies there has been no apparent difference between TTM and healthy controls. In one study, however, high

CSF 5-HIAA in TTM predicted response to a serotonin reuptake inhibitor, suggesting that in TTM, as in OCD, treatment with such an agent results in a decrease in CSF 5-HIAA levels (24).

Other neurotransmitter systems may also contribute to the mediation of hair-pulling symptoms. The dopamine system is closely linked with stereotypic behavior in animal models. Indeed, dopamine agonists can result in exacerbation of hair-pulling (25). Furthermore, dopamine blockers may have a role in the augmentation of serotonin reuptake inhibitors (SRIs) during the management of TTM (22). Finally, there is some evidence that the opioid system and hormonal factors may also play a role in hair-pulling (23).

Neuroanatomy

Obsessive-compulsive disorder is increasingly thought to be mediated by cortico-striatal-thalamic-cortical (CSTC) circuits (13). It might be hypothesized that these circuits also play a role in a range of dysfunctional repetitive motoric movements, including those that characterize TTM.

Brain imaging studies have provided some inconsistent support for a role for the CTSC circuits in trichotillomania. O'Sullivan and colleagues (26) noted decreased left putamen volume on magnetic resonance imaging of TTM patients in comparison to healthy controls. In contrast, caudate volume does not seem abnormal in TTM (26,27). These findings are consistent with current understanding of the different CSTC circuits; those involving the putamen are particularly important in mediating motoric behaviors and symptoms.

A number of neuropsychological studies have also been undertaken in TTM. Although not all research has been consistent, impairment of visual-spatial tasks has been noted by several authors (23). Such abnormalities conceivably reflect involvement of CSTC circuits in TTM. Additional work is, however, undoubtedly necessary in order to determine the way in which neuronal circuits mediate hair-pulling, and to demonstrate possible dysfunction in hair-pulling.

Neuroimmunology

An innovative hypothesis has suggested that some cases of OCD are secondary to an auto-immune process that occurs in the aftermath of streptococcal infection (28). Furthermore, there have been reports that such factors may play a role in some patients with hair-pulling (23). However, expression of D8/17, a B-lymphocyte antigen that is a marker of susceptibility to developing sequelae after streptoccocal infection, may be higher in OCD than in normal controls but does not appear to be increased in TTM (29).

Neurogenetics

There is some evidence that trichotillomania may be more common in the families of trichotillomania probands, although few studies have been rigorously controlled and those that have been done are not always consistent (1). Whether familial transmission is due to genetic or environmental factors is not known. A degree of familial association between TTM and OCD has also been found in some studies; a finding that is arguably somewhat supportive of the notion that TTM falls on an obsessive-compulsive spectrum of disorders. Recent work on an animal model of hair-pulling has strengthened the possibility of finding a molecular basis for trichotillomania (30).

Psychology

The question of what other psychological factors predispose to trichotillomania has not been well studied. The psychodynamic literature has developed a range of hypotheses about the pathogenesis of TTM (2) but has not systematically investigated them. Our group has found that scores on a measure of childhood trauma were significantly higher in subjects with trichotillomania than in normal controls (31). Clearly, the specific psychological factors that contribute to the pathogenesis of TTM require further elucidation.

PHARMACOTHERAPY

As noted earlier, clomipramine is more effective than desipramine in the treatment of trichotillomania (6). Unfortunately, however, controlled trials of the SSRIs in trichotillomania have not proven particularly persuasive (22, and initial response to these agents is not always maintained. Furthermore, there are currently no controlled trials with other agents in TTM. Given their superior tolerability, the SSRIs arguably remain the first-line choice of medication in the treatment of TTM (32).

Pharmacotherapy of trichotillomania should be particularly strongly considered when there is a comorbid condition (such as major depression, generalized anxiety disorder) known to be responsive to SSRIs. Medication is also an increasingly attractive consideration in adult patients with more severe hair-pulling. The current clinical consensus, based in part on experience with OCD, is that patients should be given a fairly long trial (up to 12 weeks), with dosage gradually increased to maximal levels in nonresponsive patients.

When a patient fails to respond to a SSRI, a different SSRI, clomipramine, or venlafaxine can be considered (22). Augmentation of a serotonin reuptake inhibitor with a dopamine blocker may be considered in adult patients who show only a partial response to these agents (22). The introduction of the new generation antipsychotics, with their relatively favorable adverse effect profile, makes them the agents of choice in this situation, despite the lack of controlled research. A number of other agents, including naltrexone and anticonvulsants, can also be considered in refractory patients (22).

PSYCHOTHERAPY

Habit reversal was early on described as a useful form of behavioral intervention for hair-pulling patients (4). This comprises a number of separate techniques including competing reaction training (replacing hair-pulling with a different motoric action), awareness training and identifying cues (increasing awareness of hair-pulling in general and of hair-pulling triggers in particular), and relaxation training (techniques to help decrease hair-pulling by enhancing relaxation). These techniques remain widely accepted; furthermore, it is not difficult for the interested practitioner to learn them and to pass them on to patients.

Current cognitive-behavioral packages have supplemented habit reversal with additional techniques including cognitive interventions focused on preventing relapse (33). Preliminary reports of the value of such intervention are extremely promising. Cognitive-behavioral therapy is a particularly attractive option in children with hair-pulling and in patients without comorbid psychiatric disorders. Although the combination of pharmacotherapy and psychotherapy has not been systematically studied in TTM, all patients on pharmacotherapy should arguably also learn the techniques of habit reversal.

Forms of psychological intervention other than cognitive-behavioral psychotherapy have not been systematically studied in TTM. However, there are a number of reports of the efficacy of hypnotherapy in TTM (34), and this is a modality that is therefore also worth considering in clinical practice. A range of additional rigorous psychotherapy research on TTM is warranted, including work on different kinds of interventions.

The growth of consumer advocacy in psychiatry in recent decades represents a major step forward for the field. The Trichotillomania Learning

Centre (TLC) is a useful resource for people with hair-pulling, who may well benefit from the information and support they obtain. There are also a number of good websites and e-mail lists devoted to trichotillomania. Patients may also be referred to various self-help resources (35).

CONCLUSION

Trichotillomania is a prevalent disorder both in the general population and in dermatology clinics. Although often considered by physicians as a minor condition, TTM is in fact a chronic medical disorder that is associated with significant morbidity and comorbidity. Inquiry about the presence of repetitive stereotypic behaviors such as hair-pulling deserves to be part of the standard psychiatric examination.

The nosological status of TTM remains unclear. Although classified as an impulse control disorder, TTM appears to have a number of features in common with OCD as well as with stereotypic movement disorder and self-injurious symptoms such as skin-picking. Although there are also considerable differences between OCD and TTM, a view of TTM as lying on an OCD spectrum of disorders has some heuristic value.

Fortunately, practitioners have a growing armamentarium of tools for the management of hair-pulling. A particularly important tool is a comprehensive psychiatric evaluation in order to exclude comorbid conditions. Additional useful tools include not only pharmacotherapy and psychotherapy, but also consumer advocacy organizations, internet resources, and self-help books. Although there is a need for much additional research on TTM, patients can already be approached with considerable hope for a good outcome (36).

ACKNOWLEDGMENTS

The authors are supported by the Medical Research Council (MRC) of South Africa.

REFERENCES

1. Christenson GA, Mansueto CS. Trichotillomania: descriptive characteristics and phenomenology. In: Stein DJ, Christenson GA, Hollander E, eds. Trichotillomania. Washington, DC: American Psychiatric Press, 1999, p. 1–42.
2. Koblenzer CS. Psychoanalytic Perspectives on Trichotillomania. In: Stein DJ, Christenson GA, Hollander E, eds. Trichotillomania. Washington, DC: American Psychiatric Press, 1999, p. 125–146.

3. Hallopeau M. Alopecia par grottage (trichomania ou trichotillomania). Ann Dermatol Venerol 10:440–441, 1889.

4. Keuthen NJ, Aronowitz B, Badenoch J, Wilhelm S. Behavioral treatment for trichotillomania. In: Stein DJ, Christenson GA, Hollander E, eds. Trichotillomania. Washington, DC: American Psychiatric Press, 1999, p. 147–166.

5. American Psychiatric Press. Diagnostic and Statistical Manual of Mental Disorders. 3rd ed, revised. Washington, DC: American Psychiatric Publishing, 1999.

6. Swedo SE, Leonard HL, Rapoport JL, et al. A double-blind comparison of clomipramine and desipramine in the treatment of trichotillomania (hair pulling). N Engl J Med 321:497–501, 1989.

7. American Psychiatric Press. Diagnostic and Statistical Manual of Mental Disorders. 4th ed, revised text. Washington, DC: American Psychiatric Publishing, 1999.

8. Christenson GA, Mackenzie TB, Mitchell JE. Characteristics of 60 adult chronic hair pullers. Am J Psychiatry 148:365–370, 1991.

9. du Toit PL, van Kradenburg J, Niehaus DJH, Stein DJ. Characteristics and phenomenology of hair-pulling: an exploration of subtypes. Comp Psychiatry 42:247–256, 2002.

10. Castellanos FX, Ritchie GF, Marsh WL, et al. DSM-IV stereotypic movement disorder: persistence of stereotypies of infancy in intellectually normal adolescents and adults. J Clin Psychiatry 57:116–122, 1996.

11. Niehaus DJ, Emsley RA, Brink PA, Stein DJ. Stereotypies: prevalence and association with compulsive and impulsive symptoms in college students. Psychopathology 33:31–35, 2000.

12. Stein DJ, Niehaus D. Stereotypic self-injurious behaviors. In: Simeon D, Hollander E, eds. Self-Injurious Behaviors: Assessment and Treatment. Washington, DC: American Psychiatric Press, 2001, p. 29–48.

13. Stein DJ. Neurobiology of the obsessive-compulsive spectrum disorders. Biol Psychiatry 47:296–304, 2000.

14. Swedo SE. Trichotillomania. In: Hollander E, ed. The Obsessive-Compulsive Related Disorders. Washington, DC: American Psychiatric Press, 1993, p. 93–112.

15. Stein DJ, Simeon D, Cohen L, Hollander E. Trichotillomania and obsessive-compulsive disorder. J Clin Psychiatry 4:28–34, 1995.

16. Stein DJ, Hollander E. Dermatology and conditions related to obsessive-compulsive disorder. J Am Acad Derm 26:237–242, 1992.

17. Chang CH, Lee MB, Chiang YC, et al. Trichotillomania: a clinical study of 36 patients. J Formos Med Assoc 90:176–180, 1991.

18. Bouwer C, Stein DJ. Trichobezoars in trichotillomania: case report and literature review. Psychosom Med 60:658–660, 1998.

19. Greenberg HR, Sarner CA. Trichotillomania: symptom and syndrome. Arch Gen Psychiatry 12:482–489, 1965.

20. Christenson GA, Ristvedt SL, Mackenzie TB. Identification of trichotillomania cue profiles. Behav Res Ther 31:315–320, 1993.

21. Muller SA. Trichotillomania: a histopathological study in sixty-six patients. J Am Acad Dermatol 23:56–62, 1990.
22. O'Sullivan RL, Christenson GA, Stein DJ. Pharmacotherapy of trichotillomania. In: DJ Stein, GA Christenson, E Hollander, eds. Trichotillomania. Washington, DC: American Psychiatric Publishing, 1999, p. 93–124.
23. Stein DJ, O'Sullivan RL, Hollander E. The neurobiology of trichotillomania. In: Stein DJ, Christenson GA, Hollander E, eds. Trichotillomania. Washington, DC: American Psychiatric Press, 1999, p. 43–62.
24. Ninan PT, Rothbaum BO, Stipetic M, et al. CSF 5HIAA as a predictor of treatment response in trichotillomania. Psychopharmacol Bull 28:451–455, 1992.
25. Martin A, Scahill L, Vitulano L, King RA. Stimulant use and trichotillomania. J Am Acad Child Adolesc Psychiatry 37:349–350, 1998.
26. O'Sullivan RA, Rauch S, Breiter H, et al. Reduced basal ganglia volumes in trichotillomania measured via morphometric magnetic resonance imaging. Biol Psychiatry 42:39–45, 1997.
27. Stein DJ, Coetzer R, Lee M, Davids B, Bouwer C. Magnetic resonance brain imaging in women with obsessive-compulsive disorder and trichotillomania. Psychiatry Res 74:177–182, 1997.
28. Swedo SE, Leonard HL, Garvey M, et al. Pediatric autoimmune neuropsychiatric disorders associated with streptococcal infections: clinical description of the first 50 cases. Am J Psychiatry 155:264–271, 1998.
29. Niehaus DJH, Knowles JA, van kradenburg J, du Toit W, Kaminer D, Seedat S, Daniels W, Cotton M, Brink P, Beyers AD, Bouic P, Stein DJ: D8/17 in obsessive-compulsive disorder and trichotillomania [lett]. S Afr Med J 89:755–756, 1999.
30. Greer JM, Capecchi MR. Hoxb8 is required for normal grooming behavior in mice. Neuron 33:23–34, 2002.
31. Lochner C, du Toit PL, Zungu-Dirwayi N, et al. Childhood interpersonal trauma in obsessive-compulsive disorder, trichotillomania, and controls. Depression Anxiety 15:66–68, 2002.
32. Vythilingum B, Stein DJ. Trichotillomania. Primary Care Psychiatry 8:58–63, 2001.
33. Rothbaum BO, Ninan PT. Manual for the cognitive-behavioral treatment of trichotillomania. In: Stein DJ, Christenson GA, Hollander E, eds. Trichotillomania. Washington, DC: American Psychiatric Publishing, 1999, p. 263–284.
34. Robiner WE, Edwards PE, Christenson GA. Hypnosis in the treatment of trichotillomania. In: Stein DJ, Christenson GA, Hollander E, eds. Trichotillomania. Washington, DC: American Psychiatric Publishing, 1999, p. 167–200.
35. Keuthen NJ, Stein DJ, Christenson GA. Help for Hair-Pullers. Oakland, CA: New Harbinger, 2001.
36. Keuthen NJ, Fraim C, Deckersbach T, et al. Longitudinal follow-up of naturalistic treatment outcome in patients with trichotillomania. J Clin Psychiatry 62:101–107, 2001.

15

Psychosocial Effects of Skin Disease on the Patient

Iona H. Ginsburg
Columbia-Presbyterian Medical Center and New York Presbyterian Hospital
New York, New York, U.S.A.

INTRODUCTION

The experience of dermatologists in clinical practice is that the majority of their patients deal with their skin disorder in an appropriate manner and do not display any undue concern or distress. However, some patients, especially those with chronic skin disease or with visible lesions, may sustain a devastating impact on their self-image, self-esteem, and self-confidence as well as on their interactions with other people. Relationships within the family, with friends, coworkers or fellow students, and with people met with in a casual context may be affected.

One of the most powerful statements about the impact of skin disease is in a short story by John Updike, who has had psoriasis since childhood (1): "Leprosy is not exactly what I have but what in the Bible is called leprosy was probably this thing, which has a twisty Greek name it pains me to write. The form of the disease is as follows: spots, plaques, and avalanches of excess skin ... expand and slowly migrate across the body like lichen on a tombstone. I am silvery, scaley. Puddles of flakes form wherever I rest my flesh. . . . My torture is skin deep . . . we lepers [are] lusty, though we are loathsome to love. Keen-sighted, though we hate to look upon ourselves. The name of the disease, spiritually speaking, is Humiliation."

Hospitalized patients with severe skin disease, mostly psoriasis, seen in consultation expressed their anguish poignantly in terms of feeling shame, anger, dirty and ugly, using such descriptions as "humiliating," "hideous," "disgrace," "furious," and "filthy" (2). With any individual person, however, the intensity of the impact of the skin disease will be very variable. Some people will be frantic with a mild, self-limited drug reaction, while others with chronic, visible disease will exhibit little concern, proceeding with their daily life in a matter-of-fact manner.

The variability of the impact of a skin disorder depends on the characteristics and implications of the skin disease itself, the characteristics of the patient and the life situation, and the characteristic attitudes of the wider society about what it "means" to have a skin disease.

CHARACTERISTICS OF THE DERMATOLOGIC DISORDER

The origin of the disease is likely to affect how patients conceptualize the disease and how they feel about it. Examples of acquired diseases include prurigo nodularis from chronic scratching or skin lesions from a sexually transmitted disease or from accidental exposure to toxic chemicals in the workplace. Clearly, the degree of responsibility the patient would be expected to feel would vary in each of these disorders and affect the psychological impact. What if the patient has a disorder that is genetically based, like psoriasis or atopic dermatitis? That response, too, is variable: the patient may feel frustration and helplessness and even blame relatives who are afflicted with it. But if the patient perceives it as a familial burden, it may be seen also as a shared misfortune for they are not personally responsible.

The timing of the onset of a skin disorder also plays an important role. If an adolescent or young adult is afflicted with a skin disease, especially one that is chronic, it may shake the person's very identity, along with self-esteem, self-image, and capacity to relate to others without undue anxiety or distress since that developmental period is focused on the consolidation of the sense of self, sexual identity, and personality. A common disorder of infancy and early childhood, such as atopic dermatitis, or one that is seen at birth, such as port wine stain, will be one determinant of the child's body image and general emotional development. One may surmise that infants with atopic eczema may feel enormous discomfort, if not pain, as they come to sense the boundaries of their bodies. In addition, their parents will often feel demoralized, frustrated, and exhausted, inadvertently creating an emotional climate dominated by anxiety and tension (3).

The objective manifestations of the lesions of the skin disease as well as their location also play an important role, since they indicate the degree of disfigurement and may also contribute to some facets of disability. Lesions may be seen as red, crusted, scaling, oozing—macules, papules, pustules, vescules, bullae, etc.; the texture and appearance may deviate from the norm, such as the leathery thickening of lichen simplex. Subjective symptoms are also of great importance. Intolerable pruritus may distort sleep patterns and cause stress, often being associated with depression (4). Pain, tenderness, and burning can be disruptive, even disabling.

The location of skin lesions can affect how patients view themselves and how the observer perceives the afflicted person. The face and hands are constantly visible and are seen, typically, by every bystander. If lesions appear on the trunk and limbs, they can be readily seen in a gym, health club, communal dressing area, and at the beach as well as during sexual activity. Lesions affecting the genitals may cause considerable torment and grief. Hair loss may be associated with embarrassment and diminished self-confidence, whether it be caused by androgenetic alopecia in both men and women or by alopecia areata (5). Women, not surprisingly, are more affected. If persons have lesions on the hands or nails, they may actually be disabled if they wrap cakes in a bakery or take money from customers as a bank teller or have any job involving transactions with other people. If a person has lesions on the soles, they cannot work as a salesclerk or a policeman walking a beat. Similarly, a person working in a job involving food preparation cannot do that work with a skin disorder affecting the hands and nails. Recreational activities can also be seriously affected: people with visible lesions are often not allowed in public swimming pools; tennis, running, softball, etc. can no longer be a part of a person's life if his skin disorder affects his feet, limbs, and trunk due to pain and soreness.

Often people worry that a skin disorder poses danger. Many people observing a person afflicted by a skin disorder fear that it is contagious, a supposition that will be discussed later. Does the disease in fact present a danger to the sufferer and/or to other people? Some skin lesions do denote an illness that is contagious, such as measles, scabies, and typhoid. And some skin diseases such as melanoma are life-threatening. The great majority of skin diseases and virtually all the common ones are neither life-threatening to those afflicted nor contagious to others, however much they may savage the quality of life.

Whether the disease is treatable and how this is to be accomplished is also a factor in the impact it may have, particularly on patients and their families. Such treatments as steroid creams, systemic steroids, cyclosporine, etretinate, accutane, etc. may have side effects that affect the health, well-being, and comfort of patients on a day-to-day basis. If a person is undergoing phototherapy, he may have to cope with problems at work because of scheduling the treatments as well as the cost.

The most common approach to treatment involves the use of topical remedies. If the prescribed preparation is too greasy or too malodorous or if it stains clothing and bedsheets, the patient will often not use it. Noncompliance is known to be an important problem in dermatology. In speaking about dealing with psoriasis, Jobling describes a "career of patienthood," with the treatment of the disease, as well as the disease itself, intruding into the patient's life and often taking over (6).

CHARACTERISTICS OF THE INDIVIDUAL PATIENT

Age and sex would intuitively be considered central in how any person copes with a chronic skin disease. A 16-year-old girl would most likely be far more distressed about her psoriasis than a 75-year-old man would be by his. One study confirming this association demonstrated that women had more psoriasis-related despair than men, and that stronger feelings of being stigmatized by psoriasis were present with younger age of onset (11).

General physical health is another variable. Skin lesions associated with a systemic illness, such as sarcoidosis, represent only one aspect of the overriding problem. Although patients may be dismayed by their skin lesions, they would probably be more affected by the underlying illness.

Personality type affects a person's experience in characteristic ways. Therefore any individual's response to a skin disorder may be influenced by personality. For example, patients with borderline personality disorder have unstable moods, intense anxiety about being alone, fear of abandonment, and identity disturbance, so they may well experience their skin disorder as a threat to their self-image and autonomy. Narcissistic personality disorder encompasses a sense of entitlement, expectation of admiration and attention, grandiose expectations of perfection, and excessive concern about how others regard them. People with this personality type may be severely shaken by a disease that changes their appearance and how they present themselves to others. If a person has an obsessive-compulsive style, he may become more anxious at not feeling in control of his body surface as well as excessive disgust at feeling unclean due to the disease as well as to topical treatments. Such a patient may be easier to treat if the dermatologist involves him in decision making more than other patients, being careful to explain the treatment alternatives and risk/benefit ratio and asking the patient to decide such matters as the frequency or timing of topical treatments.

If an Axis I psychiatric disorder exists, the patient may experience the dermatological disease in terms of depression or delusional disease. Patients with delusions of parasitosis and resulting excoriations or self-inflicted wounds will typically describe a complicated set of beliefs as to how they were exposed to the parasites, how they develop, travel through the body, reproduce, etc. A depressed person may view the skin disease as a punishment for actual or fantasized moral failings.

How a person deals with a skin disorder is strongly related to how they perceived themselves prior to the onset of the illness. The level of self-esteem and self-confidence as well as the status of the body image play important roles in determining the patient's state of mind. How a person views himself relates to early developmental experiences within the family: How was this person, as a child, seen, understood, accepted, and tended to within the family? Most people, fortunately, are the recipients of "good enough" parenting (7) and therefore come to feel that they are basically OK. They see themselves as at least reasonably good morally, reasonably intelligent, attractive, capable, and likeable. One would expect such people to be able to cope better with a skin disease than those who grew up feeling that they were ugly, incompetent, deficient, or without value.

The individual's life situation overall plays a significant role. What a person experiences in the environment of other people that inevitably enfolds him would be expected to modify the psychosocial impact of a skin disease.

Relationships with those closest to the patient are one of the most important factors determining the psychological effects of the disorder. Adults find that spouses or partners who are accepting and helpful play a vital role in their overall well-being as well as their mode of adjustment. Vitiligo (8) or atopic dermatitis (9,10) may create havoc in the psychosocial adjustment of children, depending on the attitude of their parents. If parents are affectionate and direct, if they are not secretive or ashamed, and if they don't allow the child to manipulate them, the child may well grow up to be relatively unharmed psychologically by the skin disease. When parents' unconscious resentment of their atopic children's needs and demands were explored during counseling, the dysfunctional parent-child relationship could be reversed (3).

If the patients are employed, are able to contribute to the support of the family, experience relatively harmonious interactions with colleagues and supervisors, and enjoy their work, they will experience heightened self-respect. Inevitably, the impact of the disease would be alleviated. In a study of stigma in psoriasis, it was found that patients who were employed felt less stigmatized, anticipating rejection to a lesser degree and feeling less guilt, shame, and sensitivity to others' attitudes and opinions (11).

But what is the impact of actual experiences of rejection due to their skin disease? Many afflicted patients will avoid situations where they fear rejection because of their skin and therefore may well not have experienced overt rejection, although sensitivity to how others look at them and what they may say is usually intense. A study of 100 psoriasis patients found that 20 people endured a total of 50 experiences of gross clear rejection, such as being asked to leave a gym, hairdresser, swimming pool, or job because of their skin disease. The consequences of such painful encounters entail feeling subjective emotional distress, the seeking of professional help, using tension-lessening substances such as alcohol, and experiencing interference with work (12).

THE PSYCHOLOGICAL IMPACT OF SPECIFIC SKIN DISORDERS

This section focuses on a highly selective review of recent literature relating to acne, psoriasis, and hair loss.

Acne vulgaris is a self-limited skin disease, seen primarily in adolescents, involving the pilosebaceous unit and manifested by comedones, papules, pustules, nodules, and, as sequellae to active lesions, pitted or hypertrophic scars (13). A study of 615 Turkish adolescents with acne showed higher anxiety in girls than boys even though severity of acne on the grading scale employed was similar, showing that girls are more vulnerable than boys to the negative psychological impact of this disease (14). A British study confirmed the greater impact on women (15), and also noted that although dermatological treatment produced some improvement psychologically in the men and women assessed, emotional functioning tended to be more resistant to change. Anxiety levels, as well as high levels of catecholamines, decreased when 38 patients with cystic acne were successfully treated (16). As a forceful reminder that acne, while common, is far from trivial, acne patients were found to report levels of social, psychological, and emotional problems as great as those indicated by patients with epilepsy, diabetes, chronic asthma, back pain, and arthritis (17). It is important to be aware that it is the patient's assessment of severity, not the dermatologist's, that will lead the patient to feel a greater or lesser degree of humiliation, satisfaction with appearance, and social inhibition. An uncontrolled study demonstrated that patients rated their lesions as being more severe than the assessment of the dermatologist (18).

Since acne typically and literally appears on the face one presents to the world at large, body image may be adversely affected. If an adolescent, especially a female, feels disfigured by her acne and unable to control it, she may exert mastery over her body by developing an eating disorder (19).

If a patient displays undue concern about mild or nonexistent acne, to the point of perceiving herself as monstrously disfigured, she may have body dysmorphic disorder (20,21). Such patients become intensely focused on their perceived defect, spending hours at the mirror; they may have obsessive-compulsive disorder, clinical depression, and/or social phobia and symptoms may even take on delusional intensity. Selective serotonin reuptake inhibitors may be beneficial therapy in delusional as well as nondelusional patients (22).

Employment may prove a problem for patients with visible acne. A survey of 625 patients age 18–30 showed significant differences in employment rates compared to controls: 16.2% vs. 9.2% in men (76% higher) and 14.3% vs. 8.7% in women (64% higher) (23).

There are several scenarios in which psychiatric consultation should be seriously considered for a patient with acne: the presence of clinical depression, an eating disorder, distortion of the body image, and excessive impact of acne on daily life and well-being. When dermatological treatment is successful, the emotional anguish and social avoidance may well be eradicated but if it should persist in the absence of acne lesions, consultation is also indicated.

Psoriasis is a chronic, relapsing skin disease with variable clinical features, the lesions being erythrosquamos in nature with the major morphological types being psoriasis vulgaris, psoriatic erthroderma, and pustular psoriasis. It is equally common in men and women, has a 2% incidence in the United States, with onset usually in the third decade, although it has been described as present at birth and, at the other end of the spectrum, developing at age 108 (24).

Over many decades, studies have testified to the great emotional pain, disruption of daily life, and impact on interpersonal relationships that can be associated with psoriasis (25).

A study of stigma, defined as a discrediting biological or social mark that sets a person off from others and disrupts their social interactions, found six dimensions of the stigma experience, as well as psoriasis-related despair: anticipation of rejection, sensitivity to others' opinions and attitudes, feeling flawed, guilt and shame, secretiveness, and positive attitude. The most frequent predictors were found to be age at onset, bleeding of lesions, employment status, duration, and the experience of rejection (11).

Using a measure based on the Ginsburg and Link "Feelings of Stigmatization Questionnaire," Schmid-Ott et al. (26) found that with 298 psoriasis patients and 76 with atopic dermatitis lesions in the genital area were particularly relevant for feeling stigmatized. They also concluded that a ruminative, depressive coping style measured a high level of concern about their disease.

The impact of the tendency of patients with skin disease to anticipate being evaluated in negative terms by other people is particularly significant. In a postal survey of psoriasis patients in 1976, Jobling (27) discovered that anticipation of exclusion and social avoidance was omnipresent, with 84% reporting difficulty in establishing social contacts and relationships, citing that as the worst aspect of their psoriasis. As indicated, studies of stigma found anticipation of rejection an important facet of stigma (11) as well as concealment (28). Investigation of 318 psoriasis patients' fear of negative evaluation showed that this fear, as well as disease severity, predicted their perceptions of being stigmatized, interpersonal discomfort, degree of interference with daily life and quality of life, distress at visible aspects of the disease, and worry about others' reactions (29).

Another facet of the stigma experience is a perceived deprivation of social touch: in 137 patients, 26% reported such an event in which someone made a conscious effort not to touch them. Although those patients' psoriasis was not more severe, they were significantly depressed (30). A study of pathological worrying, disease perception, and severity in 140 psoriasis patients concluded that many patients experience high levels of worrying thoughts more linked to personal and social evaluative concerns than to aspects of the disease itself (31).

Fortune et al. (32) suggest that psychosocial impact of psoriasis stems from stress associated with engaging in anticipatory/avoidance coping behavior designed to limit the sociocognitive intrusiveness of psoriasis as well as stress relating to patients' beliefs or experiences of being evaluated by other people on the basis of their skin alone.

As indicated in the prior section, it is important for the clinician to have a high index of suspicion about the presence of a clinical depression and of suicidal ideation in people with chronic dermatoses. In a survey of 480 patients with noncystic facial acne, alopecia areata, atopic dermatitis, and psoriasis (33), severely afflicted inpatients with psoriasis had the highest scores for depression and suicidal ideation (7.2%), followed by patients with mild to moderate acne (5.6%). Since general medical patients have a 2.4–3.3% prevalence of active suicidal ideation, this clearly should flag this issue for the physician. In another study (28), 8% of psoriasis inpatients were also found to have suicidal thoughts.

Androgenetic alopecia is androgen-dependent and genetically mediated, occurring in about 50% of both men and women, although the pattern and degree of hair loss differs. Women usually preserve the frontal hair line and have a progressive thinning at the top of the scalp, but it typically does not progress to frank baldness. Men commonly display bitemporal recession and vertex predominance, which may lead to total baldness (34).

As an indicator of the importance accorded hair—its length, thickness, and arrangement—one need only visit the local drugstore and note the quantity and variety of products relating to hair care. Advertising in magazines and television intensifies the societal preoccupation with youth and beauty. A total of $2 billion each year is spent on hair loss products and treatments. There is also a long history of the social and psychological significance of hair over centuries, if not millenia (5).

Although alopecia is common in men and even expected to occur by many, it is far less common in women, with an incidence of 19%. It has been found to diminish satisfaction with body image and to decrease self-esteem, especially in women and in people who seek treatment (35). Both men and women with androgenetic alopecia who sought treatment and who were found to have personality disorders experienced more distress about their hair loss than people who did not have personality disorders, suggesting that the former group might well have had difficulties with their sense of self and ineffective coping skills. Indeed, the fact that the subjects were self-selected, in that they presented for treatment of their hair loss, is an important issue in interpreting the results of various studies (35,36). Cash has noted that both men and women experienced more distress when their hair loss had an early onset and was noticeable, had heightened social self-consciousness and vulnerability regarding self-acceptance, and a more intense investment in their appearance (37). A study of 120 women from two dermatology clinics and one large worksite found wide concern focused on hair itself, such as unhappiness about appearance and worry about continued hair loss. They also reported embarrassment and self-consciousness related to others noticing their hair loss, as well as jealousy and feeling impotent regarding stopping the hair thinning (38).

CULTURAL ATTITUDES ABOUT SKIN DISEASE

The editor of a book about stigma writes in the introduction, "Most people who find themselves in an airplane next to someone with an obvious and disfiguring skin disease would find it very difficult to maintain their aplomb while conversing with the afflicted passenger" (39,40). Why is that? What are the underlying fantasies and unconscious assumptions implied by such a response (41)?

This is a very complex matter, since patients with skin disease often share these assumptions. Patients with psoriasis have told the author that they would avoid people with psoriasis if they did not have it. On an AIDS service, AIDS patients without psoriasis shunned those AIDS patients who did have it (42). It may be at times that people will project their own self-disgust onto others, but it is undeniable that other people do, in fact, avoid them or intrude with tactless comments or unwanted advice or questions.

In emphasizing the idea of "skin failure," drawing the analogy to the failure of other organ systems, such as heart or kidney failure, Ryan notes that failure of the display function of skin may lead to rejection, isolation, and marked disability (43). The extensive sociological literature which explores the widely perceived superiority of people seen as beautiful cannot be reviewed here, but it shows in general the assumption that those people have more desirable traits such as intelligence and honesty compared to people who are considered unattractive (44,45). Disfigurement of the skin distorts what is communicated about the person within that skin to society at large, as well as to the sufferers themselves.

The fears and fantasies about the "meaning" of skin disease relate to anxiety about maintaining control of the borders of the body, to narcissistic longings for perfection, and to guilt. Such issues as contagion, dirtiness, and sexuality are encompassed by these overall topics.

FANTASIES RELATING TO GUILT

When a person is afflicted by any illness, especially one that is severe or that interferes with long-treasured plans, the usual reaction would be, "What have I done to deserve this? Why is this happening to me?" These questions imply that the person feels that the disease is a punishment. Children are punished when they have been "bad" or done something "bad." Thus, the adult afflicted with a disfiguring skin disease has presumably harbored conscious or unconscious guilt about sexual feelings or behaviors or aggressive thoughts or behaviors. People often attribute skin lesions to contagion and specifically to sexually transmitted disease. The "dirt" that bursts through the skin is linked with "dirty" thoughts and wishes (46), with the skin lesions implying danger and impurity (47) as well as punishment.

CONTROL OF THE PHYSICAL AND PSYCHOLOGICAL BOUNDARIES

People afflicted by skin disease often see themselves as incapable of controlling the surface of their own bodies. Nadelson has written about skin as being the boundary of the self (46), which encloses whatever is supposed to remain closed off inside. With a skin disease, the unruly contents erupt onto the surface of the skin, of which the individual is now incapable of maintaining control. The skin, not commonly conceptualized as a bodily aperture, becomes one, and the contents, no longer properly sequestered inside, appear on the surface in the form of blotches, bumps, scales, pus, or exudates.

In unconscious terms, the skin walls off dirt, which is "anything which either symbolically or in reality emerges from the body" which is an "animated, mobile dirt factory, exuding filth at every aperture" (48), and the bodily products are perceived as dangerous and destructive. Freud refers to dirt as being "matter out of place" (49), a statement that connects subtly with what occurs with a visible skin disease. The afflicted persons have been unable to control their own inner "dirt" and by extension their own "dirty" impulses. It is pertinent that psoriasis patients, when compared to vitiligo patients, whose disorder involved only pigmentary changes rather than lesions on the skin, experience more social discrimination and embarrassment (50). Psoriasis lesions are red, raised, and covered with scales due to the rapid turnover of affected skin and are often perceived as creating "dirty" scales on carpets, clothing, etc.

Dirt implies moral judgment: dirt is bad, cleanliness and order are good. A study of attitudes about various body products disclosed that the dirtiest were considered to be blackheads, ear wax, pus, feces, nose pickings, and desquamated toe cells, in that order (51). An anthropologist contributes to this discourse (47): "Reaction to dirt is continuous with other reactions to ambiguity and anomaly [which] lead to anxiety and from there to suppression and avoidance. ... A polluting person is always in the wrong."

FANTASIES ABOUT DIRT, CONTAGION, AND SEXUALITY

A newspaper story about river blindness in Africa caused by *Onchocerea volvulus* described the dermatological aspects of the disease as even more important than blindness because "it leads to being social outcasts for many ... others avoid them for fear of infection and made it difficult for them to marry and get work" (52). The same fear exists in western culture, where the sight of a person with skin disease will cause speculation about infection. Skin lesions may well be further linked to fear of death and bodily disintegration.

The infections assumed to be the cause of a visible skin disease are almost always sexual in nature. Unconscious guilt about sexual urges and thoughts, based on distortions in thinking in early childhood, are omnipresent. Skin lesions may represent symbolically on an unconscious level the breakdown of control over one's inner dirt and over the parallel "dirty" thoughts and wishes (46), with the skin lesions implying impurity and danger (47).

FANTASIES ABOUT BEING PERFECT

A wholesome self-love is central to health, adaptation, and achievement (53). The psychological components of healthy narcissism include the ego ideals which result from introjected idealized qualities of the parents' goals and ideals as well as images of the ideal self. Skin disease will inevitably cause injury to the afflicted person's self-esteem and normal narcissism. To want to be looked at and admired is a psychological given. To be looked at with surprise, fear, horror, or disdain evokes painful shame and humiliation. "Shame then is intimately linked to the need to cover ... that which is exposed" (54).

Bodily integrity is an important facet of the integrity of the self; when it is compromised, as with skin disease, deep-seated feelings of defectiveness may be magnified and compounded. Visible skin disease, even when visible only to the patients themselves, implies imperfection. If a person is without blemish, whether the blemish is physical, moral, or psychological, that means that the person is safe from shame and humiliation (2). The repudiation of those with skin disease because of what it implies in symbolic terms is dramatized in a remarkable short story by Nathaniel Hawthorne. An alchemist prepares a potion for his beautiful young wife, noting the small birthmark on her cheek, "the visible mark of earthly imperfection, the symbol of his wife's liability to sin, sorrow, decay, and death ... this horrible stigma." As she drinks it, the birthmark disappears and she dies (55). Being perfect is apparently incompatible with being human.

There is a decided propensity for people with normal skin to turn away, physically and/or psychologically, from those afflicted with skin disease, and they may feel deeply discomfited, like the person on the airplane referred to earlier. The author believes that what happens under these circumstances is a fleeting identification with the afflicted person followed by a negative empathic response. The person with visible skin disease symbolizes how imperfect and vulnerable, how defective and helpless we all are. Aware of how embarrassed and ashamed the afflicted person is at his imperfection being so readily seen, the onlooker experiences a momentary flash of empathic identification and immediately turns away, having blotted out awareness of the sufferer's emotional pain. Compassionate warmth that might have surfaced, however briefly, has been dismissed. Instead of empathic acceptance based on knowing how fundamentally alike we all are, there is a negative twist to the empathic sensitivity, and the onlooker distances himself from the person with skin disease. There may be outright rejection and pointed withdrawal or perhaps a lesser manifestation of emotional distance, such as offering unsolicited advice. Basically it is a repudiation of those who remind us of our own inherent humanness and vulnerability.

GUIDELINES FOR MANAGEMENT OF THE PSYCHOSOCIAL IMPACT OF SKIN DISEASE

The most important methods for dealing with the impact of a skin disease include the doctor-patient relationship, education of the patient as well as the community about the actual nature of these diseases, and more specific psychological therapies, such as individual, group, or behavioral therapy.

A crucial element in the management of psychological impact is the development of a therapeutic alliance with the dermatologist. An open and empathic doctor-patient relationship leads to honest communication and the feeling that the dermatologist understands how the patient is experiencing the skin disease, thereby lessening feelings of isolation and alienation. Aspects of this relationship that have been cited as central are time, interest, information and teaching, enthusiasm and understanding, hope, candor, discussion of treatment options, and open-mindedness (56). Especially in the first appointment of a patient with a chronic disease, in which the relationship is likely to be ongoing, these issues should be addressed leading to greater rapport and the ability to assess the psychological factors that may be affecting the disease. Cultivating empathy by imaginatively projecting themselves into the patient's situation enhances both listening and communication, so that the joint task of treatment can proceed most effectively.

Dermatologists can also encourage patients to become more active on their own behalf, thereby increasing their self-esteem and sense of control. An important way to do this is to suggest that they participate in self-help groups such as the Eczema Association, the Alopecia Areata Foundation, the Trichotillomania Learning Center, and the National Psoriasis Foundation. The major function of these groups is the education of the patients, their families, and the community at large. They also give support and a sense of belonging, encourage research, advocate for patients with insurance companies and governmental agencies, and sometimes organize support groups and conferences.

An educated patient is more likely to have a positive therapeutic alliance with the physician and the office staff as well as a heightened feeling of control (57). For example, a psoriasis patient ignorant of the Koebner phenomenon will not be able to participate as fully or intelligently in his or her own care and will not be as cautious in avoiding injury to the skin.

In addition, patients who understand their disease are more likely to be able to distance themselves from it emotionally. They are less likely to identify with it; it then becomes a disease they have, not who they are (58). They are then in a position to educate family, friends, and the wider community, as when asked about their skin. Patient education should be on the physician's agenda, since it is a major modality by which the doctor-patient alliance develops.

Another focus is educating the community about the nature of skin disease (59). A wider problem is how to remove the stigma of skin disease in society at large (6). A skin disease is only a skin disease. It does not inherently mean filth, decay, promiscuity, contagion, incompetence, moral laxity, or hideousness. As Jobling points out, a skin disease means difference, not deviance or discredit.

If a patient is depressed and overwhelmed by the experience of the disease or if there is a social phobia caused or intensified by the disease, a psychiatric consultation is in order. If referral is made in a matter-of-fact fashion out of concern for the patient and if the dermatologist makes it clear that he or she will continue to provide dermatological care and is not trying to get rid of the patient, the patient is likely to follow the advice. Patients are often grateful that the intensity of their distress has been perceived and appreciated and that they have been truly heard.

Treatment modalities that might be offered would include whatever psychopharmacological treatment is appropriate to the specific disorder. Individual psychotherapy is a valuable technique for some patients which will enable them to modify the painful feelings, negative cognitive stance, and the often avoidant behavior that may occur in response to a skin disease. Group therapy, behavior therapy, and stress management may also be deemed appropriate.

Virginia Woolf wrote that "the eyes of others [are] our prisons; their thoughts our cages" (60). This is particularly relevant to the cultural attitudes about skin disorders, and clearly attacks on the prisons and cages should be launched on many fronts so that patients with skin disease can proceed with their lives free of concern about stigma.

REFERENCES

1. Updike J. From the Journal of a Leper. The New Yorker, July 19, 1976:28–32.
2. Ginsburg IH. The psychosocial impact of skin disease; an overview. Dematolo Clin 14:473–484, 1996.
3. Koblenzer CS, Koblenzer PJ. Chronic intractible atopic eczema. Arch Dermatol 124:1673, 1988.
4. Gupta MA, Gupta A, Schork NJ, Ellis CN. Depression modulates pruritus perception: a study of pruritus in psoriasis, atopic dermatitis, and chronic idiopathic urticaria. Psychosom Med: 56:36-40, 1994.
5. Knobler E. The effect of hair loss on self-image. In: Walsher RR, Beachman A, Ginsburg IH, eds. Dermatology and Person-Threatening Illness: The Patient, the Family, the Staff. Binghamton, NY: The Haworth Press, 1996:57–63.
6. Jobling R. Learning to live with it: an account of a career of chronic dermatologic illness and patienthood. In: Davis A, Horobin G eds. Medical Encounters. The Experience of Illness and Treatment. New York: St. Martin's Press, 1977:83.
7. Winnicott DW. Transitional objects and transitional phenomena. Int J Psychoanal 34:89, 1953.
8. Hill-Beuf A, Porter JDR, Children coping with impaired appearance: social and psychologic influences. Gen Hosp Psychiatry 6: 294, 1984.
9. Howlett S. Emotional dysfunction, child-family relationships, and childhood atopic dermatitis. Br J Dermatol 140(3): 381–384, 1999.
10. Gil KM, Keefe FJ, Sampson HA. The relationship of stress and family environment to atopic dermatitis in children. J Psychosom Res 31: 673, 1987.
11. Ginsburg IH, Link BG. Feelings of stigmatization in psoriasis. J Am Acad Dermatol 20: 53–63, 1989.
12. Ginsburg IH, Link BH. Psychosocial consequences of rejection and stigma feelings in psoriasis patients. Int J Dermatol 32: 587–591, 1993.
13. Strauss JS, Thiboutot DM. Acne vulgaris. In: Freedberg IM, ed. Dermatology in General Medicine. New York: McGraw-Hill, 1999, p. 769.
14. Aktan S, Ozmen E, Sanli B. Anxiety, depression, and nature of acne vulgaris in adolescents. Int J Dermatol 39: 354–357, 2000.
15. Kellett SC, Gawkrodger DJ. The psychological and emotional impact of acne and the effect of treatment with isotretinoin. Br J Dermatol. 140:273–82, 1999.
16. Schulpis K, Georgala S, Papakonstantinou ED, Michas T. Psychological and sympatho-adrenal status in patients with cystic acne. J Eur Acad Dermatol Venereol 13:24–27, 1999.
17. Mallon E, Newson JN, Klassen A, Stewart-Brown SL, Ryan TJ, Finlay AY. The quality of life in acne: a comparison with general medicine conditions using generic questionnaires. Br J Dermatol 140:672–676, 1999.
18. Medansky RS, Handler RM, Medansky DL. Self-evaluation of acne and emotion. Psychosomatics 22:379, 1981.
19. Gupta MA, Gupta AK, Ellis CN, et al. Bulimia nervosa and acne may be relaxed: a case report. Can J Psychiatry 37: 58, 1992.

20. Phillips KA. Body dysmorphic disorder: the distress of imagined ugliness. Am J Psychiatry 148:1138–1149, 1991.
21. Smith P. Body image disorders. Psychother Psychosom 58:119, 1992.
22. McElroy SL, Phillips KA, Keck Jr. PE, et al. Body dysmorphic disorder: Does it have a psychotic subtype? J Clin Psychiatry 54:389, 1993.
23. Cunliffe WJ. Acne and unemployment. Br J Dermatol 115: 386, 1986.
24. Christopher E, Mrowietz U. Psoriasis. In: Freedberg IM, Eisen AZ, Wolff K, Aussen KF, Goldsmith LA, Katz SI, Fitzpatrick TB, eds. Dermatology in General Medicine. New York: McGraw-Hill, 1999:522.
25. Ginsburg IH. Psychological and psychophysiological aspects of psoriasis. Dermatol Clin 13:793–804, 1995.
26. Schmid-Ott G, Kuensebeck HW, Jaeger B, Werfel T, Frahm K, Ruitman J, Kapp A, Lamprecht F. Validity study for the stigmatization experience in atopic dermatitis and psoriatic patients. Acta Derm Venereol 79: 443–447, 1999.
27. Jobling R. Psoriasis—a preliminary questionnaire study of sufferers' subjective experience. Clin Exp Dermatol: 233–236, 1976.
28. Schmid-Ott G, Jaeger B, Kuensebeck HW, Ott R, Lamprecht F. Dimensions of stigmatization in patients with psoriasis in a 'Questionnaire on Experience with Skin Complaints.' Dermatology 193: 304–310, 1996.
29. Leary MR, Rapp BR, Herbst KC, Exum ML, Feldman SR. Interpersonal concerns and psychological difficulties of psoriasis patients: effects of disease severity and fear of negative evaluation. Health Psychol 17:530–536, 1998.
30. Gupta MA, Gupta AK, Watteel GN. Perceived deprivation of social touch in psoriasis is associated with greater psychologic morbidity: an index of the stigma experience in dermatologic disorders. Cutis 61: 339–342, 1998.
31. Fortune DG, Richards HL, Main CJ, Griffiths CEM. Pathological worrying, illness perceptions, and disease severity in patients with psoriasis. Br J Health Psychol 5: 71–82, 2000.
32. Fortune DG, Main CJ, O'Sullivan TM, Griffiths CE. Quality of life in patients with psoriasis: the contributions of clinical variables and psoriasis-specific stress. Br J Dermatol 1997: 755–760.
33. Gupta MA, Gupta AK. Depression and suicidal ideation in dermatology patients with acne, alopecia areata, atopic dermatitis and psoriasis. Br J Dermatol 139: 846–850, 1998.
34. Olsen EA. Hair disorders. In: Freedberg IM, Eisen AZ, Wolff K, Austen KF, Goldsmith LA, Katz SI, Fitzpatrick TB, eds. Dermatology in General Medicine. New York: McGraw-Hill, 1999, p. 739.
35. Kalick SM. Psychological aspects of alopecia patients. Arch Dermatol 130: 907–908, 1994.
36. Maffei C, A Fassati, F Rinaldi, et al. Personality disorders and psychopathologic symptoms in patients with androgenetic alopecia. Arch Dermatol 130: 868–872, 1994.
37. Cash TF. The psychosocial consequences of androgenetic alopecia: a review of the research literature. Br J Dermatol 141: 398–405, 1999.

38. Girman CJ, Hartmaier S, Roberts J, Bergfeld W, Waldstreicher J. Patient-perceived importance of negative effects of androgenetic alopecia in women. J Womens Health Gend Based Med 8: 1091–1095, 1999.
39. Jones E, Farina A, Hasdorf A, et al. Social Stigma: The Psychology of Marked Relationships. New York: Freeman, 1984, p. 48.
40. Goffman E. Stigma: Notes on the Management of Spoiled Identity. Englewood Cliffs, NJ: Prentice-Hall, 1963.
41. Ginsburg IH. The psychological impact of skin disease: an overview. In: Walther R R, Beachman A, Ginsburg IH, eds. Dermatology and Person-Threatening Illness. Binghamton, NY: The Haworth Press, Inc. 1996, pp. 1–10.
42. Gregory N., personal communication, 1991.
43. Ryan TJ. Disability in dermatology. Br J Hosp Med. 46:33–36, 1990.
44. Berscheid E, Walster E. Physical attractiveness. In: Berkowitz L, ed. Advances in Experimental Social Psychology. New York: Academic Press, vol. 7, p. 157–215, 1978.
45. Alam M, Dover JS. On beauty: evolution, psychosocial considerations, and surgical enhancement. Arch Dermatol 2001.
46. Nadelson T. A person's boundaries: a meaning of skin disease. Cutis 21: 90–, 1978.
47. Douglas M. Purity and Danger, an Analysis of the Concepts of Pollution and Taboo. London: Ark, 1984.
48. Kubie LS. The fantasy of dirt. Psychoan Quart 6:388–425, 1937.
49. Freud S. Character and anal eroticism (1908). In: Riviere J, ed. Collected Papers, Vol II. London: Hogarth Press, 1956:48.
50. Porter JR, Hill-Beuf AH, Lerner A, et al. Psychosocial effect of vitiligo. J Am Acad Dermatol 15: 220–224, 1986.
51. Kurtz R, Hirt M, Ross WD, et al. Investigation of the affective meaning of body products. J Exp Res Pers 3:9–14, 1968.
52. Leary WE. River blindness disease has a devastating side. The New York Times, March 1995.
53. Kohut H. Forms and transformations of narcissism (1966). In: Ornstein PH, ed. The Search for the Self. Vol I. International University Press, 427–460, 1978.
54. Schneider CD. Shame, Exposure, and Privacy. New York: WW Norton & Co, 1997, p. 30.
55. Hawthorne N. The birthmark (1843). In: The Celestial Railroad. New York: New American Library, 1963:204.
56. Decker S, Zimmerman GM. To battle the disease, is to know the enemy. Sem Dermatol 1991; 10: 132–134.
57. Lanigan SW, Farber EM. Patients' knowledge of psoriasis: pilot study. Cutis 46:359, 1990.
58. Ginsburg IH. Coping with psoriasis: a guide for counseling patients. Cutis 57:323–325, 1996.
59. Coles RB, Ryan TJ. The psoriasis sufferer in the community. Br J Dermatol 93:111–112, 1975.
60. Woolf V. An unwritten novel. In: A Haunted House and Other Short Stories. New York: Harcourt Brace, 1972:15.

16

Depression and Dermatological Disorders

Madhulika A. Gupta
University of Western Ontario
London, Ontario, Canada

Aditya K. Gupta
University of Toronto
Toronto, Ontario, Canada

INTRODUCTION

Psychiatric and psychosocial factors are reported to play a role in at least 30% of dermatological disorders (1–6). Among the wide range of psychopathological states encountered in dermatology, depressive disease is one of the most frequently encountered psychiatric syndromes. It is important to recognize and effectively treat depressive disease that is comorbid with dermatological disorders, as depression among dermatological patients has been associated with suicidal ideation and cases of completed suicide. Furthermore, coexisting depression may prolong the morbidity associated with a dermatological disorder, e.g., in some pruritic dermatoses. Depressive disease is encountered in both the major groups of psychodermatological disorders: 1) the cutaneous associations of psychiatric disorders such as neurotic excoriations, some cases of delusions of parasitosis where delusional depression may be present, and markedly excessive concerns about cutaneous body image that are not consistent with objective clinical dermatological evaluation, and 2) the large group of dermatological disorders such as psoriasis, atopic dermatitis, chronic idiopathic urticaria, alopecia areata and acne that are both exacerbated by psychosocial stress and comorbid with a wide range of psychiatric disorders including major depressive disorder. The impact of the skin disorder on the quality of life of the patient, which results mainly from the social stigma associated with having a cosmetically disfiguring disease, can result in significant psychological morbidity including major depressive disorder. It is important to recognize, however, that depression among dermatological patients is generally a multifactorial problem, and in certain disorders like acne, the degree of depression is not always directly correlated with the clinical severity of the dermatological disorder.

It is estimated that significant psychiatric comorbidity is present in at least 30% of dermatological patients, and consideration of these factors is essential for the effective management of the skin condition (1–6). Major depressive disorder (Table 1) (7) is one of the most commonly encountered psychiatric disorders in dermatological disease. Depressive disease in encountered in both the cutaneous associations of psychiatric disorders. In this subgroup the cutaneous symptom is essentially the result of a primary psychiatric condition and effective management of the skin problem involves management of the underlying psychiatric disorder and the psychosocial and psychiatric aspects of dermatological disorders (1). This larger subgroup represents disorders that have a primary dermatopathological basis but may be comorbid with depressive disease, for example, acne, psoriasis, atopic dermatitis, idiopathic urticaria and angioedema, and alopecia areata. The social and psychological impact of having a cosmetically disfiguring condition can be a factor in a wide range of dermatological disorders and can also contribute to the development of depressive disease in the dermatological patient.

TERMINOLOGY USED IN THE DEFINITION OF DEPRESSIVE DISEASE

Depressive disease manifests as a disorder of mood. In the fourth edition of the *Diagnostic and Statistical Manual of Mental Disorders* (DSM-IV) (7), the mood disorders are categorized into the depressive disorders, the bipolar disorders, and two groups of mood disorders based on etiology—mood disorder due to general medical condition (7) and substance-induced mood disorder (7). The bipolar disorders present with hypomanic or manic episodes in addition to periods of depression. Major depressive disorder is

TABLE 1   DSM-IV Criteria for Major Depressive Episode

Five or more of the following symptoms must have been present during the same 2-week period and represent a change from previous functioning; at least one of the symptoms is either (i) depressed mood or (ii) anhedonia, i.e., loss of interest or pleasure in activities that the patient usually found pleasurable.

(1) Depressed mood most of the day, nearly every day, as evidenced by subjective report of sadness or objective evidence such as tearfulness. In children and adolescents the presentation may be different as the most prominent finding may be an irritable mood.

(2) Markedly diminished interest or pleasure in all, or almost all, activities nearly every day.

(3) Significant weight loss when not dieting or weight gain (e.g., a change of more than 5% of body weight in a month), or decrease or increase in appetite nearly every day. In growing children this may present as a failure to make the expected weight gains.

(4) Insomnia or hypersomnia nearly every day.

(5) Psychomotor agitation or retardation nearly every day.

(6) Fatigue or loss of energy nearly every day.

(7) Feelings of worthlessness or excessive or inappropriate guilt (which may be delusional) nearly every day (not merely self-reproach or guilt about being sick).

(8) Diminished ability to think or concentrate, or indecisiveness, nearly every day (either by subjective account or as observed by others).

(9) Recurrent thoughts of death (not just fear of dying), recurrent suicidal ideation without a specific plan, or a suicide attempt or a specific plan for committing suicide.

The symptoms cause significant impairment or distress in important areas of functioning, e.g., social and occupational functioning. The symptoms should not be the direct result of use of a substance or a medical disorder and should not be accounted for by bereavement.

Major depressive disorder is characterized by one or more major depressive episodes.

Source: Ref. 7.

diagnosed by the presence of one or more major depressive episodes (Table 1). A major depressive episode is characterized by at least two weeks of depression or anhedonia in association with at least four vegetative symptoms of depression. A depressed mood, however, is not always the most prominent presenting feature of depressive disease. The mood disorder in depression may manifest as prominent anxiety or increased irritability or anhedonia, which is a pervasive loss of interest in things or activities that the patient previously had found pleasurable. The term "affective disorder" is also used to denote depressive illness, but in the more current nosology (DSM-IV) (7), the term "mood disorder" has replaced this earlier terminology. Other terminologies that have been used to denote depressive illness include "involutional melancholia," "psychotic depression," and "endogenous depression." While these terms are not used in the current nosology (7), the term "melancholic features" (DSM-IV) (7) is used to denote "endogenous," "vegetative," or biological features such as a prominent disturbance in sleep, appetite, level of energy, and concentration. The terminology used to denote "neurotic depression" or "minor depression" is dysthymic disorder (DSM-IV) (7), which is an attenuated variant of major depressive disorder. Dysthymic disorder presents with chronically depressed mood that occurs for most of the day more days than not for at least 2 years (DSM-IV). The terms "neurotic" and "endogenous" depression are usually no longer used and have been replaced by dysthymic disorder (DSM-IV) and major depressive disorder (DSM-IV), respectively. This streamlining of terminologies in part reflects the fact that the newer pharmacological agents (5,6) are effective in the treatment of the psychiatric syndromes that are classified as major depressive disorder under the current nosology (7).

In cases where physical disease including dermatological disorders are present with depression, the DSM-IV (7) outlines the following criteria for assigning a diagnosis for the depression: when it is judged that the disturbance in mood is due to the direct physiological effects of a general medical condition or a substance such as ethanol or corticosteroids, the condition should be diagnosed as mood disorder due to a general medical condition (7), which must be specified, or a substance-related mood disorder (7). This approach does not take into consideration the fact that in many instances the general medical or dermatological condition such as psoriasis or acne or substances such as corticosteroids are not necessarily the primary or sole etiological factor for the depressive disorder. The dermatological condition such as psoriasis or acne is often a precipitating or triggering factor in a patient who may be otherwise predisposed genetically to develop depressive disease. Therefore, because of the very wide scope of the psychosocial and psychiatric dimension in dermatological disorders, a multidimensional biopsychosocial approach, which assesses the relative contribution of both biological and psychosocial factors (8), is probably the most appropriate when assessing the patient with a dermatological disorder who has comorbid depressive disease. Using the DSM-IV classification, the depressive disorder is specified on Axis I and the contributing dermatological condition on Axis III. The major depressive disorder in most dermatological patients represents the final common pathway of multifactorial interacting variables, both dermatological and psychiatric, and depressive disease is diagnosed independent of the presumed cause provided the diagnostic criteria for depressive disease (Table 1) (7) are present.

PSYCHOPATHOLOGY

Depressive disease is a cluster of signs and symptoms (Table 1) that typically manifests as a disturbance in mood; psychomotor activity such as excessive pacing, hair-pulling, rubbing, scratching or picking of the skin; disturbance of vegetative function such as sleep, appetite, sex drive, or, less commonly, other somatic symptoms that can involve the integumentary system; and cognition, including difficulties in concentration, memory, decision making, and excessive concerns about having a serious or life-threatening illness. In some cases psychotic symptoms are encountered where the patient can present with delusions, including delusions that their body is rotting or infested. The symptoms of depression typically cause clinically significant distress or impairment in social, occupational, or other important areas of functioning.

Primary depressive disease can have a prominent somatic component that manifests as a painful physical dysphoria, which is often described as pervasive and relentless. This physical component can be the most prominent feature of depressive disease in some cases. It has long been recognized that the vegetative disturbances associated with depressive disease are a central feature of the syndrome. For example, the term "melancholia," which means black bile, refers back to the Greeks who considered depression to be a somatic illness and ascribed it to black bile. It is well recognized that depressive disorder is accompanied by measurable alterations of circadian rhythms, for example, of cortisol secretion and the sleep-wake cycle. A commonly encountered clinical feature of circadian rhythm disturbance is the worsening of mood, energy, and psychomotor activity early in the day with an improvement as the day progresses. Another disturbance of biological rhythm encountered in mood disorders is seasonal worsening of depressive symptoms in some patients, especially during the fall and winter months. The somatic concerns related to the integumentary system, which are a feature of the underlying depressive disorder, can therefore also manifest a diurnal or seasonal pattern.

Depression is a recurrent disorder, and 50–60% of patients who have experienced one major depressive episode are expected to have a second episode (DSM-IV) (7). In about two thirds of cases the major depressive episode remits completely, and in one third the syndrome remits only partially or not at all (DSM-IV) (7). Chronic general medical conditions are a known risk factor for more persistent episodes of depression. A chronic or recurring dermatological disorder may therefore increase the risk for the persistence of depressive symptoms.

DEPRESSIVE EQUIVALENTS

Cutaneous symptoms may be depressive equivalents (1). Some depressed patients may complain primarily of physical symptoms such as pain, a burning sensation, or other cutaneous dysesthesias for which no physical basis can be identified. Some such patients lack psychological insight and may deny a depressed mood. Such symptoms have been referred to as "depressive equivalents" or "masked depression." Alternately, depressed patients may be excessively preoccupied about a dermatological problem that is minor, such as minimal hair loss, and may express feelings of low self-worth and unattractiveness in association with the relatively minor dermatological problem. More severe depression can be associated with mood-congruent delusions, which can present as a morbid preoccupation with delusions of ill health such as having cancer or acquired immunodeficiency syndrome (AIDS). Some patients may harbor the delusion that part of their body, including their skin, is rotting or disintegrating or emitting a foul odor.

SUICIDE AND PARASUICIDAL BEHAVIOR

Suicide, defined as intentional self-inflicted death, is a central feature of depressive disease. About 50% of all persons who commit suicide are depressed, and 15% of depressed patients eventually kill themselves (9). It is reported that about 35,000 individuals commit suicide every year in the United States and 250,000 individuals attempt suicide every year (9). While women attempt suicide four times more frequently than their male counterparts, men commit suicide three times more often than women (9). The suicide rate in the United States is 12 per 100,000 (9). Among men the suicide rate peaks after age 45 years and among women after age 65 years (9). Overall, suicide rates increase with age, and after age 75 the rate rises in both sexes. Currently the most rapid rise in suicide rates is among males 15–24 years of age (9). Some dermatological disorders such as acne also have a peak incidence among this age group. Therefore, suicidal behavior in the adolescent dermatological patient may not be solely attributable to the psychosocial impact of the skin disorder. The prevalence of suicidal ideation (10) and suicide (11) in certain cosmetically disfiguring dermatological disorders is high even though the disorder may not be life threatening. For example, a 5.6–7.2% prevalence of active suicidal ideation was observed among psoriasis and acne patients, higher than the 2.4–3.3% prevalence of suicidal ideation usually observed general medical patients (10).

A substance abuse disorder such as alcohol abuse in the psoriasis patient also increases suicide risk, especially if the individual is also suffering from depressive disease. Some features associated with a high risk for suicide (9) include frequent, intense, and prolonged suicidal ideation, an unambiguous wish to die, sense of hopelessness, frequent suicide attempts that are planned and/or associated with methods or situations where rescue is difficult, hoarding of pills, self-blame or tendency of the patient to internalize feelings (e.g., difficulties with the expression of anger), and availability of lethal methods such as firearms. Some demographic factors associated with high risk of suicide include male gender, single or divorced status, and unemployment.

Parasuicidal behavior is defined as repeated self-harm or self-injury. In dermatology parasuicidal behavior is encountered frequently, e.g., in the patient with dermatitis artefacta or the patient who repeatedly presents with self-injury such as superficial lacerations of the wrist. A wide range of psychiatric disorders (12) including major depressive disorder (7) may be a factor in such patients. Patients with borderline personality disorder (7), which can coexist with major depressive disorder (7), are at high risk for parasuicidal behaviors. It is important to recognize that such behaviors may lead to serious self-injury or inadvertent death and therefore should be thoroughly evaluated and managed, even when an attention-seeking component is present on the part of the parasuicidal patient.

DEVELOPMENTAL CONSIDERATIONS

The common ectodermal origins of the epidermis and the central nervous system suggest that some dermatological and psychiatric disorders may have a common origin. The skin and sense of touch play an important role in normal psychosocial development. The caregiver's touch, consisting of secure holding, hugging, and consistent caressing, is essential for mental health and social development (13). Contact clinging or care by close skin-to-skin touching is a primary factor in maternal-infant bonding. This early bonding is of considerable importance for the subsequent overall development of the infant. Failure to develop this early and primary mother-infant bond has been associated with depressive disease in later life. These findings lead one to speculate that infants with skin disorders such as infantile eczema, who sometimes experience a deprivation of tactile nurturance in early life, may also be more vulnerable to the development of depression in later life.

An overall developmental approach should be used in the assessment of the depressed dermatology patient, wherein the patient is evaluated within the context of his or her life stage. The psychosocial impact of certain cosmetically disfiguring skin disorders such as acne and psoriasis is usually greater during adolescence and young adulthood in contrast to late adulthood (14), when the patient is not dealing with the typical social and vocational demands of adolescence and young adult life.

DIAGNOSING DEPRESSION IN THE DERMATOLOGICAL PATIENT

The diagnostic criteria for major depressive disorder (Table 1) (7) can serve as a useful and standardized guideline for the dermatologist. It is important to recognize, however, that the diagnosis of depressive disease may be missed if only a one-dimensional checklist of symptoms is used (Table 1). In some patients the most prominent feature of depression can be anxiety, an exaggerated sense of frustration over minor matters, increased irritability, or outbursts of anger or persistent anger. The patient can have a sense of worthlessness or guilt that reaches delusional proportions in some instances. The patient may blame herself or himself for being sick or for having a dermatological disorder.

Following the death of a loved one, some individuals present with symptoms that meet the criteria for a major depressive episode (7). This major life event may precipitate the flare-up of a stress-reactive disorder such as psoriasis or atopic dermatitis. The psychological reaction in the bereaved individual is generally considered to be in the range of normal unless the symptoms of depression are present for 2 months after the loss of the loved one (DSM-IV) (7). However some symptoms are not considered to be characteristic of simple bereavement (DSM-IV), such as guilt about things other than actions taken or not taken by the survivor at the time of death, thoughts of death other than the survivor feeling that he or she should have died with the deceased one, morbid preoccupation with worthlessness, marked psychomotor retardation, prolonged functional impairment, or psychotic symptoms not directly related to the death of the loved one.

Some other features of a major depressive disorder (7) include a definite *change* from the patient's premorbid mental state, and the patient can usually delineate its onset. The symptoms of a major depressive disorder interfere significantly with the patient's daily functioning, for example, in the social, vocational, and/or occupational arenas. These changes are usually measurable by the patient and his or her family members or employer. There is often a past history of major depression and a family history of depressive disease. About two thirds of cases of major depression are recurrent, and patients with recurrent depression usually also have a family history of mood disorders. Patients with recurrent depression usually present with depressive disease at an earlier age than patients who experience only a single episode of depression.

Major depressive disorder can arise in the background of chronic low-grade depression or dysthymic disorder (DSM-IV) (7). This has been referred to as "double depression." Dysthymic disorder typically has an insidious onset of depression dating back to late childhood or the teens, preceding any superimposed major depressive episodes by years or even decades. A return to the low-grade depressive pattern is the rule following recovery from the superimposed acute major depressive episodes. Such patients report being depressed most or all of their lives and experience an attenuated form of major depressive disorder. In the past they were given the label of "characterological depression." Some of the features of dysthymic disorder include chronic low self-esteem or self-confidence or feelings of inadequacy, social withdrawal, subjective feelings of irritability or excessive anger, and difficulty with concentration and indecisiveness. Some of these patients eventually develop major depressive disorder. Such chronic symptoms are often encountered in the adolescent dermatology patient, such as the adolescent with acne, and may be attributed entirely to the skin disorder while the underlying mood disorder may be overlooked.

Premenstrual dysphoric disorder (7) (also referred to as premenstrual syndrome) can be associated with a markedly depressed mood, marked anxiety, and lability of mood during the last week of the luteal phase of the menstrual cycle with remission of symptoms within a few days after the onset of the menses (DSM-IV). Some patients also experience a flare-up of their acne during this period, and their depressive symptoms may be erroneously attributed to their acne.

SPECIFIC DERMATOLOGICAL DISORDERS

Cutaneous Associations of Depressive Disease

Delusions of parasitosis or bromhidrosis or delusions of disfigurement related to the skin may be the feature of a major depressive disorder with psychotic features (7). Body image disorders related to the skin presenting as dermatological nondisease (15) or dermatological complaints that are not consistent with objective findings (e.g., complaints about minimal hair loss, very minimal acne) can be the presenting feature of a major depressive disorder (7). Various cutaneous dysesthesias such as a burning sensation in the scalp or tongue can be a somatic feature of depressive disease. Self-induced dermatoses such as neurotic excoriations and *acne excoriée* are conditions in which lesions are produced as a result of repetitive self-excoriation, which may be initiated by an itch or other cutaneous dysaesthesia, or because of the urge to excoriate an acne pimple or other irregularity on the skin (12). Depressive disease and significant psychosocial stressors have been reported in 33–98% of patients with neurotic excoriations (16,17). Other self-inflicted dermatoses, such as dermatitis artefacta and trichotillomania, are a large and heterogeneous group of disorders where the patients may have wide-ranging underlying psychopathologies including major depressive disorder. Depression and self-injury may complicate the course of other dermatological conditions, e.g., exacerbation of psoriatic lesions secondary to Koebner's phenomenon.

Depression and Primary Dermatological Disorders

Psoriasis

Depressive psychopathology in psoriasis may be primary or secondary to the impact of the disease upon the quality of life of the patient. Psoriasis-related stress has been associated with greater psychiatric morbidity (18). Psoriasis patients who feel stigmatized in social situations have higher depression scores. Adult psoriasis patients who experienced greater touch deprivation in social situations as a result of their psoriasis had higher depression scores than those who did not perceive deprivation of social touch (19). A wide range of psychological characteristics have been reported in various cross-sectional surveys (20), including high depression, high anxiety, and obsessionality or difficulties with verbal expression of emotions (21–24), especially anger (23,24). Early-onset psoriasis has been associated with greater difficulties with expression of anger (24)—a personality trait that may render the patient more vulnerable to stress and depression. Severity of pruritus, which can be one of the most bothersome features of psoriasis, correlates directly with the severity of depressive symptoms (25,26) in psoriasis. The severity of depressive symptoms and suicidal ideation have been shown to correlate with psoriasis severity (27). A 7.2% prevalence of suicidal ideation was observed among severely affected psoriasis inpatients versus a 2.5% suicidal ideation reported by less severely affected psoriasis outpatients (10).

Atopic Dermatitis

School-aged children with moderate to severe atopic dermatitis (AD) are at a greater risk for developing psychological difficulties, which can adversely effect their academic and social development (28). Higher anxiety and depressive symptoms (29–32) have been reported in atopic patients, and anxiety may be a feature of an underlying primary depressive disorder in some AD patients. Adult patients were often chronically anxious and felt ineffective in handling anger in comparison to controls (30,33). Atopic patients with serum IGE > 100 IU/mL showed significantly higher levels of excitability and less adequate stress coping than patients with lower IGE levels (34). Pruritus severity was directly related to severity of depressive symptoms (25) in atopic patients. A study of 10 atopic patients showed no correlation between the severity of psychopathology and chronicity of the skin disorder (35). Chronic intractable eczema in a child may be a sign of a disturbed parent/child relationship (36); however, a major depressive disorder should be ruled out before family problems are implicated (37). Certain immune parameters such as natural killer cell activity may be affected by psychological factors such as high anxiety in atopic patients (38).

Urticaria and Angioedema

A wide range of personality characteristics was described in earlier literature (39,40), with the most frequently reported being difficulties involved with expression of anger and hostility in association with the need for approval from others. These personality traits are classically known to predispose the patient to develop depressive disease. Thirty-four patients with chronic idiopathic urticaria had lower depression scores than 34 patients with idiopathic generalized pruritus (41). However, pruritus severity in urticaria increased with increasing severity of depressive symptoms (25).

Alopecia Areata

Patients whose alopecia areata (AA) was exacerbated by stress also had higher depression scores, suggesting that comorbid depression may render the condition more stress reactive (42); 33–93% incidence of psychiatric illness has been reported in patients with alopecia areata (43). Among 31 AA patients surveyed, 74% had a lifetime prevalence of one or more psychiatric disorders with a 39% prevalence of major depression and 39% prevalence of anxiety disorder (44). Among 294 AA patients surveyed, the prevalence of major depression was 8.8%, generalized anxiety disorder 18.2%, and paranoid disorder 4.4%, with an overall 23.3% prevalence of at least one psychiatric disorder (45).

Acne

Higher anxiety levels in cystic acne have been associated with higher blood catecholamine levels (46), which decreased with treatment of the acne, suggesting that the psychosocial impact of acne can be associated with significant physiological stress for the patient. The stress resulting from the impact of acne upon the quality of life can be very disabling (47), comparable to the disability resulting from chronic disorders such as diabetes and asthma. The impact of acne upon quality of life often does not correlate strongly with the clinical severity of acne (48), as some patients with even mild acne are severely psychosocially disabled by their disorder. Mild to moderate acne has been associated with significant psychological morbidity, including depression and suicidal ideation (10) and completed suicide (11). A 5.6% prevalence of suicidal ideation was observed among patients with noncystic facial acne (10). Acne patients who experience problems at school or work and blame it mainly on their acne may be clinically depressed (48). Anxiety and anger are important factors in acne (49); treatment of both mild to moderate noncystic acne (50) and treatment of cystic acne with isotretinoin have been associated with an improvement in the psychological morbidity such as anxiety and depression (51). In some instances of chronic acne, some of the psychological morbidity may persist at the end of treatment after the acne has improved because of the impact of acne on psychosocial development and the long-term impact of acne (52,53). This finding underlines the importance of treating even mild acne aggressively if the disorder is psychosocially distressing for the patient.

Discussion

Most of the disorders described above have been associated with both psychosocial stress, which typically further exacerbates the disorder, and/or psychiatric and psychopathological factors, such as depression and anxiety. The stress resulting from the stigma experience associated with disorders like psoriasis can lead to a depressive reaction (19). Major depressive disorder (7) and suicidal ideation (10) can contribute to significant morbidity in a wide range of dermatological disorders. Completed suicide is associated with dermatological disorders (11), and disfigurement caused by the skin disorder was believed to be a major contributing factor. The relationship between depressive disease and skin disorders, however, can be complex and multidimensional. The severity of depressive symptoms correlates directly with disease severity in psoriasis (27), but this is not a consistent finding in acne, where even mild to moderate acne has been associated with depression scores that were similar to patients with more severe psoriasis (10). In contrast to psoriasis (27), some cross-sectional studies of acne patients do not consistently show a direct correlation between the clinical severity of acne and the severity of depressive symptoms. However, prospective studies involving treatment of the acne have shown that psychological morbidity in both mild to moderate noncystic acne (50) and more severe cystic acne (51) improved with treatment of the acne. Acne has a peak incidence during adolescence, a life stage when the individual is normally highly invested in his or her appearance and body image. In some vulnerable adolescents the impact of even mild acne may add to their existing psychological burden and result in significant depression, explaining the lack of a consistent correlation between acne severity and the severity of the depression scores in cross-sectional studies. This is further supported by the finding that acne and other body image pathologies, such as eating disorders, may coexist (54,55), and conditions such as *acne excoriée des jeunes filles* present with psychological dynamics that are very similar to dynamics encountered in adolescents with eating disorders, such as difficulties coping with the emerging developmental tasks of young adulthood (56). Eating disorders are often comorbid with major depressive disorder and substance abuse disorders (7).

Depression can modulate itch perception in a wide range of pruritic disorders such as psoriasis, atopic dermatitis, and chronic idiopathic urticaria (25,26). The severity of depression correlates with pruritus severity (25,26), and improvement in pruritus has been associated with an improvement in depression scores in psoriasis (26). These findings suggest that if depression is comorbid with pruritus, treatment of the depression may have a beneficial effect on the symptom of pruritus.

The impact of the skin disorder upon the quality of life of the patient can result in significant psychological and psychiatric pathology, e.g., major depressive disorder (Table 1). In some disorders like psoriasis and acne, psychological comorbidity can be one of the most bothersome features of the disorder. The psychosocial stress resulting from the impact of the skin condition upon the quality of life can in turn have an adverse impact upon the course of some stress-reactive dermatoses, such as psoriasis and atopic dermatitis. These findings suggest that when a skin condition is reported to be adversely affecting the quality of life of the patient, it should be treated aggressively, even if it is mild according to the clinical dermatological examination. Group psychotherapy (57) can help the patient to cope with the stresses of having to live with a chronic disfiguring condition while providing social support and possibly preventing the onset of depression as a result of having to live with a chronic skin disorder.

It is important to recognize the presence of clinical depression in the acne patient. As discussed earlier, while depressive symptoms in acne can be a reaction to the body image concerns caused by acne the relationship between acne and depression appears to be a multifactorial problem. In some instances the depressive symptoms are grossly out of proportion to the cosmetic problems caused by the acne. In fact, a study comparing the prevalence of depressive symptoms among patients with mild to moderate noncystic facial acne vulgaris, moderate to severe psoriasis, atopic dermatitis, and alopecia areata found a 5.6% prevalence of suicidal ideation among the acne patients, which was comparable to the 5.5% prevalence of suicidal ideation among the more severely affected psoriasis patients (10). The acne patients in this study (10) were mainly adolescents and young adults, and this finding may in part be indicative of the fact that this age group is also typically more vulnerable to the development of depressive disease, independent of whether or not they have acne. The presence of clinical depression in acne sometimes can complicate the use of isotretinoin, which has been sporadically associated with depression, suicidal behavior, and other psychiatric reactions (58). When depressive symptoms are present in the acne patient who is also using isotretinoin, the depression may or may not be related to the isotretinoin. A careful history will reveal whether or not the onset or exacerbation of depressive symptoms is temporally related to initiating isotretinoin therapy. The depressed acne patient should always be assessed for suicide risk.

REFERENCES

1. Gupta MA, Gupta AK. Psychodermatology: an update. J Am Acad Dermatol 34:1030–1046, 1996.
2. Medansky RS, Handler RM. Dermatopsychosomatics: classification, physiology, and therapeutic approaches. J Am Acad Dermatol 5:125–136, 1981.
3. Koblenzer CS. Psychosomatic concepts in dermatology. Arch Dermatol 119:501–512, 1983.
4. Panconesi P. Psychosomatic dermatology. Clin Dermatol 2:94–179, 1984.
5. Koo JYM, Pham CT. Psychodermatology—practical guidelines on pharmacotherapy. Arch Dermatol 1992; 126:381–388.
6. Gupta MA, Gupta AK. The use of psychotropic drugs in dermatology. Dermatol Clin 2000; 18:711–725.
7. American Psychiatric Association. Diagnostic and Statistical Manual of Mental Disorders. 4th ed. Washington, DC: American Psychiatric Publishing, 1994.
8. Engel GL. The clinical application of the biopsychosocial model. Am J Psychiatry 137; 535–544, 1980.
9. Sadock BJ, Sadock VA. Kaplan & Sadock's Pocket Book of Clinical Psychiatry. 3rd ed. Philadelphia: Lippincott Williams & Wilkins, 2001:261–274.

10. Gupta MA, Gupta AK. Depression and suicidal ideation in dermatology patients with acne, alopecia areata, atopic dermatitis and psoriasis. Br J Dermatol 139:846–850, 1998.

11. Cotterill JA, Cunliffe WJ. Suicide in dermatological patients. Br J Dermatol 137; 246–250, 1997.

12. Gupta MA, Gupta AK, Haberman HF. The self-inflicted dermatoses: a critical review. Gen Hosp Psychiatry 1987; 9:45–52.

13. Krueger DW. Body Self and Psychological Self. New York: Brunner/Mazel, 1989:3–31.

14. Gupta MA, Gupta AK. Age and gender differences in the impact of psoriasis upon the quality of life. Int J Dermatol 34:700–703, 1995.

15. Cotterill JA. Dermatologic non-disease: a common and potentially fatal disturbance of cutaneous body image. Br J Dermatol 104:611–619, 1981.

16. Freunsgaard K. Neurotic excoriations, a controlled psychiatric examination. Acta Psychiatr Scand 69 (suppl):1–52, 1984.

17. Gupta MA, Gupta AK, Haberman HF. Neurotic excoriations: a review and some new perspectives. Compr Psychiatry 27:381–386, 1986.

18. Fortune DG, Main CJ, O'Sullivan TM, Griffiths CE. Quality of life in patients with psoriasis: the contribution of clinical variables and psoriasis-specific stress. Br J Dermatol 137:755–760, 1997.

19. Gupta MA, Gupta AK, Watteel GN. Perceived deprivation of social touch in psoriasis is associated with greater psychological morbidity: an index of the stigma experience in dermatologic disorders. Cutis 61:339–34, 1998.

20. Gupta MA, Gupta AK, Haberman HF. Psoriasis and psychiatry: an update. Gen Hosp Psychiatry 9:157–166, 1987.

21. Vidoni D, Campiutti E, D'Aronco R, De Vanna M, Aguglia E. Psoriasis and alexithymia. Acta Derm Venereol (Stockh) 146:91–92, 1989.

22. Rubino IA, Sonnino A, Stefanto CM, Pezzarossa B, Ciani N. Separation-individuation, aggression and alexithymia in psoriasis. Acta Derm Venereol (Stockh) 146:87–90, 1989.

23. Niemeier V, Fritz J, Kupfer J, Gieler U. Aggressive verbal behaviour as a function of experimentally induced anger in persons with psoriasis. Eur J Dermatol 9:555–558, 1999.

24. Gupta MA, Gupta AK, Watteel G. Early onset (<age 40 years) psoriasis is associated with greater psychopathology than late onset psoriasis. Acta Dermato-Venereol 76:464–466, 1996.

25. Gupta MA, Gupta AK, Schork NJ, Ellis CN. Depression modulates pruritus perception: a study of pruritus in psoriasis, atopic dermatitis, and chronic idiopathic urticaria. Psychosom Med 56:36–40, 1994.

26. Gupta MA, Gupta AK, Kirkby S, Weiner HK, Mace TM, Schork NJ, Johnson EH, Ellis CN, Voorhees JJ. Pruritus in psoriasis: a prospective study of some psychiatric and dermatologic correlates. Arch Dermatol 124:1052–1057, 1988.

27. Gupta MA, Schork NJ, Gupta AK, Kirkby S, Ellis CN. Suicidal ideation in psoriasis. Int J Dermatol 32:188–190, 1993.

28. Absolon CM, Cottrell D, Eldridge SM, Glover MT. Psychological disturbance in atopic eczema: the extent of the problem in school-aged children. Br J Dermatol 137:241–245, 1997.

29. Al-Ahmar HF, Kurban AK. Psychological profile of patients with atopic dermatitis. Br J Dermatol 95:373–377, 1976.

30. White A, Horne DJ, Varigos GA. Psychological profile of the atopic eczema patient. Australas J Dermatol 1990; 31:13–16.

31. Linnet J, Jemec GB. An assessment of anxiety and dermatology quality of life in patients with atopic dermatitis. Br J Dermatol 140:268–272, 1999.

32. Hashiro M, Okumura M. Anxiety, depression and psychosomatic symptoms in patients with atopic dermatitis: comparison with normal controls and among groups of different degrees of severity. J Dermatol Sci 14:63–67, 1997.

33. Ginsburg IH, Prystowsky JH, Kornfeld DS, Wolland H. Role of emotional factors in adults with atopic dermatitis. Int J Dermatol 32:656–660, 1993.

34. Scheich G, Florin I, Rudolph R, Wilhelm S. Personality characteristics and serum IgE level in patients with atopic dermatitis. J Psychosom Res 37:637–642, 1993.

35. Ullman KC, Moore RW, Reidy M. Atopic eczema: a clinical psychiatric study. J Asthma Res 14:91–99, 1977.

36. Koblenzer CS, Koblenzer PJ. Chronic intractable atopic eczema. Arch Dermatol 124:1673–1677, 1988.

37. Allen AD. Intractable atopic eczema suggests major affective disorder: poor parenting is secondary (lett). Arch Dermatol 125:567–568, 1989.

38. Hashiro M, Okumura M. The relationship between the psychological and immunological in patients with atopic dermatitis. J Dermatol Sci 16:231–235, 1998.

39. Rees L. An aetiological study of chronic urticaria and angioneurotic oedema. J Psychosom Res 2:172–189, 1957.

40. Juhlin L. Recurrent urticaria: clinical investigations of 330 patients. Br J Dermatol 104:369–381, 1981.

41. Sheehan-Dare RA, Henderson MJ, Cotterill JA. Anxiety and depression in patients with chronic urticaria and generalized pruritus. Br J Dermatol 123:769–774, 1990.

42. Gupta MA, Gupta AK, Watteel GN. Stress and alopecia areata: a psychodermatologic study. Acta Dermato-Venereol (Stockh) 77:296–298, 1997.

43. Sandok BA. Alopecia areata: an apparent relationship to psychic factors. Am J Psychiatry 1964; 121:184–185.

44. Colon EA, Popkin MK, Callies AL, Dessert NJ, Hordinsky MK. Lifetime prevalence of psychiatric disorders in patients with alopecia areata. Compr Psychiatry 32:245–251, 1991.

45. Koo JYM, Shellow WV, Hallman CP, Edwards JE. Alopecia areata and increased prevalence of psychiatric disorders. Int J Dermatol 33:849–850, 1994.

46. Schulpis K, Georgala S, Papakonstantinou ED, Michas T. Psychological and sympatho-adrenal status in patients with cystic acne. J Eur Acad Dermatol Venereol 13:24–27, 1999.

47. Mallon E, Newton JN, Klassen A, Stewart-Brown SL, Ryan TJ, Finlay AY. The quality of life in acne: a comparison with general medical conditions using generic questionnaires. Br J Dermatol 140:672–676, 1999.

48. Gupta MA, Johnson AM, Gupta AK. The development of an Acne Quality of Life scale: reliability, validity, and relation to subjective acne severity in mild to moderated acne vulgaris. Acta Derm Venereol 78:451–456, 1998.

49. Wu SF, Kinder BN, Trunnell TN, Fulton JE. Role of anxiety and anger in acne patients: a relationship with severity of the disorder. J Am Acad Dermatol 18 (2 pt 1):325–333, 1988.

50. Gupta MA, Gupta AK, Schork NJ, Ellis CN, Voorhees JJ. Psychiatric aspects of the treatment of mild to moderate facial acne: some preliminary observations. Int J Dermatol 29:719–721, 1990.

51. Rubinow DR, Peck GL, Squillace KM, Gantt GG. Reduced anxiety and depression in cystic acne patients after successful treatment with oral isotretinoin. J Am Acad Dermatol 17:25–32, 1987.

52. Layton AM, Seukeran D, Cunliffe WJ. Scarred for life? Dermatology 195 (suppl):15–21, 1997.

53. Kellett SC, Gawkrodger DJ. The psychological and emotional impact of acne and the effect of treatment with isotretinoin. Br J Dermatol 140 (2):273–282, 1999.

54. Gupta MA, Gupta AK, Haberman HF. Dermatologic signs in anorexia nervosa and bulimia nervosa. Arch Dermatol 1987; 123:1386–1390.

55. Gupta MA, Gupta AK. Dermatological complications. Eur Eating Disord Rev 8:134–143, 2000.

56. Sneddon J, Sneddon I. Acne excoriee: a protective device. Clin Exp Derm 8:65–68, 1983.

57. Seng TK, Nee TS. Group therapy: a useful and supportive treatment for psoriasis patients. Int J Dermatol 1997; 36(2):110–112.

58. Gupta MA, Gupta AK. The psychological comorbidity in acne. Clin Dermatol 2001; 19:360–363.

17

Psychosocial Impact of Androgenetic Alopecia

Ramon Grimalt
University of Barcelona
Barcelona, Spain

INTRODUCTION

Currently available reports in the literature suggest that male pattern baldness can be associated with significant impact on quality of life, often with very serious psychological problems (1). Negative effects have been reported, which include lower self-esteem, perception of physical unattractiveness, depression, emotional distress, greater self-consciousness, anxiety, and psychosocial maladjustment, as well as dissatisfaction with appearance, preoccupation with hair loss, worry about others' reactions, and fear of social teasing. Further studies suggest that people's initial impression of men with male pattern baldness is generally less favorable than that of men without hair loss. Balding men are viewed as less desirable in a physical, personal, and social sense.

On the other hand, Maffei et al. (2) suggest that the presence of a preexisting personality disorder may determine whether a person has a psychological problem with alopecia. The same degree of alopecia will be tolerated differently depending on the preexisting personality or psychological disorder of the balding man (3). Dermatologists might be more helpful if they were aware that patients who present with the physical symptom of androgenetic alopecia may also have preexisting psychopathological symptoms. The question that arises when treating a patient with male pattern baldness is: Will he be better treated and consequently more satisfied if he receives effective antialopecia agents, or will he get more benefit if evaluated and treated for his psychological disorder?

Despite arguments that the study of its psychological and sociological implications is frivolous, hair is extremely important in our life. Another person's hair is one of the first characteristics we notice upon meeting. Our own hair is one of the first and last characteristics we attend to before a meeting or a social engagement (4).

For clinicians who treat patients with a range of diseases, many of them severe or life threatening, it may be hard to take seriously the effect of male pattern hair loss (MPHL) on the quality of life of those affected by it. But as we will discuss in this chapter, despite being so common, male pattern hair loss can still have a significant negative impact on those who experience it. MPHL, or androgenetic alopecia (AGA), is one of the most common problems that we dermatologists find among our daily patients.

It is clear that throughout history, hair on the human head has had great symbolic importance. Frequently cited examples of this include the biblical story in which Samson loses his exceptional physical strength when his hair is cut off, the scalping of defeated enemies practiced in many cultures, and the punishment of female collaborators after the liberation of occupied France by shaving off their hair (5).

Hair obviously has great importance as a social indicator, but social norms change over time within cultures. For example, hair that was considered outrageously long for an American male at the beginning of the 1940s looked conservative by the end of the same decade.

Hair growth and hair style are, of course, important elements of an individual's identity, both for the individuals themselves (as when a person refers to a new hair style as "a change of image") and their identity as perceived by others. Hair strongly influences whether or not a person is seen as physically attractive (4). Moreover, studies over the last 20 years (6) have confirmed the consistent advantage in most human interactions of being perceived as attractive (by the standards of a particular culture) and, conversely, the social disadvantage conferred by being considered unattractive, especially when it is caused by a dermatological condition (7). The consequences of such behavior can extend beyond personal isolation to extremes that include overt discrimination in employment practices.

Given the psychological and symbolic importance of hair and the fact that its removal is used as a punishment in many cultures, it is not surprising that hair loss may have a potentially adverse impact on a person's quality of life. Unfortunately, this impact is often trivialized or even ignored by those not affected by it. Many studies have verified the psychological difficulties experienced by men with AGA (5,8–19).

ANDROGENETIC ALOPECIA

Many of the cases attending a dermatological practice complaining of hair loss are due to androgenetic alopecia. Fifty percent of men aged 50 years and 40% of women in menopause have some degree of AGA. Hair loss is gradual, with miniaturization of genetically programmed hair follicles. Uptake, metabolism, and conversion of testosterone to dihydrotestosterone by 5-alpha-reductase is increased in balding hair follicles. In men with AGA, hair loss occurs in the fronto-temporal regions and on the vertex of the scalp, depending on severity. In female AGA patients hair loss is more diffuse and located centroparietally. The frontal hairline is usually intact in women (20).

Treatment is either medical or surgical. The only proven medications indicated for AGA are topical minoxidil (Rogaine®) and oral finasteride (Propecia®). Minoxidil's success for cosmetically acceptable regrowth is approximately 10% in men (4). In women, 50% show minimal regrowth and 13% moderate regrowth. Treatment is lifelong. Seven percent of patients may experience some irritation (burning, itching, redness) from the minoxidil solution. The 5% minoxidil solution has greater efficacy than the 2% minoxidil solution (21). Finasteride has recently been shown to have significant efficacy in male AGA. Finasteride reversed hair loss in 66% of men and stabilized hair loss in 83% of men after 2 years of follow-up (22). In women, the use of a systemic antiandrogen such as spironolactone (Aldactone®) 50–200 mg per day, cyproterone acetate (Androcur®), or flutamide (Eulexin®) may have some benefit in reducing the amount of hair thinning. Finasteride in not indicated in women (23). Transplantation of permanent hairs from the back and sides of the scalp to balding areas in the front is a successful procedure but usually requires three to four sessions over 2 years to fill an area with adequate density. The advent of mini- and micrografting has revolutionized hair transplantation into a more natural-looking process, eliminating clumping or tufting. Donor harvesting with strips rather than plugs has made the donor site more cosmetically acceptable. Hair transplantation is useful not only in men but also in women.

PHYSICAL ATTRACTIVENESS PHENOMENON

Selective social science data about physical attractiveness that is partially determined by hair can be reasonably generalized as social science data that specifically focus on hair. Given interdependencies between hair and physical attractiveness, these relationships reflect a straightforward extrapolation of knowledge. As a result, psychological and sociological information regarding hair exists in a robust body of social science research. In several studies performed on physical attractiveness, hair was rated as "important," "very important," and "significant" (2,3,5). We analyze here articles that have covered the physical attractiveness phenomenon regarding not only hair, but other dermatological and cosmetic issues that are highly significant and can help us to better understand the problem. The fundamental assumptions of the physical attractiveness phenomenon are: 1) physical attractiveness serves as an informational cue to infer extensive information about a person, and 2) the phenomenon is pervasive, subtle, and powerful (4).

Determinants of physical attractiveness are not restricted to physical body characteristics. Determinants identified included the face and facial features, body parts and dimensions, tangible enhancements such as clothes and cosmetics, and intangible perceptions such as reputation and accomplishments, environmental factors, and familiarity. Some rank order of facial determinants has been reported in two separate studies. In order of rated importance, the oral region, eyes, facial structure, hair, and nose were indicated in one study (24). In another interesting study (25), the mouth was the most influential component, closely followed by the eyes, hair, and nose.

HAIR

Many interesting papers have discussed non-AGA hair aspects related to psyche. Psychological research in an earlier era investigated the possible relationship between hair and psychopathy, mental deficiency, and emotionality. When no relationship was found, later efforts focused on preferences and stereotypes that are evident in conversation, folklore, and literature (4).

A very peculiar study from 1978 (26) deals with the characteristics of an "ideal" mate. Men indicated that they preferred blondes, and both sexes showed an aversion to persons of the opposite sex with red hair. Furthermore, women generally preferred men with darker hair and men generally preferred women with lighter hair. One's own hair color is of concern for both sexes, especially as an indicator of age. For men, anecdotal evidence is apparent in major marketing expenditures for hair-coloring products. It is reasonable to expect that more men will use such products in the future (27).

As with physical attractiveness, judgments related to hair revealed substantial agreement between judges (28) as well as substantial stereotypes. For example, people expect blondes to be less intelligent, redheads to be less serious (29), and men with greater hairiness to be more sexually potent (30). Also, men with relatively long hair generally make a markedly negative impression (31–35), are associated with liberal social attitudes (36), and are less compliant with instructions (37). This effect was minimized, however, when the hair length of stimulus persons was similar to that of the judges (38–40).

Having a good haircut, having pleasant smelling hair, and the impression of clean hair also seem to be extremely important. In a study performed in 1980 (41), male and female judges were asked to rate professional women used as stimulus persons in four experimental conditions: before and after cosmetic treatment and before and after hair treatment. In the post–hair treatment condition, the stimulus persons were rated as more caring, warm, sincere, reliable, poised, likely to make an effort, kind, sensitive, organized, and popular!

PSYCHOLOGICAL ASPECTS OF MALE ANDROGENETIC ALOPECIA

The motivation to avoid baldness is not unique to modern times. Trade routes and mining activities of Egyptians in 1500B.C. provide evidence of a "deep need to find ingredients to grow hair on balding heads" (42). In modern society the same attitude is readily evident from the many available remedies such as massages, creams, hormones, vitamins, hairpieces, wigs, hair weaves, suturing of synthetic fibers into bald scalps, surgical scalp reduction, and surgical hair transplants. In the United States during the 1980s, 300,000 over-the-counter products claimed to help reverse balding (37).

Despite the accepted association of psychological effects and male pattern baldness, few studies have been conducted to investigate and quantify this relationship. Of those that have been reported, most have relied on selected samples of men seeking medical attention for their hair loss and may not be representative.

Currently available reports in the literature suggest that male pattern baldness can be associated with significant impact on quality of life and often very serious psychological problems (43,44). Negative effects include lower self-esteem, perceptions of physical unattractiveness, psychological disorders, depression, emotional distress, greater self-consciousness, anxiety, and psychosocial maladjustment. In addition, dissatisfaction with appearance, preoccupation with hair loss, worry about the reactions of others, and fear of social teasing have also been reported (43–45). Results from a study by Cash (43) suggested that more than 25% of men find hair loss extremely upsetting and 62% reported modest to moderate emotional distress.

The men who may be most affected by hair loss are more self-conscious, poorly adjusted, romantically uninvolved, strongly dissatisfied with their hair, more invested in their appearance, and perhaps younger men (44) (Table 1). In a study of psychologically well-adjusted men (45), about 20% reported discomfort in the presence of women, feeling less attractive, feeling much older, and little understanding from others regarding their hair problems. Nearly one quarter of the subjects reported worrying about baldness and consideration of hair transplant, over 30% of the men were annoyed by baldness jokes, and 41% reported that others underestimated their hair problems. Surprisingly, only 37% of them had tried medical therapy for baldness. Some authors (46) have suggested that physicians should be cognizant of the psychological component as well as the physical aspects of androgenetic alopecia, and one report (2) further suggested that even partial improvement of body image through medical treatment may reduce the psychological symptoms associated with this condition.

A 1971 article (47) investigated 11 bipolar scales related to quantity of scalp hair (regular, balding, and bald) as well as color, length, and quality of scalp hair. Slides of the same stimulus person were manipulated through a modification made by a commercial artist. The results revealed that the stimulus person with a normal quantity of hair was rated as most handsome, virile, strong, active, and sharp. The balding person was rated as least potent, weak, dull, and inactive, and the baldest was rated as most unkind, bad, and ugly (47) (Table 2).

Aversion to balding is understandable in the context of the psychological and sociological dimensions of hair. In fact, any factor that

TABLE 1 Characteristics of Men Most Affected by Hair Loss

Self-conscious
Poorly adjusted
Romantically uninvolved
Strongly dissatisfied with their hair
More investment in their appearance
Younger

TABLE 2 Perception of a Stimulus Person Modified by a Commercial Artist

Regular hair	Balding	Bald
Handsome	Least potent	Most unkind
Virile	Weak	Bad
Strong	Dull	Ugly
Active	Inactive	Sharp

Source: Ref. 47.

lowers physical attractiveness by contributing to the appearance of aging is important to individuals.

De Koning et al. (18) performed a survey of general practice physicians who were requested to fill out a questionnaire on the last male and female patients who had consulted them regarding a scalp or hair problem. The questionnaire requested details of any psychological problems that were present and the treatment advice given. Forty-eight percent of the men complained about baldness and 28% about hair loss. Almost 34% consulted their physician more than once about a scalp or hair problem. Psychological problems were reported by physicians in about half of the male patients. The psychological problems most reported for men were low self-esteem (26%) and depression (9%). Regarding therapeutic options given to men, 58% of the men received information on AGA, 30% were prescribed minoxidil (this study was performed before the finasteride era), 28% were referred to a dermatologist, but no psychological referral was given to any of them. This study does point out that a large percentage of men who consult their physician about hair loss may have psychological problems, particularly low self-esteem and depression, and that there is lack of psychological support from general practitioners for these patients.

In fact, as dermatologists we have the sensation that patients affected by severe AGA are not the ones who consult more frequently. Some patients with minimal and initial fronto-temporal balding will urgently seek help from their dermatologist, and this might hide a masked depression, personal dissatisfaction, or a high degree of anxiety (6). On the other hand, patients with severe AGA (degrees IV and V in the Hamilton classification) did not always seek treatment. It is possible that only psychologically disturbed patients affected by AGA are likely to seek advice. From our point of view, and as stated by Koblenzer in regard to alopecia areata (7,48), it is not important to differentiate if the psychological disturbance present in a patient affected by hair loss was present before or appeared after the onset of the baldness: the patient is both balding and psychologically disturbed when looking for advice. The question arises whether this group of patients would respond better if treated with hair-related products (e.g., finasteride, minoxidil) or with psycho-related products (3).

On the other hand, totally opposite results have been reported. Van der Donk et al. (49) concluded that there was no indication of psychological malfunctioning in a sample of 168 men participating in a minoxidil clinical trial. Results indicated that subjects had a more positive psychological state than normative groups. The authors attributed this to the selection process of the study. Subjects volunteered to enroll at the invitation of the study centers instead of consulting a physician regarding their AGA. The authors speculate that this may have discouraged the more psychologically disturbed men from responding.

In 1992 Cash (43) performed an interesting study on the psychological effects of balding. He collected healthy males from 31 barbershops and hair salons in Virginia and classified them according to the Norwood-Hamilton classification. The sample of 145 participants was asked to answer the Hair Loss Effects Questionnaire (43), which listed 70 possible effects of AGA, including emotional, cognitive, and behavioral events. AGA patients indicated how their hair loss affected them on a 5-point rating of each item. Standardized measures were used to assess body image satisfaction, social self-esteem, social anxiety, public self-consciousness, sexual self-confidence, and locus of control (a person's belief system about his extent of control over events in his life). The results from the study are contradictory: the reported effects of balding reflected considerable preoccupation, moderate stress or distress, and copious coping efforts. These effects were especially salient among men with more extensive balding and among younger men, single men, and those with an earlier hair-loss onset. Relative to control, balding men had less body-image satisfaction yet were comparable on other personality indexes. The conclusions were that although most men regard hair loss to be an unwanted, distressing experience that diminishes their body image, balding men actively cope and generally retain the integrity of their personality function.

In 1993 Franzoi et al. (50) performed a study evaluating the relationship between public self-consciousness and perceptions of thinning hair. Ninety-one men waiting for flight departure in an international airport were asked to complete two questionnaires that were part of two separate research studies—a physical appearance study and a personal reaction study—conducted by a nearby university. Initially subjects were unaware of what the real purpose of the study was. Subjects were later debriefed after completing both surveys. The personal reaction questionnaire contained two subscales: a public self-consciousness scale (tendency to be aware and concerned about public aspects of self) and a private self-consciousness scale (tendency to be aware of nonvisible aspects of self). The physical appearance questionnaire asked questions about the subjects' hair pattern, worry and concern over hair loss, and negative consequences of thinning hair. Results indicated that 47% of the men agreed that men with thinning hair are less attractive, and 59% percent disagreed that women are less likely to date balding men.

Maffei et al. in 1994 (2) investigated the prevalence of personality disorders and psychopathological symptoms in patients who received a diagnosis of AGA when consulting an outpatient clinic. Nearly 79% of patients surveyed were diagnosed with at least one personality disorder as defined by the DSM-IIIR. Maffei's overall conclusion was that the presence of a preexisting personality disorder, but not necessarily gender, may determine whether a person has a psychological problem with alopecia.

From this paper arises once again the previously discussed issue that dermatologists should be aware that patients who present with the physical symptom of androgenetic alopecia may also have preexisting psychopathological symptoms. Furthermore, Maffei et al. stated that the restoration of a positive body image (even partially) induced by medical treatment of AGA could reduce the underlying psychopathological symptoms associated with AGA. Dawber (46) points out that by the time patients seek care for their hair loss, they tend to be highly anxious. So, once again the question arises: would these patients respond better to a psychological approach rather than a dermatological treatment?

In 1995 Wells et al. (44) performed a study on 182 men 19–73 years old divided into three groups—full head, semi-bald, and bald. The men completed a self-report questionnaire that evaluated several psychosocial domains (self-esteem, depression, psychosis, introversion, neurosis, and feelings of unattractiveness). Results indicated that degree of baldness adjusted for age was associated with lower self-esteem, higher depression, higher introversion, higher neurosis, and greater feeling of unattractiveness (Table 3). In addition, lower self-esteem, lower levels of psychosis and

TABLE 3 Traits Associated with Baldness[a]

Lower self-esteem
Higher depression
Higher introversion
Higher neuroticism
Greater feeling of unattractiveness

[a]Adjusted for age.

higher levels of introversion were also associated with increasing age independent of degree of baldness. The results also suggested that lower self-esteem, higher introversion, and greater feeling of unattractiveness were more pronounced in younger men with AGA. The authors stated that premature hair loss clearly has a major impact on intimate relationships, social life, self-confidence, self-perception of attractiveness, as well as on careers.

In 1998 Camacho (51) performed a retrospective study on 100 female AGA sufferers (FAGA) and the same number of male AGA patients (MAGA) with the objective of proving the psychological features of patients with male and female AGA. The conclusions were that anxiety is more frequent in FAGA than in MAGA (92/30%), that aggressiveness is more frequent in MAGA than in FAGA (8/6%), and that females have more aggressive tendencies than males (66/3%). Also, 89% of FAGA and 76% of MAGA improved with medical treatment, and they both attended equally follow-up sessions. Three percent of FAGA and 12% of MAGA asked for surgical treatment, and 8% of FAGA and 12% of MAGA were considered as lost to follow-up. The psychological characteristics of patients with AGA indicate an elusive person who, although accompanied to the trichology center, always enters the consultation room alone, at least for the trichological examination. Camacho reported that these patients usually try to avoid the physician obtaining hairs for the trichogram, and some MAGA even rejected this technique. They usually accept medical or surgical treatment, but they habitually telephone before the preestablished date because they did not see the good results they hoped for.

Tisher recently performed a more frivolous but interesting study (B. Tisher, personal communication, 2000) on balding men's chances of success with women. He states that men with a full head of hair have a six times greater chance of success with women than balding men (with a bald crown). This conclusion was drawn from a study in which women were questioned about their choice of partner. Three hundred and eighty-six responders between 20 and 40 years of age were shown photos of six men, two of whom had a bald crown. They were asked to choose a man as a partner for various roles. Of 1544 male candidates with a full head of hair, 23% were chosen as partners, compared to only 3.6% of the 772 balding men. The results for the choice of partner for a one-night stand (23% of men with a full head of hair chosen vs. 3.4% of balding men) and for the choice of an ideal father of the respondent's children (22% vs. 4%) were similarly devastating for balding men. Balding men had a somewhat better chance of being selected as a good friend in whom to confide without being a lover or partner. Nevertheless, only 12% of balding men were chosen as a good friend compared to 19% of men with a full head of hair (Table 4).

TABLE 4   Effect of Hair Loss on Choice of a Man as Partner for
Different Roles

Role	Percent Chosen	
	Balding	Full head of hair
Partner	4	23
Partner for a one-night stand	3	23
Ideal father for my children	4	22
Good friend in whom to confide	12	19

PSYCHOLOGICAL ASPECTS OF FEMALE ANDROGENETIC ALOPECIA

Hair loss due to androgenetic alopecia in women often begins with perceptible thinning at the crown of the head. As hair loss progresses, density of the hair in the vertex region of the scalp becomes more rarified; however, the frontal hairline is almost always retained. Women with AGA are usually hormonally normal, but if the hair loss is associated with hirsutism or hipertrichosis, hormonal studies should be started. In rare cases, hormonally normal women may express the phenotype of balding observed in men (52,53).

The negative psychological impact of hair loss has been documented in both men and women, as we have already seen. Women, however, may experience the effects of hair loss to a greater extent than men (54,55). The increased distress experienced by women may stem from social and self-imposed pressure for physical attractiveness and a concern about deviating from what is considered normal female appearance. Studies (56) have revealed that women with AGA experience increased self-consciousness, feelings of unattractiveness, social withdrawal, emotional stress, and worry as a result of hair loss compared with women without hair loss or men with hair loss (54,55).

The psychological impact of AGA is more severe for women than for men. Compared with men, about twice as many (and the majority of) women expressed that they were either "very" or "extremely upset" by their hair loss (54). The only reported effects that may be more difficult for men are the receipt of more teasing and social comments about their hair loss and men's belief that hair loss gives an aging appearance.

Relative to controls, women with AGA not only had much more dissatisfaction with their hair, but they experienced more negative overall body-image as well. In addition, they reported more social anxiety, poorer self-esteem and psychosocial well-being, less sense of control over their lives, and a less satisfying quality of life.

Physicians should recognize that AGA goes well beyond the mere physical aspects of hair loss and growth, as has been observed for other appearance-altering conditions such as acne. Cash et al. (54) reported that the patient's psychological reactions to hair loss were less related to clinicians' ratings than to patients' own perceptions of their extent of hair loss. Even in patients with slight hair loss, that loss is imbued with considerable emotional meaning that the physician should not ignore. The losses at stake and gains to be had not only pertain to hair but, from the patient's perspective, are also felt in the quality of life (54). In addition to medical or surgical treatments and nonsurgical hair replacement, psychotherapeutic assistance may be valuable in the management of certain patients' body-image difficulties, as discussed above.

CONCLUSIONS

Ours is a culture that places a premium on physical appearance. In this context, appearance-altering conditions can be psychosocially insidious, especially conditions like AGA with an uncertain course and a negative social impact (57). It is not only women who have body-image problems (58,59). Persons seeking remedies for androgenetic alopecia often anticipate experience losses beyond the loss of hair per se. An empathic understanding of these patients' concerns is essential to effective management (60,61).

Many of the studies described here were performed using samples consisting primarily of men seeking medical care for hair loss, thus limiting the generalizability of results to the overall population. To date, little or no data have been available regarding the psychosocial and quality-of-life aspects of AGA in a representative sample of men. In addition, longitudinal data in the absence of treatment are nearly nonexistent. Many of the studies described are cross-sectional in nature, and the temporal relationships between AGA and psychosocial correlates are unknown. It is unknown whether AGA is a causal factor in the development of low self-esteem, depression, introversion, and feelings of unattractiveness or whether there are underlying problems in certain patients prior to hair loss. Longitudinal studies will be important to investigate the temporal relationships between the degree of hair loss and psychosocial variables associated with AGA. To fill this void in the literature, community-based studies should be initiated in untreated men to investigate the interrelationships of quality of life, satisfaction with the appearance of one's hair, and degree of baldness with other quality-of-life constructs as well as any change in such measures over time.

The literature suggests that there is more than just a physical aspect to androgenetic alopecia. People's initial impressions of men with AGA are generally less favorable than of men without AGA. Balding men are viewed as less desirable in a physical, personal, and social sense. Given the stereotype, it is not surprising that some men with AGA appear to have a lower self-image, depression resulting in increased introversion, and increased feelings of unattractiveness.

The question posed at the beginning of the chapter—Will a patient with male pattern baldness be better treated and consequently more satisfied (better quality of life) if he receives effective antialopecia agents or get more benefit if evaluated and treated for his psychological disorder?—seems to be answered by the numerous reports here studied as follows: most patients would benefit from both approaches simultaneously.

REFERENCES

1. Cash TF. Losing hair, losing points?: The effects of male pattern baldness on social impression formation. J Appl Soc Psychol 20:154–167, 1990.
2. Maffei C, Fossati A, Rinaldi F, Riva E. Personality disorders and psychopathologic symptoms in patients with androgenetic alopecia. Arch Dermatol 130:868–872, 1994.
3. Grimalt R. Trichopsychodermatology. Dermatol Psychosom 2:41–50, 2001.
4. Patzer GL. Psycologic and sociologic dimensions of hair: an aspect of the physical attractiveness phenomenon. Psychol Sociol Dimensions 6:93–101, 1988.
5. Passchier J. Quality of life issues in male pattern hair loss. Dermatology 197:217–218, 1998.
6. Grimalt R. Cabello e imagen. Piel 21:4–7, 2001.
7. Grimalt R. Aspectos psicológicos de la alopecia areata. In: Grimalt F, Cotterill J. eds. Dermatologia y Psiquiatria: Historias Clínicas Comentadas. Madrid: Aula Médica, 277–282, 2002.
8. Trueb RM. Interrelations between physician, hairdresser and mass media in management of hair loss. Hautarzt 51:729–732, 2000.
9. Budd D, Himmelberger D, Rhodes T, Cash TE, Girman CJ. The effects of hair loss in European men: a survey in four countries. Eur J Dermatol 10:122–127, 2000.
10. Cash TF. The psychosocial consequences of androgenetic alopecia: a review of the research literature. Br J Dermatol 141:398–405, 1999.

11. Girman CJ, Hartmaier S, Roberts J, Bergfeld W, Waldstreicher J. Patient-perceived importance of negative effects of androgenetic alopecia in women. J Womens Health Gend Based Med 8:1091–1095, 1999.

12. Trueb RM. Trichodynia. Hautarzt 48:877–880, 1997.

13. Revuz J. Androgenetic alopecia and quality of life. Ann Dermatol Venereol 127:15–16, 2000.

14. Hoffmann R, Happle R. Current understanding of androgenetic alopecia. Part II: clinical aspects and treatment. Eur J Dermatol 10:410–417, 2000.

15. Rushton DH. Androgenetic alopecia in men: the scale of the problem and prospects for treatment. Int J Clin Pract 53:50–53, 1999.

16. Van Der Donk J, Hunfeld JA, Passchier J, Knegt-Junk KJ, Nieboer C. Quality of life and maladjustment associated with hair loss in women with alopecia androgenetica. Soc Sci Med 38:159–163, 1994.

17. Tran D, Sinclair RD. Understanding and managing common baldness. Aust Fam Phys 28:248–250, 252–253, 1999.

18. de Koning EB, Passchier J, Dekker FW. Psychological problems with hair loss in general practice and the treatment policies of general practitioners. Psychol Rep 67:775–778, 1990.

19. Di Prima TM, De Pasquale R, Gilotta SM, Cravotta A. Preliminary approach to the mental component in dermatologic patients. G Ital Dermatol Venereol 124:147–150, 1989.

20. Ludwig E, Montagna W, Camacho F. Alopecia androgenética femenina. In: F Camacho, W Montagna, eds. Tricologia. Madrid: Aula Médica, 1996:343–356.

21. Seidman M, Westfried M, Maxey R, Rao TKS, Friedman EA. Reversal of male pattern baldness by minoxidil. Cutis 28:551–553, 1981.

22. Kaufman KD, Olsen EA, Whiting D. Finasteride in the treatment of men with androgenetic alopecia. J Am Acad Dermatol 39:578–588, 1998.

23. Price VH, Roberts JL, Hordinsky M, Olsen EA, Savin R, Bergfeld W, Fiedler V, Lucky A, Whiting DA, Pappas F, Culbertson J, Kotey P, Meehan A, Waldstreicher J. Lack of efficacy of finasteride in postmensual women with androgenetic alopecia. J Am Acad Dermatol 43:768–776, 2000.

24. Terry RL. Further evidence on components of facial attractiveness. Percept Mot Skills 45:130, 1977.

25. Terry RL, Davis JS. Components of facial attractiveness. Percept Mot Skills 42:918, 1976.

26. Feinman S, Gill GW. Sex differences in physical attractiveness preferences. J Soc Psychol 105:43–52, 1978.

27. Waters J. Cosmetics and the job market. In: Graham JA, Kligman AM, eds. The Psychology of Cosmetic Treatments. New York: Praeger, 1985:113–124.

28. Moskowitz HR. What do women and men think of men's fragrances? Cosmet Tech 2:46–49, 1980.

29. Clayson W, Maugham M. Blonde is beautiful: status and preference by hair color. Rocky Mountain Psycological Association Convention, Phoenix, Arizona, 1976.

30. Verinis JS, Roll S. Primary and secondary male characteristics: The hairiness and large penis stereotypes. Psyco Rep 26:123–126, 1970.
31. Mace KC. The "overt-bluff" shoplifter: who gets caught? J Forensic Psychol 4:26–30, 1972.
32. Miller AG. Constrain and target effects in the attribution of attitudes. J Exp Soc Psychol 12:325–339, 1976.
33. Miller EL. Experimenter effect and the reports of Jamaican adolescents on beauty and body image. Soc Econ Stud 21:353–390, 1972.
34. Morgan WG. Situational specificity in altruistic behavior. Representative Res Soc Psychol 4:56–66, 1973.
35. Pancer SM, Meindl JR. Length of hair and beardedness as determinants of personality impressions. Percept Mot Skills 46:1328–1330, 1978.
36. Hallpike CR. Social hair. Man 4:256–264, 1969.
37. Montgomery RL, Enzie RF, Hinkle SW. Some unobtrusive measures of authoritarianism. Percept Mot Skills 35:202, 1972.
38. Alcorn DS, Condie SJ. Who picks up whom: the fleeting encounter between motorist and hitchhiker. Humboldt J Soc Relat 3:56–61, 1972.
39. Campbell MD. A controlled investigation of altruistic behavior: helping the hitchhiker. Personality Soc Psychol Bull 1:174–176, 1974.
40. Peterson K, Curran JP. Trait attributions as a function of hair length and correlates of subjects preferences for hair style. J Psychol 93:331–339, 1976.
41. Graham JA, Jouhar AJ. The effects of cosmetics on person perception. In J Cosmet Sci 3:199–210, 1980.
42. Cordwell JM. Ancient beginnings and modern diversity of the use of cosmetics. In: Graham JA, Kligman AM, eds. The Psychology of Cosmetic Treatments. New York: Praeger, 1985:37–44.
43. Cash TF. The psychological effects of androgenetic alopecia in men. J Am Acad Dermatol 26:926–931, 1992.
44. Wells PA, Willmoth T, Russell RJH. Does fortune favour the bald? Psychological correlates of hair loss in males. Br J Psychol 86:337–344, 1995.
45. Passchier J, van der Donk J, Dutree-Meulenberg ROGM, Stolz E, Verhage F. Psychological characteristics of men with alopecia androgenetica and effects of treatment with topical minoxidil: An exploratory study. Int J Dermatol 27:441–446, 1988.
46. Dawber RPR. Aetiology and pathophysiology of hair loss. Dermatologica 175:23–28, 1987.
47. Roll S, Verinis JS. Stereotypes of scalp and facial hair as measured by the semantic differential. Psychol Rep 28:975–980, 1971.
48. Koblenzer CS. Psychocutaneous Disease. Orlando, FL: Grune and Stratton, 1987.
49. van der Donk MA, Passchier J, Dutree-Meulenberg ROGM, Stolz E, Verhage F. Psychologica characteristics of men with alopecia androgenetica and their modification. Int J Dermatol 30:22–28, 1991.

50. Franzoi SL, Anderson J, Frmmelt S. Individual differences in men's perceptions of and the reactions to thinning hair. J Soc Psychol 130:209–218, 1993.
51. Camacho FM. Aspectos psicológicos de la alopecia androgenética. Monogr Dermatol 1:53–60, 1998.
52. Hamilton JB. Patterned loss of hair in man: types and incidence. Ann NY Acad Sci 53:708–728, 1951.
53. Norwood OT. Male pattern baldness: classification and incidence. South Med J 68:1359–1365, 1975.
54. Cash TF, Price VH, Savin RC. Psychological effects of androgenetic alopecia on women: comparisons wilth balding men and with female control subjects. J Am Acad Dermatol 29:568–575, 1993.
55. van der Donk J, Passchier J, Knegt-Junk C. Psychological characteristics of women with androgenetic alopecia: a controlled study. Br J Dermatol 125:248–252, 1991.
56. Dolte KS, Girman CJ, Hartmaler S, Roberts J, Bergfeld W, Waldstreichers J. Development of a health-related quality of life questionnaire for women with androgenetic alopecia. Clin Exp Dermatol 25:637–642, 2000.
57. Cash TF, Pruzinsky T. Body Images: Development, Deviance and Change. New York: Guilford, 1990.
58. Cash TF. The psychology of physical appearance: a esthetics, attributes and images. In: Cash TF, Pruzinsky T, eds. Body Images: Development, Deviance, and Change. New York: Guilford, 1990:51–79.
59. Cash TF, Brown TA. Gender and body images: stereotypes and realities. Sex Roles 21:357–369, 1989.
60. Cash TF, Butters JW. Poor body image: helping the patient to change. Med Aspects Hum Sexuality 22:67–70, 1988.
61. Van Moffaert M. Training future dermatologist in psychodermatology. Gen Hosp Psychiatry 8:115–118, 1986.

18

The Coping Challenges Facing Melanoma Patients

Andrew W. Kneier
University of California, San Francisco
San Francisco, California, U.S.A.

INTRODUCTION

It goes without saying that melanoma patients have a great deal to cope with. This is true, of course, for all patients with a life-threatening diagnosis. Many aspects of a person, and of a person's life, are threatened and disrupted by the diagnosis and treatment of a cancer such as melanoma (1). Research has found that different ways of coping with these threats and disruptions is associated with differences in one's psychological adjustment and emotional well-being over time (2). It appears that some ways of coping are generally better than others in the sense that they are more conducive to a good quality of life (physically and emotionally) when dealing with a serious illness.

This chapter addresses three topics concerned with coping. First, what has the research on coping with cancer identified as being constructive or positive ways of coping? Second, what are some of the common obstacles that make it difficult for patients to cope in these positive ways? Third, how can health care professionals help patients to overcome these obstacles and thus help them in the process of coping?

As a construct, "coping" includes attitudes and behaviors that have an adaptive intent when dealing with a threatening situation (3). That is, the person adopts ways of thinking and ways of behaving that aim to address the situation in a constructive manner and that aim to safeguard his or her emotional state and to promote adjustment. This construct is relatively new in comparison to the related construct of defense mechanism. The later construct focuses on what the person is defending against (e.g., impulses, troublesome thoughts, emotional upset), while the coping construct focuses on what the person is doing in a positive effort to meet stressful life events. Coping is also a broader construct that covers a wide range of behaviors and thoughts that are employed to deal with these events.

The issue of coping, and thus of emotional well-being, is especially relevant for the melanoma patient because the immune system is affected by one's emotional state (4–6). The link between emotions and immunity occurs because immune cells, through specific receptors, respond to many of the hormones, neurotransmitters, and neuropeptides that are affected by stress (7,8). Enzyme levels necessary for the repair of mutated DNA have also been found to be lower under stressful conditions (9). These findings suggest that melanoma patients may be able to promote a more effective immune response by virtue of how they cope with the stressful aspects of their illness.

This point was illustrated in a clinical trial with melanoma patients on the efficacy of a six-session group intervention program, which focused in part on the kind of coping strategies discussed below. Those who participated in this program showed more positive changes in their coping and greater improvement in their emotional state than the control group, and this improvement was associated with an increase in certain types of natural killer (NK) cells and an increase in the tumor-fighting potential of NK cells (10). In their follow-up study, the researchers found that these changes were associated, in turn, with improved 5-year recurrence and survival rates (11).

In this chapter an effort is made to glean 10 positive coping strategies (see Table 1) from the vast amount of research on coping with cancer and to discuss these in relation to coping with melanoma. These strategies have been associated with improved problem solving, adjustment, resilience, and emotional well-being in groups of patients. They are not applicable, however, to all individuals. The style of coping that works best for one person may not work as well for another. What works best for any one person depends on many factors related to that person's personality, current life situation, and past coping behavior (12). Moreover, a patient's coping

TABLE 1 Ten Steps Toward Emotional Well-Being When Dealing with Cancer

1.	Facing the reality of one's illness
2.	Maintaining hope and optimism
3.	Proportion and balance
4.	Expressing one's emotions
5.	Reaching out for support
6.	Adopting a participatory stance
7.	Finding a positive meaning
8.	Spirituality, faith, and prayer
9.	Maintaining self-esteem
10.	Coming to terms with mortality

strategies will be tailored to the specific demands posed by his or her diagnosis and treatment regimen, and these vary from case to case. Coping with cancer is a process that goes on over months and years, and patients use different strategies at different times, depending upon the changing situation within themselves, their relationships, and with their illness (3,13). Despite these caveats, it is nonetheless true that research on the coping strategies discussed below has shown a general association with improved adjustment.

An effort is also made to discuss these coping strategies with language and prose accessible to the general reader. The health care professionals who read this chapter may wish to share it with the melanoma patients they are caring for. A previous version of the following discussion was prepared as a booklet for patients at the UCSF Comprehensive Cancer Center. Many patients who read this booklet—"Coping: Ten Steps Toward Emotional Well-Being When Dealing with Cancer"—have commented that it helped them in dealing with their illness. Thus, the author hopes that the current chapter will prove helpful to melanoma patients.

FACING THE REALITY OF ONE'S ILLNESS

Different patients respond in different ways to their diagnosis, the initial medical work-up, subsequent tests results, and the implications of all that is happening to them. Many patients respond by confronting the full reality of their illness: they ask pointed and brave questions about the seriousness of their condition and the pros and cons of the various treatment options, and they read up on these matters on their own. They react as if they are strongly motivated to know what they are facing; this way of coping has been found to promote one's psychological adjustment (14–16).

Other patients react as if the realities confronting them are too much to deal with and they therefore retreat into a denial of these realities. It sometimes seems that a patient in denial is saying, in effect, "I can't cope with all this." Actually, the denial is a way of coping. It protects the person from being overwhelmed. But it can also prevent a person from coming to terms with the illness and getting on with other more constructive ways of coping; it is therefore associated with a poorer psychological adjustment in the long run (17,18).

In the short run, denial is often a positive coping strategy because it enables the patient to gradually face the reality of his or her illness—not all at once, in a way that might bring a flood of intense emotions, but in a step-by-step manner as the person feels in less danger of being overwhelmed or feels more supported by loved ones (19,20).

When a person is diagnosed with melanoma, the first issue confronting the person, in terms of coping, is this: How much does the person want to know about the nature of the primary lesion, the risk that it poses, and the relevant treatment options? Health care professionals can help patients to face these questions by the manner in which they relate to the patient and to the diagnosis itself. If a physician offers very little information, it can convey the message: "You don't want to know and you don't need to know." It can also convey the message: "This is too upsetting to discuss." Patients often comply with these messages by asking very few questions. Conversely, if a physician explains the seriousness of the diagnosis because of the risk of metastases and encourages a discussion about melanoma and the medical treatments, then the message is conveyed: "This is not too difficult to face. It's important that you know about the risk and about the treatments." This message helps the patient feel more capable of facing these realities and asking relevant questions.

MAINTAINING HOPE AND OPTIMISM

If the first step in coping is to face reality, the second step is maintain hope and optimism in relation to that reality. Not surprisingly, patients who are hopeful and optimistic show a better adjustment to their illness than patients who are pessimistic (21–23). In some studies, optimism has also been associated with improved medical outcomes (24,25). For example, patients with stage 4 melanoma who were optimistic about the treatment regimen were found to live longer than those who were considered to be more "realistic" (26).

Most patients tell themselves to be positive, but for many this is easier said than done. This is certainly true for patients with melanoma (27). Feeling optimistic that the disease will not recur implies that the person feels lucky. But many patients feel that getting melanoma in the first place makes them "unlucky." Therefore, they cannot expect that they would now enjoy the good fortune of a long remission or cure. For some, optimism can also seem presumptuous: after all, other patients with the same diagnosis have not done well, and a person might think, "What right do I have to expect the best?" Optimism could also make a person feel that he or she is not worrying enough about the risk posed by melanoma, i.e., is not giving melanoma the fear it deserved. Finally, if a person's prognosis is more favorable than other melanoma patients, he or she may feel that it is not right to enjoy this good fortune or to take advantage of it by being optimistic and going forward with one's life in a positive and constructive manner. The bottom line is that patients often feel that it is wrong and dangerous to be too optimistic. Sometimes patients are not fully aware that their optimism is being inhibited for these reasons.

Given these issues, how can health care professionals help patients feel an appropriate degree of optimism? The following section addresses this question.

PROPORTION AND BALANCE

For most melanoma patients, the medical situation provides a basis for hope and a basis for worry. The statistics that apply indicate a certain chance of survival, but also a certain risk that the melanoma will prove fatal. Ideally, a patient's emotional response would take both aspects into account: he or she would experience a degree of hope that was proportional to the positive survival chances that applied, but would also experience a degree of worry and emotional upset that was proportional to the mortality rate in similar cases. In other words, the patient's emotions would be mixed and (ideally) proportional to the negative and positive aspects of his or her prognosis.

A patient's emotions should also be in balance, in this sense: when he or she was feeling worried or upset, these feelings should be reduced in intensity, or tempered, by feelings of hope and optimism. Alternatively, the nature and intensity of one's positive emotions should also be tempered by, or take into account, the possibility of death. If the person is ignoring this possibility, then his or her optimism will feel false because the person will unconsciously know that it is based on denial. It is better to acknowledge the threat of death and to work through the negative emotions that stem from it (14,15). Patients then feel justified in also embracing the positive aspects of their situation, maintaining appropriate optimism, and keeping their sights set on getting better (28).

A number of studies have found that patients who maintain this kind of mixed emotional response—well proportioned to the realities of their illness and well balanced—enjoy a better psychological adjustment than patients who feel mostly pessimistic or mostly optimistic. (For a review of these studies, see Ref. 2.)

When health care professionals acknowledge that the situation is mixed and that a mixed emotional response is warranted, they are actually helping their patients to experience an appropriate degree of optimism. This is because they are not denying the negative aspects, but they are also not denying the realistic basis for hope. This helps patients to face the reality of their illness, but also supports them in feeling a valid sense of hope and optimism. And when patients do the former, they then feel entitled to do the latter as well.

EXPRESSING ONE'S EMOTIONS

Thus far we have talked about facing reality and how to feel about that reality. This section addresses the importance of emotional expression. People differ as to how good they are at this skill, and in our society women are generally better at this than men. Many studies have shown that patients who express their emotions and concerns enjoy a better psychological adjustment than those who tend to suppress their feelings or keep quiet about them (11,29–31).

Emotional expression is usually helpful because it gives the person an outlet for his or her feelings, a means of working through them, and an opportunity to obtain better emotional support. It can be an enormous help just to know that one's feelings are understood by others and seen as valid, but this requires open communication.

There are many reasons that patients keep their feelings private and try not to let on how they really feel. For many this is simply learned behavior, as when children are taught "to be seen but not heard." People also learn not to express their emotions if doing so tends to lead to negative consequences (e.g., being criticized or having one's distress trivialized). People might feel that their emotional needs are an imposition on others and that it is their role to take care of the feelings and needs of others rather than expressing their own. It is not uncommon, for example, for cancer patients to hide their true feelings as a way of protecting their loved ones.

Some people do not express their emotions because they are not very adept at even paying attention to what they are feeling. They seldom stop, check in with themselves, and try to identify the feelings and concerns that are weighing upon them. Children need permission and encouragement to develop this skill, followed by some practice and positive reinforcement. In this process, a person can learn that his or her emotions are important and valid and thus worthy of attention and expression. Some people do not have much experience with this essential ability, and even regard it as pointless or self-indulgent.

Cancer patients are consistently encouraged to "keep a positive attitude." This often makes patients feel that there is something wrong or dangerous about their "negative" emotions (32). The research evidence is just the opposite: experiencing and expressing such emotions is psychologically and immunologically healthy (11,29,30).

When health care professionals trivialize a patient's distress, the open expression of such distress is inhibited (33). Conversely, such professionals can help considerably by acknowledging the validity of a patient's distress, encouraging expression, and offering support.

REACHING OUT FOR SUPPORT

Cancer patients differ with regard to the amount of support available to them and with regard to how much they tend to reach out and take advantage of the support that is available. Those patients who have at least a few loved ones available for close emotional support *and* who call upon their support or practical help show a better psychological adjustment to cancer than patients who are largely alone or tend to "go it alone" in coping with their illness (34–36).

In a randomized clinical trial, melanoma patients who participated in a six-session support group showed an improved emotional state and coping behavior as well as better immune measures and a lower recurrence rate compared with patients in the control group (11). This group experience encouraged patients to express their emotions, gain support from each other, and cope in other positive ways.

Patients often neglect to reach out for the support they need. It may be that they are not especially adept or inclined to check in with themselves regarding their emotional needs or the practical ways that others could help. They may pride themselves in being independent and self-sufficient. A patient might feel that others would be "bothered" by his or her need for support or help or would resent being "imposed" upon. Of course, if this were really the case, it would be counterproductive to ask such people for help; more often than not, this is an assumption based on earlier experience.

An additional problem stems from the kind of support that others offer, which can be a kind of "cheerleading" to keep a positive attitude. While patients generally appreciate the positive intent behind this, it can cause them to hold back in sharing their fears or sorrows. Often, patients would rather hear that others understand how they feel, regard these emotions as valid, and will stick with them regardless of what happens.

Health care professionals can help by being attuned to a patient's emotional needs, offering support, and encouraging the patient to be aware of his or her support needs and to ask loved ones for support and practical help. Patients should also be encouraged to consider participation in a support group.

ADOPTING A PARTICIPATORY STANCE

How much initiative does a patient take to promote the best possible outcome? As with the other coping strategies discussed above, patients differ on this score. Some patients tackle their cancer head on. They have a strong fighting spirit, and they find ways of putting it into action. They go out of their way to learn about their illness and the options for treatment. They actively pursue the best treatments available and consider alternative or holistic approaches as well. In surveys, they strongly agree with the statement: "A lot depends on what I do and how I take part." Research has shown that patients who respond in this manner have less emotional distress than patients who respond in a more avoidant or passive manner (35–38).

Patients who adopt a participatory stance believe they can make a difference, and they put this belief into action. They therefore feel less helpless and vulnerable. This is a major reason that their emotional state is better. A person's belief that he or she is an active and effective agent is called "self-efficacy," and the research has consistently documented its positive emotional effects (39,40).

It is especially important for melanoma patients to actively participate in the recovery effort. Patients with metastatic disease who discuss the pros and cons of the different treatment options with the medical team, and thereby participate in decision making, feel more engaged in the treatment plan and are better able to embrace it and stick with it. This kind of proactive coping has been associated with improved mood (41), and, as mentioned at the outset, this could promote improved immunity and survival. Patients can also participate in the recovery effort by improving their overall health habits, which in turn can benefit the immune system.

Health care professionals can help by engaging patients in decision making about the treatment options and by encouraging patients to improve their health habits (if necessary) and to adopt the kind of positive coping strategies discussed here. Physicians might make the point that patients have a role to play, in concert with medical interventions, and that a collaborative effort can maximize the chances for success. This effort to engage patients as partners in promoting the best possible outcomes helps to overcome the passive, helpless stance that patients sometimes adopt and that is associated with poorer psychological adjustment (2,41).

FINDING A POSITIVE MEANING

While the diagnosis and treatment of cancer is an awful experience in many respects, it can also be a challenge and even an opportunity for positive change in a person and in a person's life. In response to their illness, many patients step back and take stock of who they are and how they have been living. They reflect on their ultimate values and priorities and often identity changes that are warranted (and perhaps overdue) in their lifestyle and personal relationships. They often comment that they are more attuned to their experience in the here and now, that they try to relish all the positive aspects of living, and they no longer take life for granted. These changes are often called the "enlightenment" or "gift" that comes with cancer, or the "wake-up call" aspect of cancer. Patients who embrace this aspect of their cancer experience have been found to be especially well adjusted and better able to deal with the many trials and disruptions caused by their illness (25,42–44).

A variety of changes can occur when patients reflect on the degree to which they are living in a way that is true to their ultimate values and goals.

These include spending more time with family members and close friends, making a greater contribution to the causes a person believes in, showing more appreciation for the positive aspects in one's life ("counting your blessings"), bringing forth aspects of one's personality that have been suppressed, pursuing life-long interests that have always been on the back burner, and seeking to be more honest with oneself and with others. These are some of the ways that a patient's illness can become an impetus for positive change. These issues are certainly relevant for many melanoma patients, especially those with metastatic disease. Even newly diagnosed patients whose primary lesion was caught early often note that the diagnosis was a kind of "tap on the shoulder" that causes them to reconsider their lifestyle and priorities.

Sometimes the idea that there is a message or lesson in one's cancer implies that the person "needed" to get cancer and perhaps even got it for a specific reason. Certain New Age writers have encouraged patients to reflect on why they "needed" their illness. Such ideas have been found to foster feelings of self-blame, guilt, and depression (45,46). A more psychologically healthy response was voiced by a patient who said: "It's too bad that it took cancer to make me see things a bit more clearly, but you know, some positive things have come out of it for me."

SPIRITUALITY, FAITH, AND PRAYER

Most people in our society have some fundamental spiritual beliefs, and these beliefs can be called upon for help in dealing with cancer. Patients who do so benefit in a variety of ways: they have a greater sense of peace, inner strength, and ability to cope and show an improved psychological adjustment and quality of life (35,47,48). These benefits derive especially from the perspective offered by one's religious faith or spirituality and from the power of prayer and religious ritual (49).

It is part of the human condition, of course, to be confronted with vulnerability to disease and with the inevitability of suffering and death. For some, these realities lead to a kind of existential despair. The world's religious and spiritual traditions offer a different perspective, one that looks beyond these realities, or that penetrates more deeply into them, to find meaning and value that transcend one's individual existence or plight. This is one reason that cancer patients often turn to these traditions, and to their personal faith, for help in dealing with their illness.

One example is the "Why me?" question. Patients often ask, either in open protest or private anguish, "Why did this have to happen to me?" Of course, the common rational answer is that it did not *have* to happen, it just did. Nonetheless, there is often an emotional poignancy to this issue that cannot be easily dismissed. The reasons for this are largely religious and cultural. It is difficult to reconcile how the God of the Bible (who is almighty, loving, and just) could allow cancer to happen to a good person. It is not uncommon for patients to wonder if the illness is a just punishment for certain wrongs or failings of character. And because of the influence of the Judeo-Christian tradition on our culture, people often assume that what happens to a person is somehow linked to what the person deserves. The nature of a malignancy, as a destructive force originating from within, also lends itself to the notion that it implies something bad about the person who has it.

The emotional turmoil and doubt that stem from these issues can be soothed by the themes of consolation and forgiveness that permeate the world's major religions. Many patients have been helped by Rabbi Kushner's popular book, *When Bad Things Happen to Good People* (50).

It emphasizes a theme in the Judeo-Christian tradition that sees God as being with those who are suffering, providing the grace needed to endure, rather than doling out suffering to those who deserve or need it. Through prayer and liturgy, patients are able to connect to their god and to their religious community and derive the solace and fortitude they need to cope with their illness. Patients often speak of the spiritual healing that comes through prayer, and there is some evidence that prayer may also have a role in bodily healing (51,52).

MAINTAINING SELF-ESTEEM

The experience of cancer can harm a person's self-esteem in many ways. One of these involves the stigma of having cancer, i.e., that it implies something bad about the person who has it. In addition, many of the sources of a person's self-esteem can be threatened by cancer and the effects of medical treatments: one's bodily appearance, physical abilities and activity level, various personal attributes (such as being healthy and independent), and one's role and identity within one's family and/or work life.

Melanoma patients must often undergo disfiguring surgery, and those with metatastic disease are often unable to carry on with their normal activities due to medical treatments or the effects of the disease itself, such as pain or fatigue. For many, the activities that are compromised or rendered impossible had been an important part of their identity and self-esteem.

Research has shown that such threats to self-esteem pose a danger and an opportunity. The danger is depression and, with that, the weakening of the will to live and the resilience the person needs (53). The opportunity lies in finding additional sources of self-esteem (44,54). For example, a person might take pride in the way he or she is coping, or have a new appreciation for being loved independent of looks or performance. For some, it has been difficult to depend on others because they had prided themselves on being self-sufficient; they might now take pride in their ability to express their needs and ask for help. A person's spirituality could be deepened by having cancer, and this could also help to renew one's self-esteem.

Research has also shown that patients who continue to do the things that are important to them, to the extent possible, enjoy a better psychological adjustment than those who too quickly abandon these roles and activities or expect too little of themselves because they have cancer (55). One study specifically noted that patients need to "deal with the cancer" but also to "keep it in its place" (28).

Health care professionals can help patients to maintain their self-esteem by encouraging them to carry on with their normal activities and roles as much as possible and to embrace new sources of self-esteem, as discussed above. A physician or nurse can help, for example, by noting that one's illness does not suddenly define them as a cancer patient, as if that is their new identity.

COMING TO TERMS WITH MORTALITY

It may seem that the major challenge in dealing with cancer is to fight against the possibility of death rather than work on coming to terms with it. Modern medicine understandably focuses on health and healing. The practitioners of alternative therapies also stress their unique healing potential. From all quarters, cancer patients hear that they must maintain hope, keep a positive attitude, and never give up. It seems that everything revolves around their getting better. And yet many patients die of cancer, and even those who do not are living with the possibility that they might. There is very little support offered to patients in coming to terms with this possibility and reaching some sense of peace about it and in not feeling that it is a failure and outrage to die (56).

This is a touchy topic. Who can say that a person should accept the possibility of dying of cancer, and therefore not rail against it and do everything possible to prevent it? Even if one's cancer progresses to a terminal stage, it would seem presumptuous to say that one's death should be accepted. Facing death is profoundly personal and inherently difficult. Nonetheless, research has shown that many patients do come to terms with death and enjoy a sense of peace that acceptance brings (57,58).

A patient can put off dealing with death until the time comes or face this possibility in the course of dealing with his or her illness. The latter approach has been found to be helpful. Facing the possibility of dying of cancer can cause more fear, desperation, and inner anguish if the person is not also striving to come to terms with it. This does not mean that the person dwells on it; it means that issues involving one's life and death are confronted, which then enables the person to go forward, living in the fullness of life, one day at a time, rather than in dread of what could possibly happen (59).

The work of coming to terms with death can draw on one's religious, spiritual, or philosophical beliefs about what is important in life, and why (60). These beliefs can provide meaning and purpose to one's life as a whole, and therefore consolation when facing death. Many people have been able to feel that their life has been about something important and of lasting value. This is one of the major ways that one's religion or spirituality can help (61).

Health care professionals who are caring for patients with metastatic melanoma can help by bringing up the issues discussed in this section and by referring patients to some of the works cited. Many patients struggle with these issues and long for a sense of peace, but feel forced to do so quietly because they have so little support for this important inner work. As one patient put it: "I can't tell anyone I'm thinking about these things, because everyone wants me to be positive."

CONCLUSION

The coping strategies discussed above are not right for everyone, but there is good evidence that they are generally helpful to patients who are dealing with cancer, including melanoma. The bottom line is that these strategies help patients feel better and stronger. They feel better because they are facing the illness squarely and working through its emotional impacts, and yet also keeping a perspective on it so that it does not define them or take over their life. Through all the trials and challenges that cancer can bring, they are keeping their wits about them and able to carry on. They feel stronger because they have support, from other people and from within themselves. They have taken stock of their most cherished reasons for living, which strengthens and sustains them in their fight against cancer. And yet they also feel that their survival is not the only important objective; the quality of their lives and relationships, the values they live by, and their spirituality also deserve attention and effort. They have the peace of knowing that their death from cancer, if it comes to that, will not obliterate the meaning, value, and joy that their life has given to them and their loved ones.

REFERENCES

1. Cassell EJ. The nature of suffering and the goals of medicine. N Engl J Med 306: 639–645, 1982.
2. Heim E. Coping and adaption in cancer. In: Cooper CL, Watson M, eds. Cancer and Stress: Psychological, Biological, and Coping Studies. Chichester: John Wiley and Sons, 1991, pp 197–235.
3. Lazarus RS. Stress and coping as factors in health and illness. In: Cohen J, Cullen JW, Martin LR, eds. Psychosocial Aspects of Cancer. New York: Raven Press, 1982, 163–190.
4. Herbert TB, Cohen S. Stress and immunity in humans: a meta-analytic review. Psychosom Med 55: 254–379, 1993.

5. Herbert TB, Cohen S. Depression and immunity: a meta-analytic review. Psychol Bull 113: 472–486, 1993.
6. Futterman AD, Kemeny ME, Shapiro D, Fahey JL. Immunological and physical changes associated with induced positive and negative mood. Psychosom Med 56: 499–511, 1994.
7. Ader R, Cohen N, Felten D. Psychoneuroimmunology: interactions between the nervous system and the immune system. Lancet 345: 99–103, 1995.
8. Sheridan JF, Dobbs C, Brown D, Zwilling B. Psychoneuroimmunology: stress effects on pathogenesis and immunity during infection. Clin Microbiol Rev 7: 200–212, 1994.
9. Kiecolt-Glaser JK, Stephens RE, Lipetz PD, Speicher CE, Glasser R. Distress and DNA repair in human lymphocytes. J Behav Med 8: 311–320, 1985.
10. Fawsy FI, Kemeny ME, Fawsy NW, Elashoff R, Morton D, Cousins N, Fahey JL. A structured psychiatric intervention for cancer patients, II: Changes over time in immunological measures. Arch Gen Psychiatry 47: 729–735, 1990.
11. Fawsy FI, Fawsy NW, Hyun CS, Elashoff R, Guthrie D, Fahey JL, Morton D. Malignant melanoma: effects of an early structured psychiatric intervention, coping, and affective state on recurrence and survival 6 years later. Arch Gen Psychiatry 50: 681–689, 1993.
12. Rowland JH. Developmental stage and adaptation: adult model. In: Holland JC, Rowland JH, eds. Handbook of Psychooncology. New York: Oxford, 1989, pp 25–43.
13. Jarrett SR, Ramires AJ, Richards MA, Weinman J. Measuring coping in breast cancer. J Psychosom Res 36: 593–602, 1992.
14. Spiegel D. Facilitatory emotional coping during treatment. Cancer 66: 1422–1426, 1990.
15. Fredette SL. Breast cancer survivors: concerns and coping. Cancer Nurs 17: 35–46, 1994.
16. Ell K, Nishimoto R, Morvay T, Mantell J, Hamovitch M. A longitudinal analysis of psychological adaptation among survivors of cancer. Cancer 36: 406–413, 1989.
17. Feigel H, Strack S, Tong Nagy V. Degree of life-threat and differential use of coping modes. J Psychosom Res 31: 91–99, 1987.
18. Carver CS, Pozo C, Harris SD, Noriega V, Scheier MF, Robinson DS, Ketcham AS, Moffat FL Jr., Clark KC. How coping mediates the effect of optimism on distress: a study of women with early stage breast cancer. J Personality Social Psychol 65: 375–390, 1993.
19. Greer S. The management of denial in cancer patients. Oncology 6: 33–36, 1992.
20. Matt DA, Sementilli ME, Burish TG. Denial as a strategy for coping with cancer. J Mental Health Counseling 10: 136–144, 1988.
21. Rustoen T. Hope and quality of life, two central issues for cancer patients: a theoretical analysis. Cancer Nurs 18: 355–361, 1995.
22. Herth KA. The relationship between level of hope and level of coping response and other variables in patients with cancer. Oncol Nurs Forum 16: 67–72, 1989.

23. Carver CS, Pozo-Kaderman C, Harris SD, Noriega V, Scheier MF, Robinson DS, Ketcham AS, Moffat FL Jr., Clark KC. Optimism versus pessimism predicts the quality of psychological adjustment to early stage breast cancer. Cancer 73: 1213–1220, 1994.

24. Segerstrom SC, Taylor SE, Kemeny ME, Fahey JL. Optimism is associated with mood, coping, and immune change in response to stress. J Personality Social Psychol 74: 1646–1655, 1998.

25. Taylor SE, Kemeny ME, Reed GM, Bower JE, Gruenewald TL. Psychological resources, positive illusions, and health. Am Psychol 55: 99–109, 2000.

26. Butow PN, Coates AS, Dunn SM. Psychosocial predictors of survival in metastatic melanoma. J Clin Oncol 17: 2256–2263, 1999.

27. Kneier AW. The psychological challenges facing melanoma patients. Surg Clin North Am 76: 1413–1421, 1996.

28. Ersek M. The process of maintaining hope in adults undergoing bone marrow transplantation for leukemia. Oncol Nurs Forum 19: 883–889, 1992.

29. Watson M, Greer S, Rowden L, Gorman C, Robertson B, Bliss JM, Tunmore R. Relationships between emotional control, adjustment to cancer, and depression and anxiety in breast cancer patients. Psychol Med 21: 51–57, 1992.

30. Spiegel D. Effects of psychosocial support on patients with metastatic breast cancer. J Psychosocial Oncol 10: 113–120, 1992.

31. Gotcher JM. The effects of family communication on psychosocial adjustment of cancer patients. J Appl Commun Res 21: 176–189, 1993.

32. Rittenberg CN. Positive thinking: an unfair burden for cancer patients? Supportive Care Cancer 3: 37–39, 1993.

33. Lazarus RS. The trivialization of distress. In: Rosen JC, Solomon LJ, eds. Preventing Health Risk Behaviors and Promoting Coping with Illness. Hanover, NH: University Press of England, 1984, pp 279–298.

34. Bloom JR, Spiegel D. The relationship of two dimensions of social support to the psychological well-being and social functioning of women with advanced breast cancer. Social Sci Med 19: 831–837, 1984.

35. Halstead MT, Fernsler JI. Coping strategies of long-term cancer survivors. Cancer Nurs 17: 94–100, 1994.

36. Dunkel-Schetter C, Feinstein LG, Taylor SE, Flake RL. Patterns of coping with cancer. Health Psychol 11: 79–89, 1992.

37. Evans DR, Thompson AB, Browne GB, Gina B, Barr RM. Factors associated with the psychological well-being of adults with acute leukemia in remission. J Clin Psychol 49: 153–160, 1993.

38. Stanton AL, Snider PR. Coping with a breast cancer diagnosis: a prospective study. Health Psychol 12: 16–23, 1993.

39. Cunningham AJ, Lockwood GA, Cunningham JA. A relationship between perceived self-efficacy and quality of life in cancer patients. Patient Ed Counseling 17: 71–78, 1991.

40. Telch CF, Telch MJ. Psychological approaches for enhancing coping among cancer patients: a review. Clin Psychol Rev 5: 325–344, 1985.

41. Aspinwall LG, Taylor SE. A stitch in time: self-regulation and proactive coping. Psychol Bull 121: 417–436, 1997.
42. Taylor EJ. Factors associated with meaning in life among people with recurrent cancer. Oncol Nurs Forum 20: 1399–1405, 1993.
43. Taylor EJ. Whys and wherefores: adult patients' perspective on the meaning of cancer. Semin Oncol Nurs 11: 32–40, 1995.
44. Ersek M, Ferrell BR. Providing relief from cancer pain by assisting in the search for meaning. J Palliative Care 10: 15–22, 1994.
45. Dirksen SR. Search for meaning in long-term cancer survivors. J Advanced Nurs 21: 628–633, 1995.
46. Burgess C, Morris T, Pettingal KW. Psychological response to cancer diagnosis II: Evidence for coping styles. J Psychosom Res 32: 263–27, 1988.
47. Stoll BA. Faith only belongs in churches? In: BA Stoll, ed. Coping with Cancer Stress. Dordrecht: Martinus Nijhoff Publishers, 1986, pp 9–20.
48. Wagner MK, Armstrong D, Laughlin JE. Cognitive determinants of quality of life after onset of cancer. Psychol Reports 77: 147–154, 1995.
49. Musick MA, Koenig HG, Larson DB, Matthews D. Religion and spiritual beliefs. In: Holland JC, ed. Psycho-Oncology. New York: Oxford University Press, 1998: 780–789.
50. Kushner HS. When Bad Things Happen to Good People. New York: Avon Books, 1991.
51. Dossey L. Healing Words: The Power of Prayer and the Practice of Medicine. San Francisco: Harper Books, 1993.
52. Creagan ET. Attitude and disposition: Do they make a difference in cancer survival? Mayo Clin Proc 72: 160–164, 1997.
53. Massie MJ, Popkin MK. Depressive disorders. In: Holland JC, ed. Psycho-Oncology. New York: Oxford University Press, 1998, pp 780–789.
54. Heidrich SM, Forsthoff CA, Ward SE. Psychological adjustment in adults with cancer: the self as mediator. Health Psychol 13: 346–353, 1994.
55. Hoskins CN. Patterns of adjustment among women with breast cancer and their partners. Psychol Reports 77: 1017–1018, 1995.
56. Holland JC, Glode LM, Gilewski T, Kushner RH. The last taboo: talking to patients about the meaning of life, death, and illness. In: Educational Book from the 32nd Annual Meeting of the American Society of Clinical Oncology, Philadelphia, 1996, pp 53–82.
57. Spiegel D, Yalom ID. A support group for dying patients. Int J Group Psychother 28: 233–245, 1978.
58. Thomas C, Turner P, Madden F. Coping and the outcome of stoma surgery. J Psychosom Res 32: 457–467, 1988.
59. Spiegel D. Living Beyond Limits: New Hope and Help for Facing a Life-Threatening Illness. New York: Times Books, 1993.
60. Nozick R. The Examined Life: Philosophical Meditations. New York: Simon & Schuster, 1989.
61. Rinpoche S. The Tibetan Book of Living and Dying. Harper San Francisco, 1992.

19

The Impact of Atopic Dermatitis on the Quality of Life of the Pediatric Patient

Jane Choi and John Y. M. Koo
University of California, San Francisco
San Francisco, California, U.S.A.

INTRODUCTION

Atopic dermatitis is a chronic skin condition characterized by inflammation, pruritus, and a multifactorial etiology. The course is a fluctuating and unpredictable one, consisting of periods of remission and exacerbation that occur throughout the patient's lifetime (1). Atopic dermatitis (AD), like other skin diseases, can be minimized in the minds of some physicians and the general public due to its smoldering, non–life-threatening nature. However, the impact of AD on patient health-related quality of life (HRQOL) is profound, affecting not only physical health, but psychological and social functioning as well. Indeed, the psychosocial morbidity associated with AD is significant and cannot be trivialized when evaluating and treating those afflicted with the disease. The influence of AD on patient overall well-being has strong implications for how the disease needs to be approached. If the impact on life quality is substantial, early and aggressive intervention is warranted no matter how mild the disease may objectively seem. Quality-of-life (QOL) measures and psychosocial therapies can be combined with traditional clinical assessments and treatments for the most successful management of the disease.

While AD can affect both adults and children, there are several reasons why special consideration needs to be given to the pediatric population when discussing the psychosocial morbidity that can result from living with AD. Children comprise a significant proportion of the AD population, and many adult patients began dealing with their symptoms in childhood. AD is the most common skin condition in children under 11 years of age and is responsible for most pediatric dermatological admissions to the hospital (2). The prevalence in children has been reported to be increasing and is estimated to range anywhere from 15.6 to 23%. Onset occurs in infancy in 50% of cases, with 80% of patients developing the disease before 5 years of age (1). One third of the time AD will extend beyond infancy, and one third of these patients will be affected in adolescence (2). It has been shown that destructive patterns of behavior are established early on and can persist even after symptoms dissipate (3). Timely intervention becomes particularly important in children, who are at an age when the disease and its associated morbidity first begin to develop. Whereas adults can lead a somewhat autonomous existence if they choose to, children are inherently and of necessity dependent upon others for survival during the crucial stages of their development. Thus, children and their social supports exert a reciprocal influence on one another. Successful management of the disease must involve the education and cooperation of these social networks along with the patient. Well-controlled AD can not only reduce the psychosocial morbidity of affected children, but also improve the QOL of their families and contacts as well.

PSYCHOSOCIAL STRESS AND AD

The purpose of this chapter is to illustrate the impact of AD on the QOL of the pediatric patient. However, it is important to note that the relationship between psychosocial stress and AD is a bidirectional one. Stress, through various mechanisms of action, exerts an effect on the physiology of the skin and immune system, and this effect can be unique to AD patients and distinct from the response seen in those who are unaffected. For example, the increase in levels of circulating CD8+ T lymphocytes and eosinophils upon acute psychosocial stress is higher in adult patients with atopic dermatitis compared to healthy controls (4). The cutaneous lymphocyte-associated antigen (CLA) molecule is thought to be involved in the migration of T cells to inflamed skin by facilitating their adherence to the endothelium of cutaneous blood vessels. The stress-induced increase in

CLA-positive lymphocytes is higher in AD subjects versus healthy subjects. Similarly, the increase in populations of helper T cells expressing IL-5, as well as CD4+ and CD8+ cells expressing interferon-γ (IFN-γ) upon mitogenic stimulation during stress, is more significant in AD patients in comparison to healthy adults. In addition, there is an earlier increase in the secretion of IL-4 by mitogen-stimulated lymphocytes during stress in AD subjects when compared to healthy controls. IL-4 is a cytokine that is increased in acute eczema, while IFN-γ and IL-5 are cytokines whose expression tends to be augmented during the chronic stage of AD (5). Psychological stress is reported to disrupt epidermal permeability homeostasis in rats (6). This effect has also been demonstrated in human subjects with AD. Higher perceived psychological stress has been correlated with reversible deterioration in permeability barrier recovery kinetics following disruption of barrier function in the skin of AD subjects (7).

Children with AD have been shown to exhibit a blunted free cortisol response to psychosocial stress. The physiological, stress-induced release of cortisol in AD children aged 8–14 years was compared to that of age- and gender-matched healthy controls (8). The induction of psychosocial stress was accomplished by having the children perform public speaking and mental arithmetic tasks in front of an audience. Salivary cortisol was measured at intervals before, during, and after the stress was introduced, and heart rate was measured continuously throughout. The stress test provoked a significant increase in the heart rate and salivary cortisol levels of the control group. Likewise, the AD children, who were all in remission and off medication for 3 weeks, displayed an increase in heart rate and cortisol levels. However, the cortisol response in the AD subjects was blunted, suggesting that their adrenocorticol response to stress is diminished.

These findings may explain in part why stress is known to be one of the variables that can influence the course of AD and why higher levels of stress are associated with exacerbations of physical symptoms (1). In a telling study performed in southern Japan, the relationship between stress and AD symptoms was examined in the aftermath of a natural disaster (9). Researchers questioned 1457 subjects about their perceived levels of stress and disease course after the Great Hanshin Earthquake of 1995. The study included children, with 12% of subjects being less than or equal to 10 years old, and 28% ranging from 10 to 20 years of age. Patients were divided into three groups depending on the extent of damage sustained by the areas they lived in. Subjects in group A resided in areas in which more than 20% of buildings collapsed, and group B patients originated from areas where less than 20% of buildings had collapsed. Group C functioned as a control group and consisted of patients who lived in areas where no damage occurred. The earthquake and resulting damage provoked stress that was reported by 63% of group A, 48% of group B, and 19% of group C subjects. Exacerbation of skin symptoms was self-reported in 38, 34, and 7% of subjects in groups A, B, and C, respectively. Higher levels of damage were associated with higher perceived levels of stress and worsening of AD. According to factor analysis, subjective distress was the factor most responsible for the exacerbation of skin symptoms.

THE IMPACT OF AD ON PATIENT HEALTH-RELATED QUALITY OF LIFE

Stress can have a negative bearing on the course of AD, leading to exacerbations or relapses of the disease. Poorly controlled AD, in turn, can exhibit a dramatic reciprocity, exerting a harmful effect on the QOL of the afflicted patient. Finlay (10) surveyed patients with different dermatological disorders using the Dermatology Life Quality Index (DLQI) to determine the impact of each on QOL. Of all the skin disorders, including psoriasis, generalized pruritus, and acne, AD was found to have the greatest impact on patient QOL. Similarly, of all the childhood skin disorders, AD has been reported to have one of the greatest impacts on a child's QOL (11). The disease, along with its associated treatments, can influence many different spheres of a patient's life. In addition to physical well-being, the psychological health, social development, and family relationships of the child can all be negatively affected.

A study of 318 AD patients, ranging from 4 to 70 years of age, examined the relationship between patient self-reported disease severity and decrement in QOL (12). Children were surveyed using the Children's Dermatology Life Quality Index (CLDQI), while the QOL impact experienced by subjects over 16 years of age was assessed using the DLQI as well as the Medical Outcomes Short Form-36 Health Survey (SF-36). The SF-36 assesses eight domains of health, including physical functioning, role functioning related to physical status, bodily pain, general health, vitality, social functioning, role functioning related to emotional status, and mental health. These categories can be combined into a Physical Component Summary (PCS) score and a Mental Component Summary (MCS) score. Lower scores are indicative of a poorer QOL (13). The psychosocial disability experienced by AD patients is comparable to that faced by patients with other chronic illnesses, such as diabetes and hypertension, as reflected in their lower scores for vitality, social functioning, and mental health. The SF-36 social functioning scores of AD patients were lower than those reported by patients with hypertension, and their mental health subscales and MCS scores were below those of patients with type II diabetes. AD patients also scored lower than psoriasis patients in role functioning related to both physical and emotional status, vitality, and social functioning. The mental health subscales and MCS scores were, again, decreased. Patients with different disease severities showed no difference in their PCS scores. However, increasing severity was correlated with a decrease in the MCS score and, with the exception of physical functioning, was associated with a greater impairment in all areas of HRQOL. This suggests that good control of disease with a decrease in the severity of symptoms can improve the QOL and mental functioning of AD patients (12).

It is important to note that the amount of subjective distress experienced by the patient does not always directly correlate with the objective clinical severity of disease. The degree of psychosocial morbidity tends to be associated more with patient perception of disease severity as opposed to physician-rated severity. The strong correlation seen in the above study was between QOL impairment and patient self-reported disease severity (12). A study of adult AD patients revealed that afflicted subjects had lower QOL and higher anxiety levels than those in the healthy control group. While a decrease in QOL was significantly correlated with higher anxiety levels and increased disease severity, anxiety levels did not directly correlate with the severity of disease as assessed by a dermatologist. The degree of disease severity is not necessarily indicative of the psychological state of the patient (14). In the case of pediatric patients, results from a study involving the Infant's Dermatitis Quality of Life Index revealed that QOL impact was poorly correlated with disease severity (15). This discussion is not meant to downplay the significance of disease severity, but rather to emphasize that aggressive treatment of even clinically mild disease is warranted if the impact on QOL is substantial as perceived by the patient.

THE PSYCHOLOGICAL SEQUELAE OF AD

One of the many ways that AD impacts HRQOL is through its negative effects on the psyche of the patient. Efforts have been made to develop a psychological profile or define the personality traits that characterize patients with AD. According to one study, which consisted of interviews and the administration of personality inventories and hostility question-naires, adults with AD scored higher on measures of anxiety and neuroticism in comparison to normative data. They also had significant problems in dealing with anger and hostility (16). Children with AD also have an increased prevalence of anxiety as well as depression (17). Another study examined the psychological traits of three sets of patients: those with AD, those with a dermatological disorder other than AD, and healthy subjects (18). Each group had 12 subjects each, ranging in age from 16 to 36 years, who were screened for anxiety, depression, hysteria, and hypochondriasis. AD patients were characterized by a higher state of anxiety, neurosis, depression, and hypochondriasis than the subjects in the other groups. They displayed a tendency to be introverted, depressed, and highly anxious. While such data offers partial insight into the mental functioning of the AD patient, psychological profiling is fraught with difficulty due to the highly individualized nature of the disease experience and cannot provide a completely accurate depiction of what is occurring within the broader AD population. The inability to confidently generalize results from qualitative research performed on smaller subsets of AD patients to the greater AD populace is a limitation of many behavioral studies. The subjective and qualitative measures often used yield data that need to be extrapolated with caution. This is even more of an issue in pediatric studies since parents often act as a proxy for their children in reporting the psychosocial impact of AD. Parental perception may not be a true reflection of what the child is actually experiencing. Nonetheless, such research still offers important and clinically significant information about QOL issues and trends in AD.

The prevalence of psychological disturbance is increased in children with AD, as demonstrated by a study of 30 children, aged 5–15 years, with varying degrees of eczema (19). Subjects were examined by a pediatric psychiatrist, and psychological disturbance was identified as an abnormality of behavior, emotions, or relationships significant enough in severity or duration to cause handicap to the child or distress to the family or community. Parents were questioned concerning behavior such as temper tantrums, frequent disobedience, and the tendency to tell lies or be fearful of new situations. The mental distress of mothers was also evaluated, and social support was assessed, including the quantity and quality of support from sources such as family and friends. The control group was comprised of 30 children with minor skin problems such as warts, benign nevi, and molluscum contagiosum. The overall rate of disturbance in AD children was nearly twice that of the control group, with 50% of the AD subjects being affected compared to 27% of the control group. The rate of disturbance increased with worsening disease severity, as seen in the 30, 53, and 80% occurrence rates in subjects with mild, moderate, and severe disease, respectively. For comparison, psychological disturbance rates have been reported in 55% of children with hemiplegia and in 58.3% of pediatric epilepsy patients. There was no difference between the two groups in terms of hyperactivity, conduct disorder, or emotional disorders. The degree of mental distress in mothers was similar in both groups, and the number of social supports did not differ. Therefore, the authors concluded that the psychological disturbance found in AD children was most likely the result of aspects of the disease experience other than a distressed maternal figure or lack of social support.

A study by Daud et al. examined the psychiatric adjustment of 30 preschoolers with AD compared to 20 healthy matched controls (20). The mean age of subjects was approximately 30 months, and at least 10% of surface area involvement was required in order for subjects to participate. The disease also had to have a degree of severity significant enough to warrant evaluation in the outpatient setting every 3 months. Psychiatric adjustment was assessed through a standardized semi-structured interview evaluating 12 areas of problem behaviors that was administered to the mothers of the subjects. A higher score reflected an increase in the presence and severity of symptoms in these areas, and a score of 10 or above was considered to be indicative of a high risk of psychiatric disturbance. AD children were reported to have considerably more psychiatric disturbance, as reflected by their higher scores. Nearly three times as many AD children as controls scored above the cut-off range, suggesting that AD is a risk factor for the development of behavioral problems. Negative behaviors that were significantly increased in AD children included clinginess, dependency, and fearfulness. More mothers of AD children described their children as being generally difficult compared to none of the controls, and AD children were seen as being poorly adaptable.

SOCIAL EFFECTS OF AD

AD is most prevalent during an age range in which critical psychological and social development is taking place. Behavioral difficulties may evolve in AD children due to the effects of the disease on this psychosocial development. It is important to address and consider the developmental issues encountered in the different stages of growth for the pediatric dermatology population. Preschoolers, or 3- to 5-year-olds, do not comprehend the concept of chance and are likely to interpret illnesses, including AD, injury, or therapeutic procedures, as a form of punishment (21). The first steps to independence, such as attending school, going to parties, or staying with relatives or friends, can be difficult to take due to parental concern about avoiding irritants and handling skin care properly. AD children also have more difficulty taking over normal routines of care and hygiene since they may require specialized maintenance. Parents are more likely to be overprotective, and consequently the AD child can become less independent (22). In terms of school life, poor performance is associated with sleep deprivation, sedation from medication, distractions from physical discomfort, and missed days due to medical visits. Participation in school activities such as sports may be limited due to physical symptoms (11). In one study, approximately 60% of school-age AD children had problems with school life, including teasing and bullying (23). Peer and teacher acceptance can be negatively affected due to concerns about appearance or infectivity. Children can be restricted in their interactions with peers due to these apprehensions (20). As children get older, peer acceptance becomes an important aspect of self-esteem. Skin symptoms can be distressing if they result in teasing or interference with activities that affect the child's image among peers. The adolescent can be particularly vulnerable to a disease that might affect personal attractiveness and sexuality (21).

THE IMPACT OF AD ON FAMILY LIFE

Because children are innately and intricately bound to their social supports, the morbidity experienced by the pediatric patient extends to include family members. The relationship between the mother and child with AD and how it may affect or be affected by the disease has been a source of great interest. Some promote the idea that the mother and infant need to be viewed as a single functional unit. It has been suggested that the symptoms of skin disease and the therapies prescribed to treat it have the potential to adversely affect maternal-infant bonding by interfering with important attachment-promoting activities such as breast feeding, resulting in the development of an anxious, insecure mother and an irritable infant (21). In one study, the maternal characteristics and attitudes of mothers of infants with AD were described (24). Two cohorts of 20 AD infants each were compared to a control group of 20 healthy infants. One cohort consisted of 3- to 4-month-old AD infants, and the second cohort contained AD infants that ranged from 10 to 12 months of age. The mothers of these infants completed standardized questionnaires concerning depressiveness, hopelessness, child-rearing attitudes, and perception of infant behavior. It was found that the mothers of AD infants characterized themselves as more depressive, hopeless, anxious, and overprotective. They tended to describe their infants as less frequently positive and more negative in their emotional behavior in comparison to the mothers in the control group. This is consistent with results from another study in which AD infants exhibited a greater tendency toward miserable mood changes (15). Parents often blame themselves for the health disorders affecting their children, and mothers can ascribe disease to unrelated events during the pregnancy. Physical imperfections in an infant can cause feelings of disappointment and loss in the caregiver (21). Classically, the clinical picture of the AD parental relationship is one of an overly anxious mother displaying negative attitudes toward an insecure child.

The psychological disturbance study by Daud et al. also observed the security of mother-child attachment in patients with AD (20). No statistical difference in attachment was found between the AD and control group, nor was there a difference in developmental assessment of the children. "Quality of parenting" evaluations as well as social stress and support assessments were additionally obtained. Mothers of AD children were found to suffer from increased global stress levels. Almost twice as many mothers in the AD group reported being highly stressed, specifically about parenting the child with AD. Two thirds felt that the disease affected the way they parented the affected child. They had poorer mean parenting scores, being more likely to feel tired, "fed up," and less effective at disciplining their child. It is thought that parents try to avoid conflict that will precipitate stress and AD exacerbation in their child. They often give in to their child's demands and, as a result, the child does not learn to cope with frustration and exhibits more emotional symptoms. Attention-seeking behavior on the part of the child led to higher-than-normal reported levels of stress in the mothers. AD further contributed to maternal stress because of its adverse effect on parental social functioning. Mothers of AD infants were less likely to be employed outside the home, had fewer friends in general, and felt less social support due to situations such as friends being afraid or unwilling to baby-sit for them. Sixty-six percent of mothers felt AD had an influence on their marriage, and this influence was most often a negative one. Eighty-six percent reported that it affected family life, and 83% stated that this effect was detrimental. Despite the higher levels of stress, the mothers of the AD children did not display significantly more negative attitudes toward their children compared to controls, nor was there a difference in their affective response to the child. In fact, more of the affected mothers reported having empathic feelings toward the child with AD, and their level of acceptance was comparable to that of the control mothers. The prevalence of maternal stress outweighed that of behavioral dysfunction, indicating that in spite of higher levels of stress, mothers were able to meet the needs of their child appropriately. This conflicts with the more traditional notions that AD results in an insecure infant and more negative maternal attitudes. Higher socioeconomic class was overrepresented in this study, and mothers were presumably more educated about the disease, possibly accounting for this discrepancy.

Lawson et al. studied the impact of AD on family life by conducting interviews of 34 families with an AD child (23). Approximately 74% described a general burden of extra care, such as household cleaning, washing, and shopping. Seventy-one percent of parents described feelings of guilt, exhaustion, frustration, resentment, and helplessness. Two-thirds reported that they did not lead a "normal" family life due to food restrictions, the inability to have a pet, and bath product restrictions. Sleeping problems were reported in 63% of families and resulted in parental frustration and exhaustion. Sleep disturbances included difficulty settling the AD child to sleep as well as frequent nighttime awakenings. Sixty-three percent of siblings were also losing sleep as a result. Behavioral disturbances such as irritability or being bad-tempered, easily bored, or hurtful to other family members during disease exacerbations occurred in 54% of families. One third of parents felt that their leisure life was affected negatively due to tiredness and difficulty in finding baby-sitters. In addition, sporting activities, especially swimming, were restricted, and 23% of families felt limited in their choice of vacationing due to climate and special needs. Surprisingly, only 29% felt that interpersonal relationships were adversely affected by caring for an AD child. While 17% reported receiving inadequate support from the teaching and medical professions, support from family members was considered good (23). The problems associated with AD can lead to dysfunctional family relationships. The parent who is the primary caregiver often has to spend more time with the AD child, resulting in jealousy or resentment on the part of the other parent as well as siblings (25).

According to a study performed by Su et al. (2), the effects of AD on the family can be as profound as those faced by families of children with other chronic debilitating disease. Subjects included 48 children with AD who were categorized as mild, moderate, or severe according to the total body surface area (BSA) involved, severity of itching, and course of the illness. They ranged from 4 months to 15 years of age, with a mean age of 4.5 years. Comparisons were made between AD subjects and a control group consisting of children with insulin-dependent diabetes. Impact on family QOL was measured by utilizing a survey that determines the effects that chronic illness has on families and has been used to assess diseases such as spina bifida, posttraumatic brain injury, and ventilator dependence. The areas evaluated include the perceived financial burden of disease, familial/social impact, personal strain, and mastery of illness. A high score correlated with a high impact on family life. Direct financial costs included the cost of medication and medical care such as doctor visits and admissions. Indirect financial costs included time taken off work to care for the child, the effect of eczema on employment, and the time needed for treatment. Non-financial costs included sleep deprivation and marital problems. The average daily time needed to treat a child with AD was 2–3 hours, and the mean amount of sleep lost by the parents and the AD child amounted to 1–2 hours per night. Subjects with moderate to severe AD reported significantly higher impact scores than the diabetic controls, while those with mild disease had equivalent scores. The cost of treatment was similar in the AD and diabetes groups. Thus, the higher family impact scores in AD seem to reflect stressors other than financial burden. These can include sleep deprivation, parental feelings of guilt, child behavioral problems, and the psychological and developmental effects of the illness.

Just as AD can affect family life, the family environment can also influence the child's disease course in either a positive or negative way. Gil et al. (26) performed a study in which stress and family environment were found to be important predictors of symptom severity. The mean age of the 44 subjects was 6.9 years, and most had severe disease with a history dating back to infancy. Stress measures included a life events checklist that recorded major life occurrences such as moving or the birth of a new sibling. A chronic problems checklist was also administered to assess ongoing daily problems. These included problems specifically relating to skin disease, such as applying medications or taking frequent baths, as well as those that all children in general encounter, such as trouble getting along with siblings or getting bad grades in school. The Family Environment Scale provided information on the cohesion, expressiveness, conflict, independence, organization, control, achievement orientation, active-recreational orientation, intellectual-cultural orientation, and moral-religious emphasis of families. A standard symptom score sheet covering dimensions such as the intensity of scratching, use of antibiotics and antihistamines, and course of disease was used to assess symptom severity. The BSA affected was also recorded. Chronic problems related to AD were correlated with disease severity, whereas major life events and general chronic stressors were not. These results are in contrast to previous studies that used more global measures of stress instead of AD-specific measures. Higher levels of distress from AD were associated with more BSA involvement, a more continuous course of disease, greater intensity of scratching, and the increased use of antibiotics and antihistamines. In terms of family types and their relation to symptom severity, families high on independence and organization were associated with fewer symptoms, lower BSA involvement, a less continuous course, and less scratching. Encouraging regular routines, independent thinking, self-reliance, planning, and the clear designation of family responsibilities may promote a reduction in symptoms. These familial traits may buffer against the effects of stress and are associated with higher compliance. Such families are likely to provide clear instructions regarding the consequences of scratching and give the child more responsibility for care. The other significant finding was that families high on the religious/ moral factor who were characterized by strict views of right and wrong, regular participation in religious activities, and the belief in punishment for wrongdoing used more medications. The reasons for this were not clear.

Fritz (27) proposed a cycle in which a demanding irritable infant, combined with the amount of required care and physical imperfection from the disease, results in parental resentment, embarrassment, and withdrawal. Children respond to this with a deterioration of their condition. Parents blame themselves or the child, with the end effect being a preoccupation with the skin that is reinforced by both positive and negative attention. As the child grows, so do the issues faced by the patient and parents, including social rejection, impaired school performance, and sleep deprivation. These patterns can become fixed and persist even when the symptoms have resolved.

FINANCIAL IMPACT

Although in the Lawson study (23) only 11% of families felt that their financial lifestyle was impacted by AD, it is clear that there is substantial cost involved in caring for the AD child (2). A 1993 study conservatively estimated the annual cost of treating AD in the United States to be $364 million (28). In a cross-sectional survey of the parents of 290 AD children aged 1–5 years old, the most significant costs were incurred from medical consultations, prescription medications, and additional family costs. In the previous year, 96% of the children had visited their general practitioner for treatment of their disease. Family costs included miscellaneous expenses such as the purchasing of special bedding or clothing, transportation costs, private specialists and alternative medicine consultations, and income loss due to time missed from work. Transportation costs were incurred by 48% of families, and 5% had taken time off work in the previous year to care for their child with AD (29). Su et al. (2) reported that the direct financial cost of treating a child with moderate to severe AD was found to be substantially higher than the cost of treating the average child with asthma. The direct cost of caring for a child with severe AD was higher than for a child who required hospitalization for asthma. The cost of AD was similar to the cost of treating a child with diabetes. Time off work was significant in the AD groups, although unemployment due to AD was only found in those with moderate to severe disease. AD can result in a societal loss of productivity and an individual loss of income. It is important to note that lower socioeconomic groups are at higher risk for psychosocial morbidity. Psychosocial dysfunction has been shown to be strongly associated with socioeconomic status, with lower status being a potent predictor of dysfunction (30).

SLEEP DIFFICULTIES ASSOCIATED WITH AD

Children with AD are known to suffer from sleep disturbances with lasting effects that spill over into daytime behavior. In a study of AD infants, nighttime awakenings occurred in almost 90% of subjects. Along with itching, scratching, and mood changes, sleep disturbance was an area in which AD exerted a great effect with negative consequences for patient QOL (15). Night waking in preschoolers is a common finding in AD. In one study of preschool-aged children, sleep problems characterized by waking at night more than three times a week were twice as common in AD subjects compared to healthy controls (20). Reid and Lewis-Jones (31) performed a retrospective study in which they surveyed the parents of 39 AD patients with differing severities of eczema. Subjects had an average age of 25 months and disease duration of 19.8 months. When flaring, 86% of parents reported sleep disturbance, with an average of 2.7 wakings per night and a mean parental sleep loss of 2.6 hours per night. During remissions, the frequency of sleep disturbance settled into the upper range of that reported in the general preschool population. The sleep of siblings was disrupted 28% of the time. When the disease was not well controlled, 76% reported difficulty with the child settling to sleep, and the average time it took to settle the child was 49 minutes. During remission, 26% reported difficulty in settling the child to sleep, and the time it took to do so decreased to 17 minutes. Interestingly enough, 26% of subjects continued to have difficulty settling to sleep and 41% continued to wake during the night even after the disease was brought under control. This occurred more frequently when parental strategies involved behaviors that contributed to the maintenance of disrupted sleep patterns, including taking the child into the parent's bed. The most common strategies employed to help the child get back to sleep included treatments to control the itching and close physical contact.

Sleep difficulties continue to occur in older AD children as well. A study of subjects aged 5–15 years found sleep disturbance to be present in 67% of AD children versus 13% of healthy controls (19). The specific way in which AD affects sleep was researched by Reuveni et al. in a study involving 14 mild to moderate AD children in clinical remission with a mean age of 6 years (32). The control group consisted of seven children with mild "benign" snoring and without evidence of respiratory disturbance during sleep. One month prior to the study, AD treatment was restricted to emollients, topical steroids, and oral antihistamines. Medications were limited to emollients alone one week before the study. Patients were evaluated by overnight polysomnography, scratch electrodes, and parental self-reported questionnaires including information on demographics, medical history, sleep hygiene, and sleep quality. There was no difference between the groups in self-reported sleep habits or sleep latency. Polysomnography confirmed no differences in sleep latency, total sleep time, sleep efficiency, or percentage of time spent in each of the sleep phases. The most marked difference was found in sleep fragmentation. AD patients experienced 24.1 arousals and awakenings per hour compared to 15.4 in the control group. The mean duration of the arousals was approximately 4.5 seconds for both groups.

Scratching is thought to be a strong contributing factor in decreasing the quality of sleep in AD patients. In a study of parents of 59 AD children with a mean age of 8 years and mostly mild to moderate disease, AD children were reported to suffer from more restless sleep, frequent waking during the night, difficulty falling asleep, difficulty waking up in the morning, and fewer hours of sleep compared to normal values. Active skin involvement was significantly positively correlated with waking during the night, difficulty falling asleep due to itching and scratching, observed scratching of the skin during sleep, and waking at night due to itching and scratching. Active skin involvement was negatively correlated with ease of falling asleep and ease of waking up in the morning. Subjects in remission also reported sleep difficulties, reinforcing the idea that sleep patterns and behaviors established during flares can be perpetuated beyond the symptoms of active AD (3). Home polysomnography results for 20 school-age AD children compared to a group of matched healthy controls revealed that AD children suffered from reduced sleep efficiency as well as sleep disruption due to both brief and extended awakenings associated with episodes of scratching (33). Bartlett et al. (34) studied the sleep behavior was of 44 AD children and 18 children with other skin conditions including warts, nevi, hair loss, and psoriasis. Parents of subjects between 5 months and 13 years of age answered questionnaires regarding sleep behavior. A reported 73% of AD children had night waking problems compared to 22% of the non-AD children. There was a strong correlation between sleep difficulties and nighttime scratching. Thirty percent of AD subjects versus 11% of controls regularly spent time in a parental bed. Interestingly enough, approximately 85–90% of the observed arousals in the Reuveni et al. study (32) were spontaneous in that they were not associated with a specific event such as apnea, scratching, or muscle jerks. In fact, scratching could only account for 15% of the arousals and awakenings, occurring at a frequency of 1.8 bouts per hour (32). Perhaps the itching sensation results in brief arousals but is not strong enough to induce scratching behavior.

The effects of sleep deprivation on the AD child as well as the parents can be pronounced (31). Sleep disturbance is associated with difficulty staying awake during the day, disruption of family activities due to irritability or aggressive behaviors on the part of the sleep-deprived child, complaints about sleep by the child, and major discipline problems.

Difficulty falling and staying asleep due to itching results in difficulty waking in the morning, difficulty staying awake in the afternoon, and behavior problems due to daytime sleepiness and irritability (3). Sleep deprivation can lead to hyperactivity and poor concentration and interfere with school performance (34). While AD can cause sleep disturbance that results in daytime behavior problems, it must be recognized that children may have psychological problems unrelated to AD that may be the source of sleep difficulties (17).

Negative sleep patterns often continue even during remission due to behaviors that are instituted when the disease is active. Therefore, the early establishment of good sleep hygiene becomes important in minimizing difficulties with sleep (3). Methods of coping such as taking the child into the parent's bed have been associated with the persistence of sleep disturbance and are not encouraged. Medications to help with sleep latency have not shown long-term efficacy in children and have untoward side effects. They are not generally recommended for the management of sleep disturbance in the pediatric AD patient (32).

SCRATCHING BEHAVIOR IN AD CHILDREN

Repetitive trauma to the skin in the form of scratching is the single most amplifying factor in AD and is part of the destructive "itch–scratch" cycle that perpetuates the disease. Scratching can become a learned behavior that does not necessarily have to be triggered by itch after a certain point (35). Although one study comparing a group of 15 AD children where scratching was reported by the mother as a severe problem to 15 AD children without severe scratching revealed no difference in child morbidity or maternal distress between the two groups, scratching is known to be a source of distress for the patient as well as the parent (20). Gil et al. (36) systematically examined parental response to scratching in 30 AD children with a mean age of 5.6 years and 16.5% bodily involvement. Parent-child interactions were videotaped, and results showed that parents almost always paid attention to scratching behavior. Regardless of whether or not this attention was positive or negative, the end result was increased scratching behavior in the children. As the scratching increased, so did the parent's attempt to stop the scratching. Structured tasks led to decreased scratching behavior by engaging the parent and child in distracting activities. Parents and children were observed for 5 minutes while occupied with building a model and then subsequently observed for another 5 minutes without any specified task to do or any toys in the room. Scratching was significantly decreased during the period of time in which the parent and child were busy performing their task. It can be concluded that decreasing parental attention to scratching as well as giving positive reinforcement when the child is not scratching might lead to decreased scratching behavior. Distraction in the form of structured tasks may also lead to a decrease in scratching.

Parents can become anxious about provoking scratching behavior and, as a result, children may unconsciously begin using scratching as a manipulative behavior. Psychological dimensions should be addressed in the clinical setting to avoid negative patterns of behaviors (22). A combined approach of topical medications and behavior modification can be successful at reducing scratching behavior. Education about the function and use of emollients and steroids is crucial. Habit reversal can be encouraged through registration, a process in which patients are made aware of their unconscious behavior by keeping a record of their scratching, and replacement of scratching with a safe habit, such as clenching of the fists. Families and patients need to be taught to manage their disease beyond the point where the skin may appear well. Vigilance and the immediate treatment of problem areas are necessary to prevent relapses. A reduction in scratching and the resulting decrease in AD symptoms can endow patients with feelings of self-efficacy and ability to control their disease (35).

IMPLICATIONS FOR MANAGEMENT OF AD

The impact of AD on HRQOL necessitates intervention that is effective and timely. Behavior problems and parental distress tend to be associated with the severity of AD, indicating that well-controlled disease can lead to a reduction in psychosocial morbidity (20). Aggressive treatment is warranted even in cases where disease may be clinically mild if the impact on QOL is perceived to be high by the patient. Prompt intervention is essential in order to prevent the establishment of negative behavioral patterns that may persist even after the physical symptoms dissipate. Patient education is paramount, as is allowing the patient to be a vocal and active participant in their care and the establishment of goals (27).

The effect of education on the management of disease was examined by Staab et al. (37) in 204 families of AD children with moderate to severe disease. Subjects were recruited to participate in a study evaluating the effectiveness of a parental education and training program. Ninety-three families participated in the training, and 111 were assigned to the control group, which was scheduled to undergo training one year later. The QOL of the parents was assessed using a disease-specific questionnaire focusing on psychosomatic well-being, the social effects of disease, confidence in medical treatment, emotional coping, and acceptance of the disease. A more general

QOL survey was also administered along with an assessment of treatment habits, therapeutic costs, and coping strategies. The training consisted of six 2-hour educational sessions conducted weekly with a multidisciplinary team of pediatricians, psychologists, and nutritionists. Severity of AD was not different between the two groups after one year, but there were significant differences in the parental management of AD. Before intervention, the regular use of skin care products was similar in both groups. Posttraining, the educated group still regularly used products while there was a significant decline of use in the control group. Education was the strongest predictor of regular skin care product use. Use of antiseptics rose from 10 to 19% in the intervention group, while it fell from 19 to 7% in the control group. At baseline, approximately one third of both groups used topical steroids to treat inflammation of the skin. After training, this number nearly doubled in the intervention group, while it remained the same in the control group. More than 50% of parents in both groups used unconventional therapy before training. This fell to 26% in the educated group and remained at 51% in the control group, perhaps reflecting a greater confidence in the ability to self-manage disease. This is also seen in the increase in confidence in medical treatment captured on the disease-specific QOL questionnaire in the intervention group. Rumination is characterized by withdrawal and cognitive avoidance of problems in managing disease, as well as a fixation on the past and wrongs that might have been done. A decrease in rumination as a coping strategy was detected in the education group, signifying movement from a passive to more active, healthy forms of coping. Cost reduction in treatments, measured in terms of expenses covered by public health insurance, was significant in the intervention group despite an increase in the use of topical medications. This might be explained by the need for less frequent visits to the physician due to better management of disease.

Establishing a strong therapeutic relationship with the patient and caregiver can have a positive effect on patient compliance and management of disease. In one study, 258 mothers of AD children under 20 years of age with a mean age of 6.9 were surveyed regarding demographic data, adherence to treatment measures such as skin care and allergen avoidance, psychosocial items such as the doctor-patient (mother) relationship, perceived severity of illness, and attitudes toward steroids (38). The quality of the doctor-patient relationship, spousal cooperation, social support, maternal worry about the child's eczema, and perceived severity of disease were strongly correlated with skin care adherence. Anxiety about using topical steroids had no significant effect on the reported use of steroids. It seems that apprehension about using steroids can be overcome by a strong doctor-patient relationship. Also, a strong therapeutic relationship seems to be correlated with an increased sense of self-efficacy and confidence in the ability to self-manage the disease. Mothers who begrudged the cost of treatment reported poorer doctor-patient relationships. Concern over cost was not related to income level, but to the mother's personality and attitudes about money. Mothers who felt the most financial concern felt less supported socially and tended to have negative attitudes toward the disease. For example, they reported feelings that their life was sacrificed in order to care for their child. Maternal personality and social support can influence the doctor-patient relationship and, consequently, influence adherence to treatment advice.

It is important to address issues that may affect patient compliance with treatment. Dysfunctional families show poor treatment compliance and poor control of symptoms (25). Intervention on a familial level may be necessary in order to improve adherence to treatment advice. Since stress is known to exacerbate symptoms, psychotherapies aimed at reducing distress may prove to be useful supplements to traditional therapies. In one study, a group of children with AD were treated with standard topical care and, in addition, were administered 20 minutes of daily massage by their parents (39). The control group received topical treatment alone. There was an improvement noted in the children's affect and activity level immediately following the massage therapy sessions. Throughout the one-month duration of the study, parents of the massaged children reported lower levels of anxiety in their children. The parents themselves also reported decreased anxiety following massage therapy. There was significant improvement in clinical measures as well, including a decrease in erythema, scaling, lichenification, excoriation, and pruritus. In contrast, the control group improved in scaling only. Massage therapy could be a useful and cost-effective adjunct to traditional therapy, with parental training in massage technique being an economical, one-time expense. Psychiatric referral may need to be obtained in some cases and is most useful for patients with evident psychological symptoms, whose symptoms are related to emotional stress, and who are motivated to obtain therapy. Factors influencing successful psychiatric referral include optimal preparation of the patient and family through education regarding the reasons for referral, expectations, physician support of therapy, assurance of continuity of care, and the physician's firm belief in the necessity of psychiatric involvement (27).

PSYCHOSOCIAL ISSUES IN PEDIATRIC DERMATOLOGY PRACTICE

Although AD is one childhood skin disorder in which the reciprocal influence of physical and psychosocial health is clearly apparent, there needs to be an overall increased awareness of the impact skin disease can have on the QOL of the pediatric patient. In 1986, a literature review of 15,000 articles written on skin disease yielded only 25 that addressed the psychological impact of skin disease on children (21). Rauch et al. (30) surveyed 377 pediatric dermatology patients ranging from 6 to 12 years of age using the Pediatric Symptom Checklist (PSC), a 35-item parental questionnaire that screens for psychosocial dysfunction in pediatric practice. A higher score reflects a higher level of dysfunction, and a cut-off score of 28 is considered positive and indicative of dysfunction serious enough to require further evaluation. Of the AD patients, 12.7% received positive PSC scores. In a comparison group of 300 subjects drawn from general pediatric practice, 14% scored positive on the PSC. The overall rates of psychosocial dysfunction in patients found in pediatric dermatology practice are similar to those found in the general pediatric population. Approximately half of the PSC-positive group subjects were reported by their parents to have skin disorders that significantly affected their physical appearance. Over one quarter of patients, regardless of PSC score, reported their skin disorder as seriously affecting appearance. This demonstrates a strong correlation between psychosocial dysfunction and the perceived impact of skin disease on appearance. Children with disease that affects their appearance are at higher risk of having psychosocial dysfunction, underscoring the important role appearance may have in a child's psychosocial health. Physicians should not underestimate the degree of impact, as perceived by both patient and parent, that skin disease has on a child's appearance and overall well-being.

The large volume of patients, the fast pace required to see such a volume, and extended periods between visits pose a challenge in terms of dealing with psychosocial issues (21). In the Rauch study, only 26% of subjects in the high-risk positive PSC group had received counseling during the previous year, demonstrating the need for dermatologists to improve at capturing and treating those with psychosocial dysfunction (30). Education is paramount in alleviating the psychological strain of disease burden. Despite time constraints, such efforts can result in facilitating the patient-doctor relationship and increasing compliance with treatment strategy (21).

CONCLUSION

The impact of skin disease on the QOL of the pediatric dermatology population can be dramatic and just as profound as that seen in children with other chronic debilitating diseases. The overall decrement in life quality not only affects the patient but also has consequences for the social supports that surround the patient. Prompt and aggressive intervention is essential in order to prevent the formation of negative behavioral patterns that can result in psychosocial morbidity that may persist beyond the duration of the disease. Effective treatment of AD takes the patient's perception of illness into account and, along with the medical treatment of physical symptoms, incorporates the management of psychosocial issues. The concept of assessing QOL impact and aiming therapy at improving overall QOL is not specific to AD, but has implications for general pediatric dermatology practice as well.

REFERENCES

1. Leung DYM, Tharp M, Boguniewicz M. Psoriasis. In: Fitzpatrick TB, Freedberg IM, Eisen AZ et al., eds. Dermatology in General Medicine. 5th ed. New York: McGraw-Hill, 1999:1464–1465.
2. Su JC, Kemp AS, Varigos GA, et al. Atopic eczema: its impact on the family and financial cost. Arch Dis Child 1997; 76(2):159–162.
3. Dahl RE, Bernhiesel-Broadbent J, Scanlon-Holford S, et al. Sleep disturbances in children with atopic dermatitis. Arch Pediatr Adolesc Med 1995; 149(8):856–860.
4. Schmid-Ott G, Jaeger B, Adamek C, et al. Level of circulating CD8 + T lymphocytes, natural killer cells, and eosinophils increase upon acute psychosocial stress in patients with atopic dermatitis. J Allergy Clin Immunol 2001; 107(1):171–177.
5. Schmid-Ott G, Jaeger B, Meyer S, et al. Different expression of cytokine and membrane molecules by circulating lymphocytes on acute mental stress in patients with atopic dermatitis in comparison with healthy controls. J Allergy Clin Immunol 2001; 108(3):455–462.
6. Denda M, Tsuchiya T, Elias PM, Feingold KR. Stress alters cutaneous permeability barrier homeostasis. Am J Physiol Regul Integr Comp Physiol 2000; 278(2):367–372.
7. Garg A, Chren MM, Sands LP, et al. Psychological stress perturbs the epidermal permeability barrier homeostasis: the implications for the pathogenesis of stress-associated skin disorders. Arch Dermatol 2001; 137(1):53–59.
8. Buske-Kirschbaum A, Jobst S, Psych D, et al. Attenuated free cortisol response to psychosocial stress in children with atopic dermatitis. Psychosom Med 1997; 59(4):419–426.

9. Kodoma A, Horikawa T, Suzuki T, et al. Effect of stress on atopic dermatitis: investigation in patients after the Hanshin earthquake. J Allergy Clin Immunol 1999; 104(1):173–176.

10. Finlay AY. Dermatology Life Quality Index (DLQI)—a simple practical measure for routine clinical use. Clin Exp Dermatol 1994; 19(3):210–216.

11. Lewis-Jones MS, Finlay AY. The Children's Dermatology Life Quality Index (CDLQI): initial validation and practical use. Br J Dermatol 1995; 132:942–949.

12. Kiebert G, Sorenson SV, Revicki D, Fagan SC, et al. Atopic dermatitis is associated with a decrement in health-related quality of life. Int J Dermatol 2002; 41:151–158.

13. Ware JE, Snow KK, Kosinski M, et al. SF-36 Health Survey Manual and Interpretation Guide. Boston: The Health Institute, New England Medical Center, 1993.

14. Linnet J, Jemec GBE. An assessment of anxiety and dermatology life quality in patients with atopic dermatitis. Br J Dermatol 1999; 140:268–272.

15. Lewis-Jones MS, Finlay AY, Dykes PJ. The Infant's Dermatitis Quality of Life Index. Br J Dermatol 2001; 144(1):104–110.

16. White A, Horne DJ, Varigos GA. Psychological profile of the atopic eczema patient. Australas J Dermatol 1990; 31:13–16.

17. Bender BG. Psychologic dysfunction associated with atopic dermatitis. Immunol Allergy Clin North Am 2002; 22(1): 43–54.

18. Ahmar H, Kurban AK. Psychological profile of patients with atopic dermatitis. Br J Dermatol 1976; 95(4):373–377.

19. Absolon CM, Cottrell D, Eldridge SM, et al. Psychological disturbance in atopic eczema: the extent of the problem in school-aged children. Br J Dermatol 1997; 137(2):241–245.

20. Daud LR, Garralda ME, David TJ. Psychosocial adjustment in preschool children with atopic eczema. Arch Dis Child 1993; 69(6):670–676.

21. Rauch PK, Jellinek MS. Developmental and psychosocial considerations in pediatric dermatology practice. Pediatr Dermatol 1986; 3(5):380–383.

22. Howlett S. Emotional dysfunction, child-family relationships and childhood atopic dermatitis. Br J Dermatol 1999; 140(3):381–384.

23. Lawson V, Lewis-Jones MS, Finlay Ay, et al. The family impact of childhood atopic dermatitis: the dermatitis family questionnaire. Br J Dermatol 1998; 138(1):107–113.

24. Pauli-Pott U, Darui A, Beckmann D. Infants with atopic dermatitis: maternal hopelessness, child-rearing attitudes and perceived infant temperament. Psychother Psychosom 1999; 31(1):13–136.

25. Lapidus CS. Role of social factors in atopic dermatitis: the US perspective. J Am Acad Dermatol 2001; 45(1 suppl):S41–43.

26. Gil KM, Keefe FJ, Sampson HA, et al. The relation of stress and family environment to atopic dermatitis symptoms in children. J Psychosom Res 1987; 31(6):673–684.

27. Fritz GK. Psychological aspects of atopic dermatitis. Clin Pediatr 1979; 18(6):360–364.
28. Lapidus CS, Schwartz DF, Honig PJ. Atopic dermatitis in children: Who cares? Who pays? J Am Acad Dermatol 1993; 28:699–703.
29. Emerson RM, Williams AC, Allen BR. What is the cost of atopic dermatitis in preschool children? Br J Dermatol 2001; 144(3):514–522.
30. Rauch PK, Jellinek MS, Murphy JM. Screening for psychosocial dysfunction in pediatric dermatology practice. Clin Pediatr 1991; 30(8):493–497.
31. Reid P, Lewis-Jones MS. Sleep difficulties and their management in preschoolers with atopic eczema. Clin Exp Dermatol 1995; 20(1):38–41.
32. Reuveni H, Chapnick G, Tal A, et al. Sleep fragmentation in children with atopic dermatitis. Arch Pediatr Adolesc Med 1999; 153(3):249–253.
33. Stores G, Burrows A, Crawford C. Physiological sleep disturbance in children with atopic dermatitis: a case control study. Pediatr Dermatol 1998; 15(4):264–268.
34. Bartlett LB, Westbroek R, White JE. Sleep patterns in children with atopic eczema. Acta Derm Venereol 1997; 77(6):446–448.
35. Staughton R. Psychologic approach to atopic skin disease. J Am Acad Dermatol 2001; 45(1):53–54.
36. Gil KM, Keefe FJ, Sampson HA, et al. Direct observation of scratching behavior in children with atopic dermatitis. Behav Ther 1988; 19:213–227.
37. Staab D, Von Reuden U, Kehrt R, et al. Evaluation of a parental training program for the management of childhood atopic dermatitis. Pediatr Allergy Immunol 2002; 13(2):84–90.
38. Ohya Y, Williams H, Steptoe A, et al. Psychosocial factors and adherence to treatment advice in childhood atopic dermatitis. J Invest Dermatol 2001; 117(4):852–857.
39. Schachner L, Field T, Hernandez-Reif M, et al. Atopic dermatitis symptoms decreased in children following massage therapy. Pediatr Dermatol 1998; 15(5):390–395.

20

Health-Related Quality-of-Life Instruments for Psoriasis

Paula S. Lin and John Y. M. Koo
University of California, San Francisco
San Francisco, California, U.S.A.

INTRODUCTION

Psoriasis is a chronic, cosmetically disfiguring and psychosocially disabling dermatological disease which affects 2.6% of the U.S. population (1). Traditionally, outcome measures of various medical treatments have utilized physical assessment of the severity of psoriasis (e.g., assessment of surface area involvement, erythema, thickness, amount of scales) (2). However, more and more healthcare providers have come to realize the psychosocial and occupational impact that psoriasis can have on the patients. For example, 19% of the patients in Ginsburg and Link's study (3) reported incidents of blatant rejection, most often from a gym, pool, hairdresser, or job. In Koo's study (1), 51% felt that the worst or second worst thing about psoriasis was appearance-related (mostly unsightly physical appearance or noticeable flakes). A significant proportion of psoriasis inpatients studied by Ramsey and O'Reagan (4) reported interference with sexual relationships. The physical, social, and psychological aspects all affect a person's quality of life. Given that the usual goal of dermatological care is to improve a patient's quality of life rather than survival, the adequacy of physical outcome measures has been questioned in recent years, with increasing awareness of the importance of quality-of-life measures.

DEFINITION OF QUALITY OF LIFE

A person's quality of life (QoL) is an inclusive concept that encompasses all factors that impact a person's life, including physical, social, and psychological well-being (5). Health-related QoL (HRQoL) is more narrow; it is QoL associated with a disease and its symptoms (5). HRQoL for psoriasis encompasses the following (1,2,6–8):

> *Physical disability*: e.g., itching, irritation, pain, insomnia, interference with walking/using hands/doing housework
> *Psychological impact*: e.g., self-consciousness, embarrassment, helplessness, anger/frustration, depression, stigmatization, anticipation of rejection, preoccupation with psoriasis, peer acceptance, family acceptance
> *Social impact*: e.g., making friends, forming relationships, going to social functions, going to a beach/pool/gym, participating in sports, shaking hands, wearing different types or colors of clothing to cover affected areas, going to a hairdresser
> *Sexual impact*: e.g., less sexual activity (because of feelings of physical unattractiveness)
> *Occupational impact*: denied promotions, not hired for jobs, lost time from work/school
> *Daily burdens*: e.g., changing clothes frequently, taking more baths, vacuuming frequently, encountering problems at the hairdresser's, wearing specific clothing to cover affected skin
> *Treatment impact*: e.g., time demands, money, side effects of treatment, messiness of treatment

HRQoL INSTRUMENTS

Various health questionnaires have been designed to address patients' HRQoL, including generic, specialty-specific (e.g., dermatology-specific), and disease-specific (e.g., psoriasis-specific) instruments (9). In order for such an instrument to be useful, it would:

1. Have validity (i.e., it measures well what it purports to measure)
2. Have reliability (i.e., it is reproducible over time)

3. Be sensitive enough to measure HRQoL in the entire spectrum of psoriasis severity
4. Be applicable to a wide variety of patients in different settings
5. Be quick and easy for patients to take

The validity of an instrument is a crucial element. It tells how well an instrument measures what it purports to measure. There are three types of validity: content validity, criterion validity, and construct validity (10). *Content* validity indicates the degree to which the items on the test are representative of knowledge being tested (10). For example, by giving surveys to a small focus group of sample patients to ascertain the psychosocial and occupational issues they consider relevant, one can compile the results of these surveys and use these results to design a questionnaire that can claim content validity. *Criterion* validity is ideally established by comparing the measurement to a gold standard, if one exists (10). For example, questionnaires with high correlation to well-established instruments would have criterion validity. *Construct* validity involves testing explicit hypotheses about dimensions that comprise the construct being measured and about their expected interrelationships (11). For instance, an instrument has construct validity if there is confirmation of the hypothesis that patients with widespread skin lesions have higher scores on the instruments (i.e., higher negative impact on QoL) than patients with isolated skin lesions.

Reliability, or reproducibility, of an instrument is another crucial element. Measures of reliability include internal consistency and test-retest. The internal consistency reliability indicates how strongly the items are related to each other, i.e., whether they are measuring a single characteristic (10). Internal consistency is measured by Cronbach's alpha coefficient. Test-retest reliability is an instrument's ability to give consistent measurements on different occasions (10) and is measured by Spearman's rank correlation coefficient or Pearson's correlation coefficient. Correlation coefficients for both validity and reliability measurements can range from 0 to 1.00, with 0 being no correlation and 1.00 being very high correlation (10).

In this chapter we review the current state of psoriatic HRQoL instruments for dermatologists. We will present an overview of two psoriasis-specific instruments (Psoriasis Disability Index and Psoriasis Life Stress Inventory) and four dermatology-specific instruments (Dermatology Life Quality Index, Dermatology Quality of Life Scales, Skindex-61, and Skindex-29), with emphasis on the five characteristics discussed previously.

Quality-of-life instruments may enable dermatologists to better tailor the aggressiveness of the treatment to each individual patient's level of HRQoL impairment. The findings from these instruments may also help detrivialize psoriasis in the eyes of the general public, mass media, insurance companies, the government, nondermatological physicians, and even some dermatologists. With the increasing emphasis on evidence-based medicine, HRQoL instruments also help make outcome studies in the field of dermatology more evidence-based.

A systematic literature review of all available information published between 1985 and 1999 in English on HRQoL instruments for psoriasis was performed. In order to keep the scope of the review and the discussion manageable, only instruments that were purposely developed for dermatological use were reviewed.

MAJOR HRQoL INSTRUMENTS UNDER DEVELOPMENT

Psoriasis-Specific Instruments

Psoriasis Disability Index

The Psoriasis Disability Index (PDI), developed by Finlay and Kelly (2), was a 10-item instrument designed to quantify functional lifestyle disability within 4 weeks before treatment and 4 weeks after discharge. Fifty-four psoriasis patients in the United Kingdom (35 inpatients, 19 outpatients) completed a 28-item questionnaire; 18 items were later discarded to form a 10-item instrument [6 items had too weak a correlation (i.e., ambiguous or inconsistent; $r < 0.32$, $p > 0.01$) and 12 items had too strong a correlation (i.e., measuring similar or redundant information; $r > 0.4$, $p < 0.002$)] (2). The final 10-item instrument had five questions on daily activities—one on work, three on leisure, and one on treatment—with a visual analog scale from 1 to 7 for each question (maximum score of 70) and a question time base of 4 weeks. Content validation consisted of literature review and modified responses from 54 patients. Construct validation via correlation with percent of affected body surface area was significant but small ($r = 0.29$, $n = 54$, $p < 0.003$) (2,5). Internal consistency reliability was moderate, with correlation $rs = 0.32$–0.40 (2,5).

Finlay et al. (12) added items to the 10-item version to create the 15-item version: daily activities (5 items), work/school (3 items), relationships (2 items), leisure (4 items), and treatment effects (1 item). Unchanged were the scale of 1–7 for each question and the question time base of 4 weeks. This version was given to 32 psoriasis patients in the United Kingdom (23 inpatients, 9 outpatients) and validated against the following:

1. **Psoriasis Area and Severity Index (PASI)**: Moderate correlation: $rs = 0.40$, $p < 0.05$, $n = 32$ (5,12). The PASI is an assessment of the

clinical severity of psoriasis by area of involvement, erythema, infiltration, and desquamation.

2. **United Kingdom Sickness Impact Profile (UK SIP)**: Moderate correlation: $rs = 0.47$, $p < 0.01$, $n = 32$ (5,12). The UK SIP is a generic instrument with 136 items in three dimensions and 12 categories: physical dimension (body care/movement, mobility, ambulation), psychosocial dimension (emotional behavior, social interaction, alertness behavior, communication), and independent categories (sleep/rest, home management, work, recreation/past-time, eating). The UK SIP determines the impact of disease on patients' functional behavior and has been used in hypertension, angina, other diseases, and assessment of medication side effects (12).

In other studies, the 15-item PDI was validated against the following:

1. **General Health Questionnaire (GHQ)**: High correlation: $rs = 0.71$, $p < 0.001$, $n = 22$ tested in PUVA patients in the United Kingdom (5,13). The 28-item GHQ is a widely used generic instrument to assess psychological distress (13).

2. Two **Medical Outcomes Study 36-Item Short Form Health Survey (SF-36) tests**: low to moderate correlation: $r = -0.17$ to -0.45, $p < 0.001$, $n = 644$ (5), and $r = -0.29$ to -0.44, $p < 0.0001$, $n = 404$ (5,14). SF-36 is a generic instrument that fulfills stringent criteria of reliability and validity (14) and was designed to survey health status in the Medical Outcomes Study. It is composed of 36 items in eight areas: physical functioning, social functioning, role limitations due to physical problems, role limitations due to emotional problems, general mental health, bodily pain, energy/fatigue, and general health perceptions (15).

3. **Dermatology Life Quality Index (DLQI)**: High correlation: $r = 0.82$, $p < 0.001$, $n = 644$ for mild to moderate psoriatic outpatients at University Hospital of Wales (5). DLQI is a dermatology-specific instrument that will be discussed below.

PDI showed significant decline in scores after inpatient treatment. Before inpatient treatment, PDI $= 34.1$ (± 11.1); 4 weeks after treatment, PDI $= 22.3$ (± 10.9) ($n = 20$, $p < 0.002$) (2). This suggests that PDI is sensitive to changes in severity of psoriasis. However, one must keep in mind that the improvement in scores may be partly attributable to adaptation over time to a chronic disease. A major limitation of PDI is the exclusion of psychological disability. According to Koo (1), PDI may be a useful instrument for people with severe psoriasis (e.g., patients who are referred to dermatologists by primary care providers in the United Kingdom), who have more physical disability and limitations on lifestyle. However, for psoriasis patients who have mild to moderate disease, a psychometric instrument may provide a better HRQoL measurement. Koo's idea was supported by a Finlay study which found that, when the 15-item PDI was given to those with mild to moderate disease as well as those with severe disease, there was no correlation of the PDI with the PASI or UK SIP (1).

Psoriasis Life Stress Inventory

The Psoriasis Life Stress Inventory (PLSI) is a 15-item psoriasis-specific instrument designed by Gupta and Gupta (6) to provide an index of psoriasis-related stress. An original 41-item questionnaire, compiled from clinical experience with 50 patients, was given to 217 patients with mild to moderate psoriasis at the University of Michigan (139 inpatients, 78 outpatients). Fifteen of the original 41 items were included in the final version. Of the 15 items, 11 were stress associated with cosmetic disfigurement/social stigma and 4 were stress associated with symptoms of the disease/inconvenience of treatment. The PLSI had a scale from 0 to 3 for each question, with a maximum score of 45. Question time base was one month.

Content validation consisted of experiences with 50 patients and modification from a 41-item version. Criterion/construct validity was evaluated with the following:

1. Comparison of PLSI with **global patient self-ratings** of psoriasis severity showed significant but small correlation ($r = 0.15$–0.24, $p = 0.001$–0.04) (6). PLSI score of 10 delineated a subgroup of patients with greater overall psoriasis severity ($p = 0.007$), greater involvement of cosmetically disfiguring areas ($p < 0.01$), greater number of psoriasis flare-ups ($p = 0.009$), and great pruritis ($p = 0.001$).
2. Comparison of PLSI with **PASI** (psoriasis severity determined by a clinician) showed no difference between high-stress (PLSI > $10, n = 116$) and low-stress (PLSI < $10, n = 34$) reactive groups (16).
3. Comparison of PLSI with **SF-36** and **PDI** showed that the high-stress group (PLSI > $10, n = 116$) had poorer mental health by SF-36 ($p = 0.001$) and experienced more disability in all areas of PDI ($p = 0.001$) than the low-stress group (PLSI > $10, n = 34$) (16).

Internal consistency was high. The Cronbach's alpha coefficient was 0.90 in the United States (5,6) and 0.88 in the United Kingdom (5). Test-retest reliability was not reported. Sensitivity to change in HRQoL over time was not assessed. Compared with the PDI, the PLSI may be a better measurement of HRQoL, especially in patients with mild to moderate psoriasis, given PLSI's emphasis on psychosocial stressors. Limitations include having only modest correlation with global patient self-rating and no correlation with PASI.

Dermatology-Specific Instruments

Dermatology Life Quality Index

The Dermatology Life Quality Index (DLQI) is a 10-item dermatology-specific instrument designed by Finlay and Khan (7) to provide a simple, practical method of measuring the disability of patients with any skin disease. The DLQI was developed from the answers of 120 dermatology outpatients at the University Hospital of Wales and subsequently given to 200 consecutive new dermatology outpatients there. The 10 items focused on symptoms (1 item), feelings (one item), daily activities (two items), leisure (two items), work/school (one item), relationships (two items), and treatment (one item). There was a scale of 0–3 for each item, with a maximum score of 30. Patients answered questions concerning the previous 7 days.

Content validity consisted of modification of answers from 120 dermatology outpatients. Construct/criterion validity was evaluated by the following:

1. Comparison of DLQI scores in 200 dermatology outpatients and 100 controls: DLQI scores of patients with psoriasis, atopic eczema, generalized pruritus, viral warts, and acne all were significantly higher ($p < 0.0001$) than those of control. Overall mean DLQI was 7.3(± 6.3) for patients and 0.5(± 1.1) for controls (5,7).

2. Comparison with **PDI**: There was high correlation ($r = 0.82$, $p < 0.001$, $n = 644$ patients with mild to moderate psoriasis) (5).

3. Comparison with **SF-36**: There were small to moderate negative correlations ($r = -0.13$ to -0.43, $p < 0.001$, $n = 644$ patients with mild to moderate psoriasis) (5).

Internal consistency had a wide range ($rs = 0.23$–0.70, $p < 0.002$) (7). Test-retest reliability ($n = 53$, 1-week interval) was very high ($rs = 0.99$, $p <$

0.0001) (7). DLQI has shown sensitivity to changes in QoL after inpatient treatment (17). Overall DLQI on admission was 13.2 ($\pm$ 7.6), which decreased to 7.7 ($\pm$ 6.8) 4 weeks after discharge ($n = 181$ inpatients at Wales, $p < 0.001$) (7). Similarly, for psoriasis patients, DLQI on admission was 13.9 (6.5); 4 weeks after discharge, 6.7 ($\pm$ 5.6) ($n = 63$, $p < 0.001$) (7). DLQI has the advantages of being short and practical, highly reliable, and applicable to many dermatologic disorders. However, only 1 of the 10 items addressed psychological disability, and the time base of 7 days may be too short.

Dermatology Quality of Life Scales

Dermatology Quality of Life Scales (DQOLS) is a 41-item dermatology-specific instrument (8) designed to complement the DLQI, with greater emphasis on the psychosocial aspect. The 41 items were compiled from the written answers of 50 dermatological outpatients in London and subsequently given to 118 dermatological outpatients in London. Items were divided into four psychosocial subscales [embarrassment (five items), despair (five items), irritableness (three items), distress (four items)], four activity subscales [everyday (six items), summer (three items), social (two items), sexual (one item)], and 12 symptoms. Each item was rated 0–4, with scores standardized to 100. Question time base was 4 weeks.

Content validity consisted of modification of the answers from 50 outpatients to develop the questionnaire. Construct/criterion validity was evaluated by the following:

1. Ability of scales to detect clinically expected differences in patients with acne and psoriasis ($n = 66$ acne $+ 66$ psoriasis): acne had more psychosocial impact (not significant) but less activities impact ($p = 0.004$) compared with psoriasis. Also, there was a greater psychosocial impact of acne for women than for men ($p = 0.01$) (5,8).
2. Comparison with the Nottingham Health Profile (NHP): DQOLS demonstrated greater sensitivity (compared to the NHP) to psychosocial and activity subscales experienced by acne and psoriasis patients (5,8). NHP is a widely used generic health status instrument consisting of 38 items in six categories.

Internal consistency was high, with Cronbach's alpha coefficient of 0.92 (psychosocial) and 0.83 (activities) (8). Test-retest reliability ($n = 41$ phototherapy patients, 7- to 10-day interval) was also high, with correlation coefficient of 0.84 for both psychosocial and activities subscales (5,8). Sensitivity to change in HRQoL after treatment was not assessed. DQOLS has emphasis on psychosocial aspect and would complement DLQI for general dermatological conditions. However, DQOLS is too long to be practical for use in the clinical setting. DQOLS can benefit from additional validation against well-established instruments, correlation of psychosocial/ activity scores with symptom scores, and modification/elimination of redundant questions.

Skindex-61

Skindex-61 (11) is a 61-item dermatology-specific instrument with 8 scales: cognitive (15 items), social (10 items), depression (7 items), fear (7 items), embarrassment (4 items), anger (5 items), physical discomfort (4 items), and physical irritation (9 items). Its purpose was to measure comprehensively the effects of skin conditions on patients' HRQoL and to compare this measure with physicians' judgments of clinical severity. Two hundred and one dermatology outpatients in Ohio answered the questionnaire with regards to the previous 4 weeks. Scores were standardized to 100.

Content validity consisted of literature search and directed focus sessions with patients, physicians, and dermatology nurses. Construct/ criterion validity was evaluated by the following:

1. Comparison of scores in patients with inflammatory skin conditions (eczema, psoriasis, and acne) and in patients with isolated skin lesions (nevi, malignancies): higher Skindex-61 scores in all eight scales in the inflammatory skin group, as hypothesized (5,11).
2. Exploratory factor analysis: seven factors were identified that correlate with Skindex-61 scores (5,11).
3. Comparison of scores with physician's judgment of clinical severity: no correlation ($p > 0.3$), except for acne (5,11).
4. Convergent validity with SF-36: moderate correlations ($r = 0.44$– 0.56) between both instruments (using comparative scales) (18).

Internal consistency was high, with Cronbach's alpha coefficient of 0.76–0.86 (5,11). Test-retest reliability was also high, with correlation coefficients of 0.68–0.90 ($n = 40$, 72-hour time interval) (5,11). Three of the eight scales demonstrated responsiveness to clinical change after 6 months (11). Skindex-61 is comprehensive but takes too long to complete (15 min).

Skindex-29

Skindex-29 (19) is a modification of Skindex-61, developed in an effort to improve discriminative capability, improve evaluative capability, and reduce the time for completion of the test. It has 29 items with three factors:

emotions (10 items), symptoms (seven items), and functioning (12 items). The test was taken by 591 outpatients in Ohio with regard to the previous 4 weeks. Scores were standardized to 100.

Content validity consisted of modification of Skindex-61 and examination of the responses of the same patients to open-ended questions. Construct validity was evaluated by the following:

1. Comparison of Skindex-29 scores in patients with psoriasis/ eczema and patients with isolated lesions: patients with psoriasis or eczema had higher mean Skindex scores ($p < 0.001$) than patients with benign/non-melanoma skin malignancies (19).
2. Exploratory factor analysis: three factors were identified that correlated with *a priori* scales (19).
3. Comparison of Skindex-29 scores with physician's judgment of clinical severity for inflammatory dramatoses (including eczema, acne, psoriasis, rosacea, tinea, etc): significant but small correlations ($r = 0.15$, 0.24, 0.14, for the functioning, emotion, and symptom scales, respectively; $p \leqslant 0.001$ for each) (19).

Internal consistency was high, with Cronbach's alpha coefficient ranging from 0.87 to 0.96 (19). Test-retest reliability (72-hr interval) was also high, with correlation coefficient ranging from 0.88 to 0.92 (19). Skindex-29 compared with Skindex-61 showed the following (19):

1. Shorter test-taking time (5 vs. 15 min)
2. Improved discriminative capability: >70% of patients chose the same response in only 3 (10%) of 29 items [compared with 17 (28%) of 61 items]
3. Improved evaluative capability: three of three scales were significantly responsive to clinical change after 3 months (compared with three of eight scales)

See Table 1 for a generalized summary of the six HRQoL instruments previously discussed.

REVIEW OF ACTUAL FINDINGS OF HRQoL STUDIES ON PSORIASIS

In addition to evaluating the various HRQoL instruments, it is interesting to see what studies to date have shown about psoriatic patients' HRQoL. Unfortunately, the studies mentioned so far have focused on how valid and reliable their instruments were, instead of what the instruments actually showed about the various aspects of HRQoL in patients with psoriasis.

TABLE 1 Overview of Six Health-Related Quality-of-Life Instruments for Psoriasis

Name of instrument No. of items; time base	Validity/correlation with clinical severity	Reliability	Sensitivity to change	Comments
Psoriasis Disability Index (PDI) 15 items; 4 weeks	Good/moderate correlation for severe psoriasis No correlation for mild to moderate psoriasis	Good	Good	Does not address psychosocial impact Specific for psoriasis Short; practical for quick evaluation
Psoriasis Life Stress Inventory (PLSI) 15 items; 1 month	Good/no correlation	Good	Not tested	Addresses psychosocial impact Specific for psoriasis Short; practical for quick evaluation No correlation with clinical severity
Dermatology Life Quality Index (DLQI) 10 items; 7 days	Good/correlation not tested	Good	Good	1/10 items addresses psychosocial impact Time base may be too short Not specific for psoriasis Short; practical for quick evaluation
Dermatology Quality of Life Scales (DQOLS) 41 items; 4 weeks	Good/correlation not tested	Good	Not tested	Addresses psychosocial impact Not specific for psoriasis May be too lengthy for quick evaluation
Skindex-61 61 items; 4 weeks	Good/no correlation	Good	Moderate	Comprehensive questionnaire Addresses psychosocial impact May be too lengthy for quick evaluation Not specific for psoriasis No correlation with clinical severity
Skindex-29 29 items; 4 weeks	Good/modest correlation	Good	Good	Addresses psychosocial impact Not specific for psoriasis Short; practical for quick evaluation Significant (although modest) correlation with clinical severity

Other studies will be discussed instead to give us a better perspective of what psoriatic patients experience.

Gupta and Gupta (20) studied 215 psoriasis inpatients and outpatients in the United States and found that, regarding appearance/socialization, patients most often reported being self-conscious among strangers (53% reported this), avoiding public places like swimming pools, health clubs, or restaurants (50%), wearing unattractive/uncomfortable clothes to cover affected areas (46%), and avoiding sunbathing (44%). Least common were people not wanting to be seen in the patient's company (4%), being rejected by opposite sex (7%), friends/family making rude remarks (10–12%), and hairdresser reluctant to cut the patient's hair (15%). Regarding occupation/finances, patients most often reported having inadequate money to pay for medical bills (22%), having fear of losing jobs (15%), and losing wages/income (13%). Lastly, regarding symptoms/treatment, patients most often were inconvenienced by shedding of skin (66%), had to set aside a large amount of time for psoriasis care (51%), and feared the side effects of medical treatments (31%). The 18–29 and 30–45 year age groups had more problems with appearance/socialization and occupation/finances. Men had more work-related stress than women, but there was no gender difference in appearance/socialization.

Another study by Gupta and Gupta (6), the PLSI study on 217 psoriasis patients in the United States, found that the most commonly reported negative impact of psoriasis can be classified into two categories. The first category is stress from cosmetic disfigurement, especially self-consciousness among strangers (52% reported this), avoidance of public place (e.g., swimming pool, health club, restaurant) (50%), wearing certain clothes to cover affected areas (46%), and avoidance of sunbathing (44%). Less common were stress from having a hairdresser reluctant to cut the patient's hair (15%) and people making a conscious effort not to touch patient (18%). The second category is stress from coping with the physical aspects of the disease, especially inconvenience from the shedding of skin (66%), time commitment to the care of psoriasis (51%), fear of medication side effects (31%), and not enough money for medical bills (22%).

Dooley and Finlay (21) evaluated social adjustment of 43 respondents with psoriasis in the United Kingdom in 12 social situations. These authors defined social adjustment as the relationship between constructs (i.e., psychological parameters), such as confidence, embarrassment, self-consciousness, aggression, body awareness, and shyness for psoriasis patients. They found that psoriasis patients are less well socially adjusted in highly visible situations, especially on the beach and at the hairdressers. There was no difference in social adjustment between men and women, but women have elevated body awareness at work and at home, which correlates with the severity of their illness.

Ginsburg and Link (3), in a study involving 100 psoriasis patients in the United States, found that 19% of patients experienced 50 episodes of gross rejection, most often from gym/health clubs, hairdressers, and swimming pools. They concluded that rejection experiences led to feelings of stigmatization, which is then associated with help seeking and, to some degree, with interference with work.

Koo (1) performed a nationwide, population-based epidemiological study of psoriasis, with emphasis on psychosocial impact and impact on day-to-day living. Overall, there was good correlation between self-rated severity of psoriasis and the extent of impact on psychosocial factors. The emotions most affected were self-consciousness, helplessness, embarrassment, and anger/frustration, whereas interference with peer/family acceptance and wish to be outgoing were least affected. Itching, physical irritation, and physical pain/soreness had the most physical impact; difficulty with housework, walking, or using hands had the least physical impact. The day-to-day activities most affected were going to a pool/beach/gym, wearing swimming suits, and going to a hairdresser; whereas being interviewed, shaking hands, and going to school were least affected. Regarding body image and social acceptability, respondents were concerned about the extent to which psoriasis makes physical appearance unsightly. In the overall psychosocial impact, the question "How disturbing is your psoriasis?" received the highest rating and correlated most closely with self-rated psoriasis severity. Respondents tended to agree that people in general and doctors underestimate the psychological and social impact of psoriasis. Respondents were least likely to feel that psoriasis has negatively affected their career or caused them to experience rejection by the opposite sex. Seventy-four percent of the respondents felt that the worst or second worst thing about psoriasis was symptom-related, especially itching or scratching, whereas 51% felt it was appearance-related, with unsightly physical appearance and flaking most often mentioned.

Ramsay and O'Reagan (4) evaluated the social and psychological effects of psoriasis in 140 inpatients in the United Kingdom. Regarding social activities, the most common effects were avoidance of swimming (72%)/sunbathing (60%), avoidance of hairdressers (34%), avoidance of sports (40%), and avoidance of communal baths/showers (64%). Emotional impact included getting constant stares (57%), feeling embarrassed (55%), feeling "unclean" (56%). 50% reported sexual impact, of whom 65% had genital plaques. The majority (86%) felt that psoriasis did not affect their career choice, but 37% missed work for 1–8 weeks in the previous 12 months and 11% missed work for even longer. Regarding clothes, 64% avoided buying short-sleeved summer clothes, 33% avoided dark-colored clothes (because of scalp scales), and 25% avoided buying clothes altogether. When asked about the worst aspect of psoriasis, 48% reported general appearance of skin and 31% reported itching. Eighty-six percent felt that problems with psoriasis would markedly decrease if the general public were educated about psoriasis.

DISCUSSION

From the various HRQoL studies it appears that the worst aspects about psoriasis are pruritis and the general appearance of skin (1,4). Most of the physical impact is from itching/irritation/pain and less from difficulty with using hands/walking/doing housework (1). Psychological impact is attributed mostly to self-consciousness and embarrassment, with peer/family acceptance playing minor roles (1,4,6,20). Avoiding beaches, swimming pools, gyms, and hairdressers and wearing unattractive/uncomfortable clothes to cover affected areas have great social impact on psoriatic patients, whereas shaking hands, forming relationships, making friends, and going to social functions have less social impact (1,4,20). Psoriasis also has some sexual impact, especially if it involves the groin (1,4). In terms of occupational impact, there is loss of time from work with loss of wages and there is fear of losing jobs, but career choice is not usually affected (1,4,20). There appears to be no gender difference in appearance/socialization (20,21).

So what purposes can HRQoL instruments serve? According to Finlay (9), HRQoL measures can be used for clinical, research, audit, and political/financial purposes. Clinical uses include giving the physician and patient more insight into the patient's problems, monitoring progress after therapy, informing clinical decisions, and helping the patient understand and cope with the impact of his or her skin condition (e.g., referral to support groups or psychiatric counseling). Research use includes demonstrating the effectiveness of a specific therapy. Audit use includes giving a patient-based view of service effectiveness. Political/financial use includes comparing the impact of skin diseases to other diseases in order to convince the funding sources that patients with skin diseases matter and that treatments can make a difference in a patient's quality of life.

However, at least three studies (1,11,16) have shown no correlation of psoriasis severity (as assessed by clinicians) with various HRQoL instruments. This brings into question the usefulness of these HRQoL measurements for the aforementioned purposes, as these scores do not correlate with physical outcome measures. Two other instruments (DLQI and DQOLS) were not specifically tested for correlation with clinically determined disease severity. Skindex-29 appears to be the only instrument with significant (although only modest) correlations with clinical assessments of inflammatory skin conditions (e.g., eczema, acne, psoriasis, rosacea, tinea). With the knowledge that, among individuals, there may be vastly different HRQoL responses to a given degree of disease severity (e.g., some individuals with a few spots are devastated; others with extensive disease are well adjusted to it), HRQoL measures may not correlate with objective measures of disease severity yet still be valid measures of the impact of the disease on individual patients. Thus, the lack of correlation to disease extent in no way reduces the validity of HRQoL measurements; however, it diminishes the usefulness of these measurements. Therefore, there is a still a need to modify existing HRQoL instruments or design new instruments to create one that can demonstrate better correlation between the overall HRQoL and average clinical severity in a group of psoriatic patients, even if such correlation may be unattainable for individual patients. Only then can HRQoL instruments be fully utilizable for clinical, research, audit, and political/financial purposes. For now, dermatologists can utilize the existing instruments to determine the most appropriate level of aggressiveness of treatment based on each individual patient's level of HRQoL impairment. They can use the instruments to gain insight into their patients' problems and to help their patients cope with their disease. These instruments, as they become more refined, will hopefully help detrivialize psoriasis in the eyes of the insurance companies, the government, the general public, mass media, nondermatological physicians, and even some dermatologists.

CONCLUSION

Much progress has been made in designing and validating various HRQoL instruments. However, in order to enhance the usefulness of these instruments, there is still a need for future efforts at refining them to achieve better correlation between HRQoL measurements and the clinical severity of psoriasis.

REFERENCES

1. Koo J. Population-based epidemiologic study of psoriasis with emphasis on quality of life assessment. Psychodermatology 1996; 14:485–496.
2. Finlay AY, Kelly SE. Psoriasis—an index of disability. Clin Exp Dermatol 1987; 12:8–11.

3. Ginsburg I, Link B. Psychosocial consequences of rejection and stigma feelings in psoriasis patients. J Invest Dermatol 1993; 32:587–591.

4. Ramsay B, O'Reagan M. A survey of the social and psychological effects of psoriasis. Br J Dermatol 1988; 118:195–201.

5. Ashcroft D. Quality of life measures in psoriasis: a critical appraisal of their quality. J Clin Pharm Ther 1998; 23:391–398.

6. Gupta M, Gupta A. The Psoriasis Life Stress Inventory: a preliminary index of psoriasis-related stress. Acta Derm Venereol 1995; 75:240–243.

7. Finlay AY, Khan GK. Dermatology Life Quality Index (DLQI)—a simple practical measure for routine clinical use. Clin Exp Dermatol 1994; 19:210–216.

8. Morgan M, McCreedy R, Simpson J, Hay RJ. Dermatology quality of life scales—a measure of the impact of skin diseases. Br J Dermatol 1997; 136:202–206.

9. Finlay AY. Quality of life measurement in dermatology: a practical guide. Br J Dermatol 1997; 136:305–314.

10. Dawson-Saunders B, Trapp R. Summarizing Data. Basic and Clinical Biostatistics. Norwalk, CT: Appleton and Lange, 1994:41–63.

11. Chren MM, Lasek RJ, Quinn LM, Mostow EN, Zyzanski SJ. Skindex, a quality-of-life measure for patients with skin disease: reliability, validity, and responsiveness. Soc Invest Dermatol 1996; 107:707–713.

12. Finlay AY, Khan GK, Luscombe DK, Salek MS. Validation of Sickness Impact Profile and Psoriasis Disability Index in psoriasis. Br J Dermatol 1990; 123:751–756.

13. Root S, Kent G, Al-Abadie MSK. The relationship between disease severity, disability and psychological distress in patients undergoing PUVA treatment for psoriasis. Dermatology 1994; 189:234–237.

14. O'Neill P, Kelly P. Postal questionnaire study of disability in the community associated with psoriasis. Br Med J 1996; 313:919–921.

15. Ware J, Sherbourne C. The MOS 36-Item Short-Form Health Survey (SF-36). Med Care 1992; 30:473–481.

16. Fortune DG, Main CJ, O'Sullivan TM, Griffiths CEM. Quality of life in patients with psoriasis: the contribution of clinical variables and psoriasis-specific stress. Br J Dermatol 1997; 137:755–760.

17. Kurwa H, Finlay AY. Dermatology in-patient management greatly improves life quality. Br J Dermatol 1995; 133:575–578.

18. Chren MM, Lasek RJ, Quinn LM, Covinsky KE. Convergent and discriminant validity of a generic and disease-specific instrument to measure quality of life in patients with skin disease. J Invest Dermatol 1997; 108:103–107.

19. Chren MM, Lasek RJ, Flocke SA, Zyzanski SJ. Improved discriminative and evaluative capability of a refined version of Skindex, a quality-of-life instrument for patients with skin diseases. Arch Dermatol 1997; 133:1433–1440.

20. Gupta M, Gupta A. Age and gender differences in the impact of psoriasis on quality of life. Int J Dermatol 1995; 34:700–703.

21. Dooley G, Finlay AY. Personal construct systems of psoriatic patients. Clin Exp Dermatol 1990; 15:401–405.

21

Cutaneous Sensory Disorder

Roger S. Lo*
UCLA Medical Center
Los Angeles, California, U.S.A.

John Y. M. Koo
University of California, San Francisco
San Francisco, California, U.S.A.

INTRODUCTION

Cutaneous sensory disorder (cutaneous dysesthesia syndrome) refers to cases in which the patients present with idiopathic, abnormal skin sensations such as itching, burning, stinging, crawling, or biting without apparent primary skin lesions associated with a diagnosable dermatological, mental, or medical condition. In certain cases, more specific diagnostic terms have been used to refer to specific anatomical locations of involvement (e.g., vulvodynia, glossodynia) or if the pathogenesis were understood (e.g., notalgia paresthetica, postherpetic neuralgia). The average practicing dermatologists are well trained to make dermatological diagnoses based on skin morphologies and to elucidate an underlying systemic etiology for a

---

* *Current affiliation*: Weill Medical College of Cornell University, New York, New York, U.S.A.

cutaneous sensory complaint such as pruritus. However, in situations where no primary skin lesions can be visualized and an exhaustive medical work-up has failed to reveal underlying organic diseases such as lymphoma or renal insufficiency, they are frequently at a loss as to what to pursue next. In such situations, the patient is often assumed to have a cutaneous sensory disorder as a diagnosis of exclusion.

As the diagnostic strategy outlined in this chapter will make evident, the diagnosis of cutaneous sensory disorder should not be reached hastily without a thorough and systematic consideration of the differential diagnoses, some of which may be treatable. Even when a diagnosis of cutaneous sensory disorder is entertained, certain cases may still warrant further diagnostic work-up. For instance, one subtype of cutaneous sensory disorder involves patients with chronic pruritus without evidence of primary skin lesions, underlying systemic disorder, or documentable mental illness. These cases have been termed central pruritus as the patients respond poorly to peripherally acting (nonsedating) antihistamines. Among these patients, there has been a growing recognition that at least some of these cases of chronic idiopathic pruritus may involve specific central nervous system (CNS) lesions (e.g., CNS tumors, stroke). These lesions may be treated surgically, and/or the symptoms (i.e., intractable pruritus) may be treated using agents that aim to target potentially relevant neurotransmission pathways for CNS-mediated itch.

ON THE ROAD TO DIAGNOSING A CUTANEOUS SENSORY DISORDER: NEUROGENIC VERSUS PSYCHOGENIC PRURITUS

Besides the absence of primary skin lesions, certain clinical findings suggest that the pruritus can be CNS mediated. Frequently, pruritus is associated with an observable psychiatric problem, especially anxiety and/or depression, but occasionally obsessive-compulsive disorder and psychosis with delusional ideations. In this context, a chronological association where the onset of psychological stress or disorder precedes the onset of pruritus can be suggestive of psychogenic pruritus. However, in real-life practice, it is often very difficult to ascertain whether the observed psychopathology (such as anxiety of depression) is primary or secondary to the pruritus. In actual management, this distinction is not as critical as it appears since it is well established that even secondary psychopathologies can enhance itch perception (1–4). Therefore, associated psychopathologies should be treated whether thought to be primary or secondary in relation to pruritus. In fact, in cases where the temporal relationship between the onset of psychopathology and pruritus is difficult to ascertain, it is better not to make an issue out of whether pruritus is primary or secondary to psychopathology.

At times, the clinical clue comes directly from the patient suffering from psychopathologies where insight is intact. For instance, patients suffering from neurotic excoriation, which is associated with obsessive-compulsive disorder, may acknowledge the self-inflicted nature of the excoriated lesions, leading to a cycle of itch–compulsive scratch–itch (5). In addition, the symptoms of neurotic excoriation reportedly worsen at night or when the patient is alone (6).

Another important clue to the possible psychogenic origin of pruritus comes from its paroxysmal nature. Paroxysmal pruritus is usually intense with sudden onset and sudden resolution, with no pruritus in between the episodes. However, paroxysmal pruritus can be either neurogenic or psychogenic, and it is of paramount importance to try to distinguish between the two. Although rare in the literature (reviewed in Refs. 2 and 7), pruritus can present as the predominant symptom of central or peripheral nervous system lesions. The reported etiologies of neurogenic pruritus are summarized in Fig. 1. These "real" neurogenic causes of pruritus most often occur in the absence of primary skin lesions and should be considered in the differential diagnoses of psychogenic pruritus (Fig. 2). The prominent characteristics of neurogenic pruritus, which can be helpful in distinguishing neurogenic from psychogenic pruritus, are outlined in Table 1.

According to conventional wisdom, psychogenic pruritus should not wake the patient at night, while "real" organic or neurogenic pruritus can awake the patient at night. This may relate to the generalization that organic

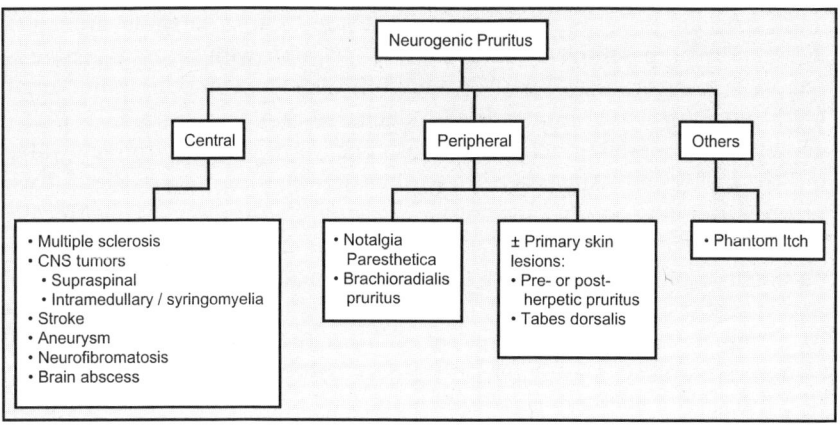

FIGURE 1 Etiologies of neurogenic pruritus.

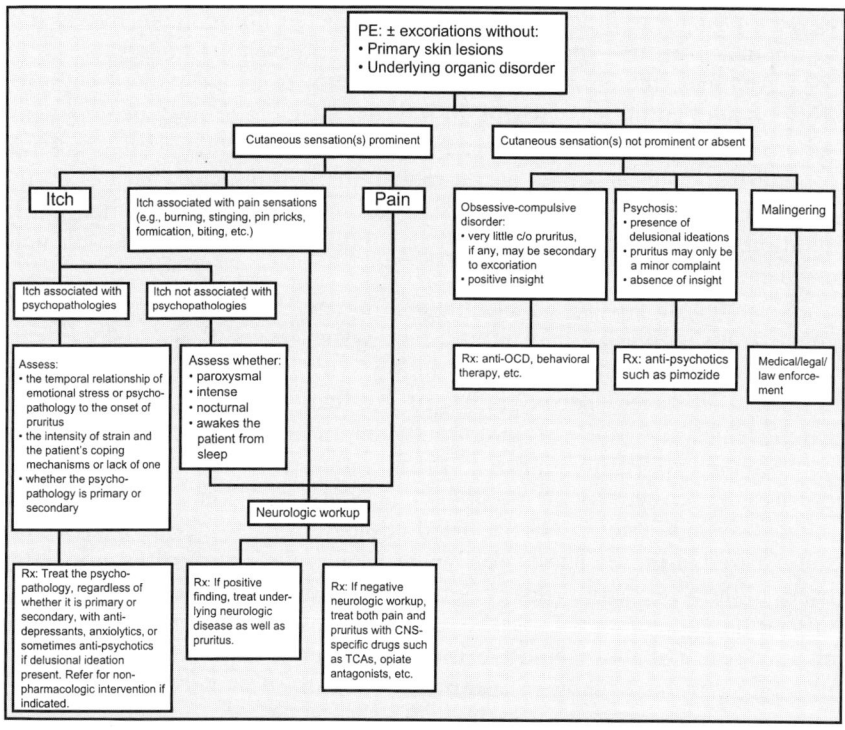

FIGURE 2 Differential diagnosis of cutaneous sensory disorder.

or neurogenic pruritus is simply more severe or to a possible differential interaction of psychogenic and organic pruritus with sleep-related CNS factors. However, there exists some controversy about this point in the literature. Work by Gupta et al. (8) concluded that psychiatric factors (e.g., depression) underlying itchy dermatosis (i.e., psoriasis) determine awakening from sleep and suggested that arousal from sleep in association with pruritus is not always because of increased afferent sensory input from the skin. In other words, the CNS may play a role in the initiation and modulation of itch perception. However, a correspondence (9) in response to this report argued that since only patients with primary skin disease with underlying psychopathologies were studied, the findings of Gupta et al. cannot be applied to patients with generalized pruritus without a primary skin disease. At the very least, the findings of Gupta et al. (8) showed that "there exists at least one exception to the clinical adage that 'psychogenic' pruritus does not interfere with sleep" (10). In other words, a psychogenic

TABLE 1 Characteristics of Neurogenic Pruritus

Onset is usually not immediate, i.e., within hours.
Course of disease is usually chronic but can be reversed with treatment of the CNS lesion.
Pruritus can be extremely intense.
Pruritus may be localized to one side of the body (i.e., sidedness) contralateral to the CNS lesion or bilateral, in which case the onset is usually unilateral.
Pruritus may be accompanied by other sensory deficits.
Pruritus may be accompanied by anomalous sensory phenomenon such as dysesthesia, allodynia, allokinesis, and hyperpathia. As a corollary, itch attacks may be precipitated by touch (allokinesis) or high temperature.
Pruritus is generally in cutaneous areas but may be restricted to the nostril and throat.
Pruritus is often paroxysmal. Each episode starts and ends abruptly, lasting seconds to minutes, and can recur frequently (>5–6 times per day). Paroxysmal pruritus can be successfully treated by antiepileptic drugs such as carbamazepine and phenytoin. However, EEG studies do not support an epileptic mechanism in the cortex for central neurogenic pruritus.
The location of itch may be segmental or dermatomal.
The attacks of pruritus can awake the patient from sleep and even cause insomnia.
Paroxysmal pruritus may be accompanied by paroxysmal or constant pain (burning and aching) in the same area.

etiology may not be ruled out automatically just because the pruritus is associated with nocturnal wakening.

DIFFERENTIAL DIAGNOSIS OF CUTANEOUS SENSORY DISORDER

This section outlines a general diagnostic strategy for patients who 1) are complaining of a variable degree of abnormal skin sensations such as itch or pain, 2) may or may not reveal the presence of excoriation on physical examination, 3) have neither primary skin lesion nor any underlying organic disorder, and 4) have not had a neurological work-up (Fig. 2). Among the patient population thusly defined, separate the cases into those in whom cutaneous sensations are a more prominent part of the clinical presentation and those in whom cutaneous sensations are either minor or entirely absent relative to the chief complaint (e.g., delusion of parasitosis, neurotic excoriation). Among the former cases, further separate them into three subgroups: 1) those cases where the reported cutaneous sensations consists mostly of itch, 2) those cases where the cutaneous sensation of itch is associated with pain sensations of all types such as burning, stinging, pin pricks, formication, biting, etc., and 3) those cases where pain turns out to be the most prominent cutanous sensation.

When itch presents as the most prominent cutaneous sensation, it is useful to categorize these patients into those whose itch is or is not associated with psychopathologies. Among those patients with psychological disturbances, the most commonly encountered psychopathologies are depression, anxiety, and a mixture of the two, albeit delusional ideations may be an occasional concomitant finding. For a detailed discussion of the diagnosis of psychopathologies common in the dermatological setting, the reader is referred to a review on psychodermatology (11). In addition, it is important to elicit a temporal relationship between the onset of pruritus and the timing of emotional stress. It is even more important to evaluate the degree of strain in response to stress. As constitutional personalities and coping strategies vary greatly from one individual to another, the resultant strain in response to stressors in life also varies immensely from one person to another. Thus, a knowledge of the intensity of strain on a patient and the coping mechanism (or the lack of it) in response to stress may be especially helpful in determining the need for adjunct, nonpharmacological intervention. Finally, whether the psychopathologies are primary or secondary, it is important to treat them anyway with antidepressants, antianxiety agents, and sometimes antipsychotics if delusional ideation is present (see below) (Fig. 3). In this context, it is noteworthy that among patients suffering from psychogenic pruritus, a major depressive disorder often presents with prominent symptoms of anxiety and agitation, leading often to misdiagnosis as a primary anxiety disorder. Furthermore, prescription of anxiolytic medications instead of antidepressants can actually exacerbate the underlying depressive disorder (12), as most anxiolytics such as benzodiazepines generally have a depressant effect (11).

On the other hand, for those patients with itch but without associated psychopathologies, it may be helpful to determine whether their itch is intense, paroxysmal, nocturnal, or capable of awakening the patient at night. In some cases, pruritus can be severe enough to cause insomnia. In this group of patients, neurological screening work-up should be considered, and clinical treatment starting with CNS-specific options such as doxepin and naltrexone may be considered (see below) (Fig. 3).

Patients whose itch is associated with other cutaneous sensations such as pain (e.g., burning, stinging, pinprick) or formication should definitely be referred for screening neurological evaluation. General characteristics of neurogenic pruritus are summarized in Table 1. However, as with any

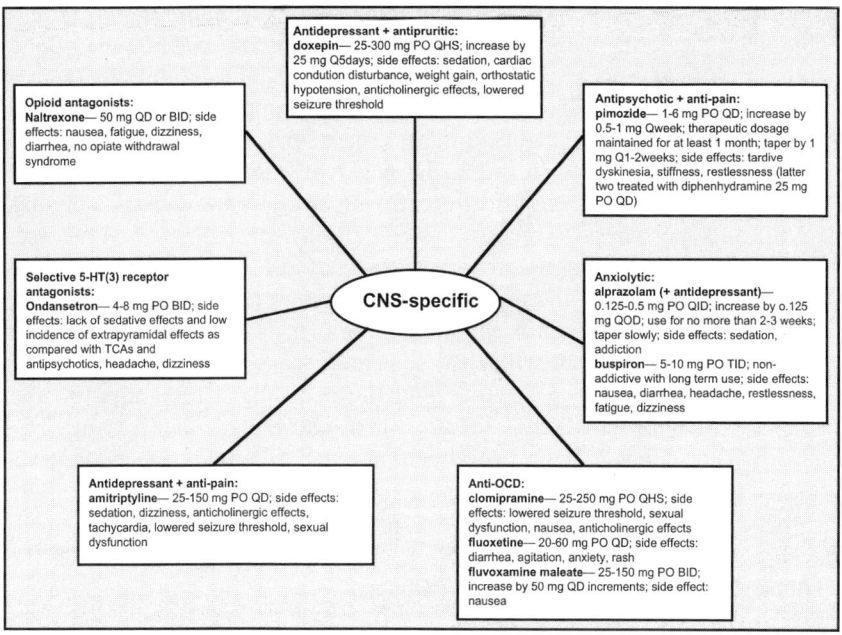

FIGURE 3   CNS-specific therapeutic options.

generalization, further specifications can be made. For instance, the anatomical area of pruritus does not necessarily have to be dermatomal or segmental. In cases of CNS tumor (3,13,14), brain abscess (15), stroke (16–18), aneurysm (19), and neurofibromatosis (7,13) (see Fig. 1), the pruritus can be generalized, dermatomal, or localized to the nostrils [pruritus in the nostrils occurs in patients with advanced tumors spreading to the base of the fourth ventricle (14)]. In cases of neurogenic pruritus associated with multiple sclerosis (MS), the anatomical pattern of involvement can involve more than one dermatome. As a further specification, the paroxysmal nature of pruritus may vary widely. In all 26 reported cases of MS-associated pruritus in the literature to date (1,20–25), paroxysmal pruritus has been found to last from seconds to minutes each time and to recur up to 20 times a day. In contrast, pruritus associated with brain tumors typically lasts hours at a time and recurs once every few weeks (13,14). In a case of lichen simplex chronicus presenting as the initial manifestation of intramedullary neoplasm, pruritus associated with occasional prickly pain was found to be constant for a period of 7 years (3).

These examples underscore the importance of being familiar with the characteristics of neurogenic pruritus when one is confronted with a patient complaining of itch associated with dysesthesia and presenting with no primary skin lesions. They also underscore the importance of a careful and thorough neurological work-up for these patients. If, however, the neurological work-up turn out to be negative, the neurologist often loses interest. In this case, empirical treatment by dermatologists using both CNS- and peripheral nervous system (PNS)-specific as well as other nonspecific treatment strategies are warranted even if the precise diagnosis could not be made by the neurologist (see below) (Fig. 3; Tables 2 and 3).

Cases in which pain is the most prominent complaint also deserve a careful and thorough neurological screening work-up. If the neurological work-up turns out to be negative and the neurologist loses interest, these patients often benefit from the use of the tricyclic antidepressant (TCA) amitriptyline (Elavil). If amitriptyline is not well tolerated, newer TCAs such

TABLE 2 PNS-Specific Therapeutic Options

Treatment	Proposed mechanisms	Side effects
Doxepin cream (5%)	Antihistamine	Localized burning or stinging; transient, mild drowsiness (decrease with use)
EMLA cream, paramoxine lotion (1%)	Local anesthetics	Mild and localized edema, erythema
Capsaicin solution (1%) ± EMLA pretreatment	Neuropeptide depletion	Mild burning, erythema, and itch (lasting 20–60 min after treatment and limited to initial 3–5 days)
Nedocromil sodium solution (2%) by ionophoresis	Sensory nerve depolarization	Localized inflammation
Topical steroids	Inhibition of prostaglandin synthesis	Not noted
Topical aspirin (3%)		Not noted
Cutaneous field stimulation (4 Hz, 1 ms pulse, 0.4–0.8 mA, 25 min duration)	Mimicking the reflex antipruritic effect of scratch (spinal presynaptic inhibition)	Mild pinprick, burning, and buzzing sensations

TABLE 3 Nonspecific Therapeutic Options

Cold compresses with moisturization
Mentholated compounds, e.g., Sarna lotion
Oral and topical antibiotics if secondary infection
Occlusion, e.g., Unnaboot, Duoderm, boxing gloves
Laser
Cryotherapy
Intralesional steroid injection
Phototherapy (UVA, PUVA)
Goeckerman

as doxepin (Sinequan, Adapin), desipramine (Norpramine, Pertofrane), or nortriptyline (Aventyl, Pamelor) should be tried before resorting to nontricyclics such as selective serotonin-reuptake inhibitors (SSRIs). Amitriptyline has the best documentation in the literature of its analgesic property followed by the newer TCAs; SSRIs have the least documentation regarding their efficacy as an analgesic (26,27). This said, more recent studies in experimental animals appear to suggest that both tricyclics and the SSRI antidepressants have an analgesic property via overlapping mechanisms involving serotonin (26), α_2-adrenoceptors (28), and opiate receptor stimulation and peptide release (29,30). The other major "branch" of the diagnostic strategy presented in Fig. 2 consists of those patients without cutaneous sensations as the most prominent clinical presentation. Cutaneous sensations such as itch may be secondary, may be entirely absent, and, when present, are much less prominent as a complaint relative to delusional ideation or obsessive-compulsive picking. Obsessive-compulsive disorder (OCD), psychosis, and malingering should be considered as the possible differential diagnoses.

OCD patients frequently present with excoriations with very little or no complaint of pruritus (or pruritus only secondary to excoriations). A classic example is neurotic excoriation where the patient is driven to scratch, pick, or rub the skin compulsively in areas within the reach of hands. Although the activity does not make sense to the patient, he or she is usually fully aware of maladaptive activity but powerless to stop it. In general, OCD patients typically have good insight into their own suffering. Classically, both obsession and compulsion should be observed, but among skin patients obsessive ideation may be missing. The main treatment involves anti-OCD medications (Fig. 3) such as clomipramine (Anafranil), fluoxetine (Prozac), and fluvoxamine maleate (Luvox) as well as behavioral therapy. In contrast, psychotic patients are diagnosed by the presence of delusional ideation. Pruritus is often absent and, when present, constitutes only a very minor part of the complaint. Commonly encountered psychotic patients in the dermatological setting are not those with schizophrenia but rather those with monosymptomatic hypochondriacal psychosis (MHP), a common example of which is delusion of parasitosis. Antipsychotics such as pimozide (Orap) are the treatment of choice (Fig. 3). Finally, malingering patients who present with excoriations present a very difficult situation to manage, since malingering is officially not considered a psychiatric illness (as opposed to a moral and ethical deficit) and the patient knows exactly what he or she wants to achieve from having a medical illness. Needless to say, these patients would never voluntarily admit that they are malingering. If malingering were suspected, apart from supportive care to minimize secondary complications such as skin infection, the management involves more legal and law enforcement personnel as opposed to medical personnel.

THERAPEUTIC OPTIONS

The multitude of therapeutic options for pruritus suspected of having a psychogenic origin is divided into the following three categories: 1) CNS-specific pharmacological therapy (Fig. 3), 2) PNS-specific pharmacological and nonpharmacological therapy (Table 2, and 3) nonspecific and supportive therapy (Table 3). Specific information on dosage and prominent side effects can be found in Fig. 3 and Table 2.

CNS-Specific Therapeutic Options

Pharmacological therapies directed at psychopathologies such as depression, anxiety, OCD, and psychosis have been alluded to earlier, discussed in depth elsewhere (11), and summarized in Fig. 3. Briefly, for psychogenic pruritus with underlying depression, the newer TCA doxepin is recommended for both its antidepressive and antihistamine action profiles. In fact, doxepin is 775 times more potent as an H1 antagonist than diphenhydramine and 56 times more potent than hydroxyzine (31). For psychogenic pruritus provoked by underlying anxiety, one can resort to one of two types of antianxiety medications: a quick-acting benzodiazepine that can potentially be sedating and a slow-acting nonbenzodiazepine that is not dependency producing or sedating. Among the former, the newer benzodiazepine alprazolam (Xanax) is recommended; among the latter, buspirone (BuSpar) is the preferred choice. Unlike most other benzodiazepines, alprazolam also has an antidepressant effect; this feature proves especially helpful since most psychodermatological patients have the agitating subtype of depression. Anti-OCD medications have been alluded to earlier and consist of antidepressant medications. For MHP, pimozide is the treatment of choice. Notably, pimozide also has an antiopiate effect in addition to its antidopamine effect (32), suggesting that it may also be helpful in treating pruritus secondary to self-induced trauma to the skin.

In practice, treatment of potential psychopathologies underlying psychogenic pruritus may not be successful, may be met with only partial success, or may have a slow onset of efficacy for much-needed symptomatic relief. Hence, effective treatments aimed directly at the symptom of itch are often needed. In fact, most of the medications cited above for psycho-pathologies are recommended for their cross-acting efficacy directly against itch: doxepine for its potent antihistamine action, alprazolam for its sedating effect, and pimozide for its antiopiate effect. Interestingly, sedation has been found to be critical in the antipruritic action of conventional H1 antihistamines (e.g., diphenhydramine, tripelennamine, chlorpheniramine, cyproheptadine, and hydroxyzine). For instance, astemizole and terfenadine (nonsedating H1 antihistamines) have been shown to have no effect on itch, whereas trimeprazine (sedating but less potent H1 antihistamine) as well as nitrazepam (a sedating benzodiazepine) were shown to be antipruritic (33). It was thus concluded that H1 receptor antagonists have a peripheral antipruritic action only when the itch is due to histamine release (as in whealing disorders such as chronic idiopathic urticaria) (34,35). In this context it is noteworthy that doxepin (10 mg TID) has been shown to be much more effective in the treatment of chronic urticaria than diphenhy-dramine (25 mg TID) (36). Thus, although conventional H1 antihistamines are effective in many patients with chronic urticaria (urticaria and pruritus lasting >6 weeks), a sizable fraction of these patients does not obtain adequate relief of symptoms from these medications. It has been shown that as much as 70% of chronic urticaria is idiopathic and 16% is associated with severe depression or other psychiatric problems (37).

While there are potentially many mediators and modulators of itch, the central mechanism(s) of itch remains largely unknown and a common final pathway elusive. CNS-specific therapeutic options are available, targeting some promising targets. These options include opiate antagonists (e.g., naloxone, nalmefene, and naltrexone) and selective serotonin 5-HT3 receptor antagonists (i.e., ondansetron, tropisetron). Clinical and experi-mental observations indicate a role for central opiates in evoking or intensifying itch independent of their histamine-releasing effect (38,39). Naltrexone, an oral opiate antagonist, was first shown to ameliorate intractable cholestatic pruritus and uremic pruritus in double-blind and placebo-controlled trials (40,41). More recently, in open-label pilot studies, naltrexone was shown to be highly antipruritic (i.e., improvement of 50% or more), with a total response rate of 70% within a week of administration and well tolerated in a variety of internal and dermatological diseases and among a patient population, the majority of whom did not respond to other therapeutic options (42,43). In particular, naltrexone was found to be highly antipruritic among patients with prurigo nodularis (PN) (9/17); among the 17 patients with PN, 7 were diagnosed with psychogenic pruritus.

In addition to opiate antagonists, serotonin type 3 receptor antagonists such as ondansetron and tropisetron may be a potential addition to the armamentarium against psychogenic pruritus (44–46). These drugs are well known as antiemetics for anesthesia- and especially chemotherapy-induced nausea and vomiting. However, there are indications that this group of agents has novel applications ranging from anxiety disorders to pain disorders and pruritus. In particular, ondansetron has been shown to be highly effective against cholestatic and uremic pruritus in placebo-controlled trials, with a success rate approaching 100% within 30–60 minutes and an effect lasting up to 6 hours among a small group of intractable patients. Severe pruritus following intrathecal administration of morphine has also been successfully treated with ondansetron, suggesting a central mechanism of action for its antipruritic effect. However, there has hitherto been no report in the literature regarding the potential efficacy of serotonin type 3 receptor antagonists specifically in the management of psychogenic pruritus. Whether ondansetron also acts peripherally against the generation and/or sensation of itch remains to be seen.

PNS-Specific Therapeutic Options

As mentioned earlier, doxepin exerts both central (i.e., antidepressant, sedative) and peripheral (i.e., H1 histamine receptor antagonistic) actions against pruritus. Thus, it is not surprising that the peripheral antipruritic action profile of doxepin has been capitalized upon for the management of pruritic skin conditions. In experimentally induced (i.e., histamine-induced) pruritus, a 5% topical solution of doxepin was found to be more efficacious than topical amitriptyline, diphenhydramine, and the vehicle control (47). In addition, doxepin cream 5% (Zonalon) has been found to relieve pruritus in patients with atopic dermatitiis in a double-blind, vehicle-controlled, multicenter study (48). Because psychogenic pruritus represents a hetero-geneous diagnostic group of patients, it is not clear whether topical doxepin has specific role in the management of patients with psychogenic pruritus.

EMLA (eutectic mixture of local anesthetics) cream, like topical doxepin, has been shown to be effective in increasing the threshold to experimentally induced pruritus (using histamine, cowage, and papain) as compared to placebo (49). It contains both lidocaine and prilocaine ointments, effective topical analgesics. Other topical anesthetics shown to be effective in experimental itch include pramoxine (1% lotion) (50). Topical pramoxine was shown to decrease both itch magnitude and duration while having no effect on thermal and pain thresholds. Notably, the anti-itch effect of these topical analgesics appears to be unrelated to their analgesic properties (50,51). Furthermore, EMLA may have a role together with other topical agents in the management of pruritus. It has recently been shown that pretreatment with EMLA significantly blocked the side effects of topical capsaicin (see below) such as burning and hyperalgia in experimental subjects (52). It is unknown whether EMLA and capsaicin might have synergistic therapeutic effects on pruritus, especially that of psychogenic or neurogenic etiologies.

Capsaicin (Zostrix), the pungent agent of red pepper, has been proposed to be effective in a wide variety of pruritic conditions by excitation of C-fiber afferents and the subsequent neuropeptide (such as SP) depletion, leading to skin desensitization to pruritic stimulation (53). In clinical pruritus, it has been shown to be efficacious for notalgia paresthetica (54,55), brachioradial pruritus (56,57), and PN. In the latter study, the etiologies of PN included psychogenic pruritus and generalized idiopathic pruritus in cases that were recalcitrant to previous therapeutic attempts. Capsaicin cream 0.025% was administered BID under occlusion for the initial 3 days and subsequently raised in steps of 0.025% up to 0.3% every 3–5 days until total relief. Strikingly, complete remission of PN and pruritus was observed in all patients (58). However, capsaicin use in clinical practice appears to be limited by its side effects such as burning and hyperalgia.

The cromones, including nedocromil sodium, appear to inhibit peripheral sensory nerve function and have also been shown to be effective against histamine-induced itch in the experimental setting (59). This group of agents is better known for its mast cell–stabilizing effect. However, recent studies have made apparent its anti-inflammatory action as well as its ability to modulate peripheral sensory nerve functions. Specifically, it has been shown that nedocromil sodium can induce a long-lasting chloride-dependent nerve depolarization, thereby reducing the sensitivity of the nerve to subsequent action potentials. However, the use of nedocromil sodium at present appears to be limited by its poor penetration into the skin; development of an appropriate vehicle should facilitate efficacy testing in the clinical setting.

Topical steroids have long been used to ameliorate inflammatory dermatosis. More recently, in double-blind trials, topical steroids (clobetasol ointment 0.05%, hydrocortisone 1% and 2.5%) were shown to reduce both histamine-induced itch intensity and duration (60,61). Similarly, in a small vehicle-controlled trial, topical aspirin was shown to reduce histamine-induced experimental itch (62). Interestingly, neither topical steroid nor aspirin modulates thermal or pain threshold. It was presumed that the antipruritic action of both topical steroid and aspirin is mediated by inhibition of prostaglandin production. Prostaglandin, together with serotonin, is known to cause experimental itch (63), but blockade of its production for the management of clinical pruritus still awaits validation.

Last but not least, another potentially promising therapeutic option lies in cutaneous field stimulation (CFS), which stimulates peripheral sensory nerves, but its mechanism of antipruritic action may lie centrally (64). CFS aims to mimic the beneficial, antipruritic effect of scratching without damaging the skin, which aggravates itch over time, leading to a scratch-itch-scratch vicious cycle. It uses a flexible plate with 16 needle-like electrodes to electrically stimulate nerve fibers in the superficial skin. In contrast to transcutaneous nerve stimulation (TNS), which preferentially activates large myelinated fibers with no effect on nociceptors, CFS activates nociceptive C fibers. TNS has been studied for its potential antipruritic effect based on the presumptive theory that stimulation of large, myelinated afferent fibers should exert a presynaptic inhibition of the impulses in itch-carrying fibers (i.e., the so-called gate control theory). However, studies of TNS in treating experimental pruritus have so far been disappointing, making a role of TNS in the management of clinical pruritus unlikely (65,66). CFS, however, has been shown to have a robust itch inhibitory effect as compared to TNS (64). This effect is long-lasting and presumably occurs via activation of an antipruritic spinal reflex normally activated by scratching.

Nonspecific Therapeutic Options

Many nonspecific treatment options exist to be used concomitantly with other more specific treatment agents or, unfortunately in some cases, as measures of last resort. In all cases, one cannot ignore the fundamental importance of supportive care such as cold compresses with liberal moisturization. Such supportive care is soothing, provides hydration, and facilitates debridement of crusts and reduces xerosis, which may exacerbate itch. Mentholated compounds such as Sarna lotion may also be helpful for symptomatic relief. When present, secondary bacterial infection must be treated aggressively with antibiotics. Moreover, occlusion using methods such as Unnaboot, Duoderm, or boxing gloves can be helpful, given the cooperation of the patients. Pruritic lesions such as NP resulting from chronic itch may be removed by laser, cryotherapy, or even intralesional triamcinolone injection. Other measures that may play a role in the management of psychogenic pruritus include Goeckerman therapy and phototherapy with UVB or PUVA (the former of which should be tried first).

CONCLUSION

It has been estimated that one third to more than three fourths of dermatology patients have a significant psychogenic component to their skin complaints (67). Among these, those complaining of abnormal cutaneous sensations such as itch and pain without a primary skin lesion often present a real diagnostic and therapeutic challenge to the average dermatologist. This chapter considered diagnostic and therapeutic strategies available when one considers the array of pathophysiology on the road to diagnosing a cutaneous sensory disorder, which by definition excludes a known dermatological, medical, or psychiatric illness. It is the hope of the authors that the readers will find this chapter to be clinically relevant and helpful in their day-to-day practice of dermatology.

REFERENCES

1. Khan OA. Treatment of paroxysmal symptoms in multiple sclerosis with ibuprofen. Neurology 1994; 44:571–572.
2. Canavero S, Bonicalzi V, and Massa-Micon B. Central neurogenic pruritus: a literature review. Acta Neurol Belg 1997; 97:244–247.
3. Kinsella LJ, Carney-Godley K, and Feldmann E. Lichen simplex chronicus as the initial manifestation of intramedullary neoplasm and syringomyelia. Neurosurgery 1992; 30(3):418–421.
4. Schmelz M. A neural pathway for itch. Nat Neurosci 2001; 4(1):9–10.
5. Arnold LM, McElroy SL, and Mutasim DFea. Characteristics of 34 adults with psychogenic excoriation. J Clin Psychiatry 1998; 59:509–514.
6. Fruensgarrd K. Neurotic excoriations. A controlled psychiatric examination. Acta Psychiatr Scand 1984; 312:1–52.
7. Johnson RE, Kanigsberg ND, Jimenez CL. Localized pruritus: a presenting symptom of a spinal cord tumor in a child with features of neurofibromatosis. J Am Acad Dermatol 2000; 43(5):958–961.
8. Gupta MA, et al. Pruritus associated with nocturnal wakenings: organic or psychogenic? J Am Acad Dermatol 1988; 21(3):479–484.
9. Bernhard JD. Nocturnal wakening caused by pruritus: organic or psychogenic? J Am Acad Dermatol 1990; 23:767.
10. Gupta MA. Nocturnal wakening caused by pruritus: organic or psychogenic? J Am Acad Dermatol 1990; 23:767.
11. Koo J. Psychodermatology: a practical manual for clinicians. Curr Probl Dermatol 1995; (Nov/Dec):204–232.

12. Gupta MA. Evaluation and treatment of "psychogenic" pruritus and self-excoriation. J Am Acad Dermatol 1995; 32(3):532.

13. Summers CG, MacDonald JT. Paroxysmal facial itch: a presenting sign of childhood brain stem glioma. J Child Neurol 1988; 3:189–192.

14. Andreev VC Petkov I. Skin manifestations associated with tumours of the brain. Br J Dermatol 1975; 92:675–678.

15. Sullivan MJ, Drake ME. Unilateral pruritus and nocardia brain abscess. Neurology 1984; 34:828–829.

16. King CA, Huff FJ, Jorizzo J. Unilateral neurogenic pruritus: paroxysmal itching associated with central nervous system lesions. Ann Int Med 1982; 97(2):222–223.

17. Massey EW. Unilateral neurogenic pruritus following stroke. Stroke 1984; 15(5):901–903.

18. Shapiro PE, Braun CW. Unilateral pruritus after a stroke. Arch Dermatol 1987; 123:1527–1530.

19. Vuadens P, et al. Segmental pruritus and intramedullary vascular malformation. Schweiz Arch Neurol Psychiatr 1994; 145(3):13–16.

20. Yabuki S, Hayabara T. Paroxysmal dysesthesia in multiple sclerosis. Folia Psychiatr Neurol Jpn 1979; 33:97–104.

21. Mathews WB. Symptoms and signs. In: Mathews WB et al., eds. McAlpine's Multiple Sclerosis. Edinburgh: Churchill Livingstone, 1991.

22. Osterman PO, Westerberg C-E. Paroxysmal attacks in multiple sclerosis. Brain 1975; 98:189–202.

23. Osterman PO. Paroxysmal itching in multiple sclerosis. Br J Dermatol 1976; 95:555–558.

24. Yamamoto M, et al. Paroxysmal itching in multiple sclerosis: a report of three cases. J Neurol Neurosurg Psych 1981; 44:19–22.

25. Koeppel MC, et al. Paroxysmal pruritus and multiple sclerosis. Br J Dermatol 1993; 129:597–598.

26. Tura B, Tura SM. The analgesic effect of tricyclic antidepressants. Brain Res 1990; 518(1–2):19–22.

27. Egbunike IG, Chaffee BJ. Antidepressants in the management of chronic pain syndromes. Pharmacotherapy 1990; 10(4):262–270.

28. Gray AM, Pache DM, Sewell RD. Do alpha2-adrenoceptors play an integral role in the antinociceptive mechanism of action of antidepressant compounds? Eur J Pharmacol 1999; 378(2):161–168.

29. Isenberg KE, Cicero TT. Possible involvement of opioid receptors in the pharmacological profiles of antidepressant compounds. Eur J Pharmacol 1984; 103:36–57.

30. Gray AM, Spencer PSJ, Sewell RDE. The involvement of the opioidergic system in the antinociceptive mechanism of action of antidepressant compounds. Br J Pharmacol 1998; 124:669–674.

31. Richelson E. Tricyclic antidepressants block antihistamine H1 receptors of mouse neuroblastoma cells. Nature 1978; 274:176–177.

32. Boublik JH, Funder JW. Interaction of dopamine receptor ligands with subtypes of the opiate receptor. Eur J Pharmacol 1984; 107(1):11–16.

33. Krause L, Shuster S, Mechanism of action of antipruritic drugs. Br Med J 1983; 287(6400):1199–1200.

34. Monroe EW, et al. Relative efficacy and safety of loratadine, hydroxyzine, and placebo in chronic idiopathic urticaria. Arzneimittelforschung 1992; 42(9):1119–1121.

35. Brostoff J, et al. Efficacy of mizolastine, a new antihistamine, compared with placebo in the treatment of chronic idiopathic urticaria. Allergy 1996; 51(5):320–325.

36. Green SL, Reed CE, Schroeter AL. Double-blind crossover study comparing doxepin with diphenhydramine for the treatment of chronic urticaria. J Am Acad Dermatol 1985; 12(4):669–675.

37. Juhlin L. Recurrent urticaria: clinical investigation of 330 patients. Br J Dermatol 1981; 104:369–381.

38. Bernstein JE, et al. Antipruritic effect of an opiate antagonist, naloxone hydrochloride. J Invest Dermatol 1982; 78:82–83.

39. Fjellner B and Hagermark O. Potentiation of histamine-induced itch and flare response in human skin by the enkephalin analogue FK 33-824, beta-endorphin, and morphine. Arch Dermatol Res 1982; 274:29–37.

40. Peer G, et al. Randomized crossover trial of naltrexone in uraemic pruritus. Lancet 1996; 348:1552–1554.

41. Wolfhagan FH, et al. Oral naltrexone treatment for cholestatic pruritus: a double-blind placebo-controlled study. Gastroenterology 1997; 113:1264–1269.

42. Metze D, Reimann S, Luger TA. Effective treatment of pruritus with naltrexone, an orally active opiate antagonist. Ann NY Acad Sci 430–432.

43. Metze D, et al. Efficacy and safety of naltrexone, an oral opiate receptor antagonist, in the treatment of pruritus in internal and dermatological diseases. J Am Acad Dermatol 1999; 41:533–539.

44. Ye JH, Ponnudurai R, Schaefer R. Ondansetron: a selective 5-HT(3) receptor antagonist and its application in CNS-related disorders. CNS Drug Rev 2001; 7(2):199–213.

45. Weisshaar E, et al. The anti-pruritic effect of 5-HT3 receptor antagonist (tropisetron) is dependent on mast cell depletion-an experimental study. Exp Dermatol 1999; 8(4):254–260.

46. Wilde MI, Markham A, Ondansetron: a review of its pharmacology and preliminary clinical findings in novel applications. Drugs 1996; 52(5):773–794.

47. Bernstein JE, Whitney DH, Soltani K, Inhibition of histamine-induced pruritus by topical tricyclic antidepressants. J Am Acad Dermatol 1981; 5(5):582–585.

48. Drake LA, et al. Relief of pruritus in patients with atopic dermatitis after treatment with topical doxepin cream. J Am Acad Dermatol 1994; 31(4):613–616.

49. Shuttleworth D, et al. Relief of experimentally induced pruritus with a novel eutectic mixture of local anaesthetic agents. Br J Dermatol 1988; 119(4):535–540.

50. Yosipovitch G, Maibach HI. Effect of topical pramozine on experimentally induced pruritus in humans. J Am Acad Dermatol 1997; 37(2):278–280.
51. Bjerring P, Nielsen A. A quantitative comparison of the effect of local analgesics on argon laser induced cutaneous pain and on histamine-induced wheal, flare, and itch. Acta Derm Venereol 1990; 70:126–131.
52. Yosipovitch G, Maibach HI, Rowbotham MC. Effect of EMLA pre-treatment on capsaicin-induced burning and hyperalgesia. Acta Derm Venereol 1999; 79(2):118–121.
53. Lynn B. Capsaicin: actions on C fiber afferents that may be involved in itch. Skin Pharmacol 1992; 5:9–13.
54. Cappugi P, et al. Capsaicin treatment of different dermatologic affections with itching. Skin Pharmacol 1989; 2:230.
55. Wallengren J. Treatment of notalgia paresthetica with capsaicin (Zostrix). Skin Pharmacol 1989; 2:229–230.
56. Knight TE, Hayashi T. Solar (brachioradial) pruritus: response to capsaicin cream. Int J Dermatol 1994; 33:206–209.
57. Goodless DR, Eaglstein WH. Brachioradial pruritus: treatment with topical capsaicin. J Am Acad Dermatol 1993; 29:783–784.
58. Stander S, Luger T, Metze D. Treatment of prurigo nodularis with topical capsaicin. J Am Acad Dermatol 2001; 44:471–478.
59. Ahluwalia P, McGill JI, Church MK, Nedocromil sodium inhibits histamine-induced itch and flare in human skin. Br J Pharmacol 2001; 132:613–616.
60. Yosipovitch G, et al. High-potency topical corticosteroid rapidly decreases histamine-induced itch but not thermal sensation and pain in human beings. J Am Acad Dermatol 1996; 35(1):118–120.
61. Zhai H, et al. Antipruritic and thermal sensation effects of hydrocortisone creams in human skin. Skin Pharmacol Appl Skin Physiol 2000; 13(6):352–357.
62. Yosipovitch G, et al. Topically applied aspirin rapidly decreases histamine-induced itch. Acta Derm Venereol 1997; 77(1):46–48.
63. Hagermark O. Peripheral and central mediators of itch. Skin Pharmacol 1992; 55:1–8.
64. Nilsson H-J, Levinsson A, Schouenborg J, Cutaneous field stimulation (CFS): a new powerful to combat itch. Pain 1997; 71:49–55.
65. Ward L, Wright E, McMahon SB, A comparison of the effects of noxious and innocuous counterstimuli on experimentally induced itch and pain. Pain 1996; 64:129–138.
66. Fjellner B, Hagermark O. Transcutaneous nerve stimulation and itching. Acta Dermatovenerol (Stockh) 1978; 58:131–134.
67. Fried RG. Evaluation and treatment of "psychogenic" pruritus and self-excoriation. J Am Acad Dermatol 1994; 30:993–999.

22

Psychological Aspects of Acne

Ernest Lee and John Y. M. Koo
University of California, San Francisco
San Francisco, California, U.S.A.

INTRODUCTION

Psychological factors may play a significant role in acne (1). First, emotional stress can exacerbate acne. Second, as a consequence of their acne, patients may develop psychiatric problems related to depression, social phobias, and low self-esteem. Third, patients with primary psychiatric illnesses such as obsessive-compulsive disorder and psychosis may focus on their acne. In this chapter there will be a discussion of how acne and emotional factors connect to help the clinician identify potential psychiatric problems contributing to or resulting from acne.

EMOTIONAL FACTORS EXACERBATING ACNE

Disorders characterized by demonstrable physical pathology that can be worsened by emotional stress are termed psychophysiological disorders. Peptic ulcer disease, migraine headaches, and Crohn's disease are all examples of these types of disorders. It is generally accepted that acne probably falls into this category as well since patients frequently complain of acne flares when they experience frustration, stress, or anxiety (2). For example, college students often report exacerbation of their acne during exam periods.

From interviews with 4576 patients with various dermatological problems, 55.3% of those with acne reported a close chronological association between exacerbation of their condition and episodes of emotional stress (3). Two days was the average latency period between the onset of emotional stress and clinical changes (e.g., papules). Intense anger may also aggravate acne. A study performed in the 1950s showed an increase in the number of lesions within days after "stress" interviews in which anger was deliberately induced (4).

Several hypotheses have been advanced concerning the mechanism underlying exacerbation of acne by emotional distress. Certain stress hormones, such as glucocorticoids, are released in greater quantity with psychological stress (5). In response to emotional stress, adrenal androgens are also secreted in increased quantities. It is postulated that stress is linked to acne flares by inducing higher blood levels of androgens (6) and glucocorticoids (7), which can exacerbate acne. In fact, one study by Goulden et al. (55), of 200 patients over the age of 25 with acne showed that postadolescent acne was more prevalent in women than men (76% women, 24% men). Also, true late-onset acne, defined as onset after the age of 25 years, was seen in 18.4% of women and 8.3% of men. One hypothesis is that these older women have an increased sensitivity to androgens (8).

While certain disfiguring skin diseases, such as acne, may lead to depression (see below) and even suicidal ideation (9), depression may also contribute to acne. In a case report on several acne patients, Monssavian (10) found improvement in the acne of at least seven depressed patients treated with 10–20 mg daily of paroxetine. However, other serotonin reuptake inhibitors [e.g., fluoxetine (Prozac®), setraline (Zoloft®)] used by the patients did not have similar benefits in terms of either treating the depression or improvement in acne. It is uncertain whether it was the indirect benefit of reduction in depression or some more direct effect of paroxetine that produced the clinical improvement in acne in this particular study.

Given the contribution of emotion and stress to acne, treatments aimed at reducing stress, anger, anxiety, and depression are of potential benefit. Adjusting one's expectations, lifestyle, and work demands can reduce emotional stress and help manage the psychophysiological aspect of acne. Pscyhopharmacology, progressive relaxation, and self-hypnosis may all be helpful. Cognitive imagery and biofeedback relaxation have already been studied as adjuncts to medical treatment of acne. Compared to only medical means, these methods were found to significantly improve acne in

30 study patients. Treatment consisted of 12 sessions over 6 weeks. In addition, treatment group patients who continued home practice until follow-up maintained their gains, whereas a relapse in severity occurred with discontinuation of these psychological interventions (11). Similar interventions such as hypnosis may also be beneficial in reducing potential complications of acne (12). Using posthypnotic suggestion, Hollander (13) had success in controlling acne excoriée, in which patients habitually pick their lesions, in two patients. Whenever either patient wanted to pick her face, the patient was instructed to remember the word "scar" and refrain from picking by saying "scar" instead. The underlying acne did not resolve, but the excoriations did. For minimizing excoriation of acne, hypnosis may be a useful treatment.

PSYCHIATRIC DISORDERS RESULTING FROM ACNE

The general psychosocial impact of acne is comparable to the psychosocial impact of many chronic diseases, such as diabetes, asthma, and arthritis (14). In a study of 111 acne patients referred to a dermatologist in England, quality of life was measured using the Dermatology Life Quality Index, Rosenberg's measure of self-esteem, a version of the General Health Questionnaire (GHQ-28), and the Short Form 36 (SF-36). Population quality-of-life data for the SF-36 instrument were measured from a random sample of adult local residents ($n = 9334$), some of whom reported a variety of longstanding disabling diseases. All quality-of-life instruments showed substantial deficits for acne patients that correlated with each other but not with clinically assessed acne severity. The acne patients (a relatively severely affected group) reported levels of social, psychological, and emotional problems as great as those reported by patients with chronic disabling asthma, epilepsy, diabetes, back pain, or arthritis. While the relationship between psychiatric morbidity and acne is generally accepted (15), there is some conflicting data as to whether certain characteristic types of emotional dysfunction are consistently associated with acne. In an uncontrolled study of 145 men and women, Medansky et al. (16) were unable to show a relationship between acne and anxiety. Other controlled studies have successfully demonstrated that acne patients have increased anxiety levels (17,18). It is clear that the worse the acne, the greater the anxiety (19).

Disfigurement from acne can have serious emotional consequences. More specifically, acne may lead to depression, social phobia, anger, and low self-esteem (Table 1). In a study of 317 pupils aged 14–16 years in Nottingham, England, participants with significant acne (12+ lesions) had higher levels of emotional and behavioral difficulties than those with

TABLE 1   Psychological Morbidity Associated with Acne

Anger
Anxiety
Depression
Impaired self-image/self-esteem
Less satisfaction with general appearance
Lower quality of life
Social impairment

minimal acne (20). Participants with acne were nearly twice as likely (32% vs. 20%; odds ratio 1.86) as those without acne to score in the abnormal/borderline range of the Strengths and Difficulties Questionnaire, an age-appropriate, validated measure of emotional well-being. Acne is psychologically debilitating even in comparison to other skin diseases. In Peshawar, Pakistan, a comparison of 50 patients with acne and 50 patients with seborrheic dermatitis (all patients in the study were 13–25 years in age) showed a statistically significant higher prevalence of depression and anxiety in the acne group compared to the seborrhea group (21).

With regards to depression, the principal hypothesis is that symptoms are a reaction to the body image concerns caused by acne (22). Depression is usually manifested by one or more signs or symptoms, such as withdrawal from social and occupational activities, loss of concentration, spontaneous crying spells, insomnia or hypersomnia, anorexia or hyperphagia, and suicidal ideation (23). In addition, since acne primarily affects teenagers, clues that an adolescent may be significantly depressed include social withdrawal, truancy, delinquent behavior, and deterioration in academic performance (24). There has been renewed interest in the concept of depression caused by the physical manifestations of acne with the recent high-profile cases of suicide in acne patients on isotretinoin (Accutane®). From the beginning of isotretinoin's introduction into the market, there have been very rare concerns about its possible relationship to depression (25–27). However, a recent large population study of acne patients using isotretinoin versus oral antibiotics showed a relative risk of approximately 1.0 for depression or psychosis with isotretinoin use and a relative risk of 0.9 for suicide and attempted suicide when comparing current isotretinoin exposure with nonexposure (28). Despite this negative result showing no increased risk with isotretinoin, it is imperative for the clinician to be cognizant of the signs and symptoms of depression in an acne patient to be able to make an early detection of depression because adolescents are at notoriously high risk for suicide and depression whether these emotional difficulties have any relationship to isotretinoin or not.

Social phobia is an exaggerated fear of social contact. Teenagers can be extremely sensitive to issues of peer acceptance and tend to be overly self-conscious regarding their appearance. Hence, they are vulnerable to developing a social phobia that may inhibit their lifestyle (29). The negative influence of acne on social interactions extends also to older individuals (30). Motley and Finlay studied 100 patients with acne and found that their disease interfered with social interactions such as sports, eating out, and dating for both school-age and older persons (31). Patients with severe acne were also shown to have poorer academic functioning (30). In addition, there is a highly significant positive association between the severity of acne and poor self-image (32). Acne can also impact an individual's ability to function in society. Cunliffe found that patients with acne had significantly higher unemployment levels than controls: 16.2% versus 9.2% in males and 14.3% versus 8.7% in females, respectively (33). The social morbidity associated with acne is summarized in Table 2.

A quantification of the negative social impact of acne can be found in a decreased quality of life. Sixty patients with acne vulgaris in a cross-sectional and longitudinal questionnaire study were evaluated with respect to quality-of-life measures (34). Skindex, a validated 29-item instrument to measure the effects of skin disease on patients' quality of life in regard to three scale scores (functioning, emotions, and symptoms), was used. Higher Skindex scores indicate greater effects on quality of life. Findings indicated that patients with acne experienced functioning and emotional negative effects from their skin disease comparable with those of patients with psoriasis, despite experiencing fewer symptoms (not specifically stated what symptoms were experienced). The Skindex scores (acne and psoriasis patients) were 14.9 and 22.8 ($p = 0.08$) for functioning, 39.2 and 38.9 ($p = 0.95$) for emotion, and 29.5 and 42.1 ($p < 0.05$) for symptoms. Patients 40 years or older were less likely to report improvement in their acne after 3 months (43% vs. 85%; ($p < 0.05$), and Skindex scores were higher for older

---

TABLE 2 Social Morbidity Associated with Acne

Decreased dating
Decreased eating out
Decreased participation in sports
Increased unemployment
Impaired academic performance

patients versus younger patients. Among patients reporting no improvement in their acne, surprisingly, older patients reported greater negative impact of acne on their quality of life. Even after controlling for sex and acne severity as judged by the dermatologist, older adults reported more impact of acne on their quality of life than younger adults in multivariate analyses.

The patient often perceives even an insignificant case of acne as repulsive, leading to a desire to avoid social contact (17). In one published study, patients consistently rated their acne as more severe than did clinicians (14). A study by Newton et al. (35) showed a discrepancy not only between the patients' and dermatologists' assessment of acne severity, but also that patients' satisfaction with treatment outcome was less than that of the treating dermatologist. When asked to make a hypothetical choice between a large sum of money and a cure for their acne, 87% of patients, most of whom had minimal acne, would choose the cure (29). The patient's perception of his or her acne can reach delusional proportions. Seaton et al. (36) described a case in which a patient's "delusions of dysmorphosis" were so powerful that her beliefs were transferred to her own daughter. Such individuals usually resist referral to a psychiatrist, feeling that their perception of their acne is accurate and that they do not require psychiatric evaluation, and they respond poorly to most psychological and pharmacological treatments, with the possible exception of serotonin reuptake inhibitors (37). There is, of course, a wide range of perceived psychological morbidity from acne. Koo examined the nature of the psychological distress experienced by patients with acne with several illustrations of patients' perceptions of their own disease (38).

Aggressive medical treatment may be at least as important as addressing psychiatric issues for patients who have developed a psychiatric disorder from the disfigurement of acne. Women who were severely distressed about their acne had significantly improved mental status when successfully treated with isotretinoin (39). Patients treated with isotretinoin also have significantly decreased levels of anxiety and depressive symptoms after treatment versus before treatment. In addition, the most significant reduction in anxiety and depression occurred in those patients with the greatest dermatological improvement (40). Even improvement in patients with mild to moderate facial acne treated with erythromycin and benzyl peroxide (Benzamycin®) causes an improvement in mental state, a decrease in self-consciousness, greater satisfaction with general appearance, and decreased concern about losing weight (41). However, not all study results demonstrate psychological benefit from the treatment of acne. A recent study by Mulder et al. (42) involving 50 females with mild to moderate facial acne assessed these patients by questionnaires and clinical assessments before and after a 9-month treatment with oral contraceptives. The results of the study showed great variability in psychosocial impairment between individuals. After 9 months a significant reduction in clinical severity in acne was seen overall. However, this did not correlate with the significant improvements in self-esteem, stability of self-esteem, and acceptance of appearance.

One of the difficulties of discussing the psychological impact of acne is the fact that attempts to quantify the nature and intensity of psychopathological effect of this disease have yielded inconsistent results. Even widely accepted psychometric instruments (43,44) such as the Pier-Harris self-concept scale and the Hopkins' Symptoms Checklist have been found to be unsuitable for use in the acne patient population. This may be because variables such as anxiety, depression, sociability, and self-esteem are influenced by other real-life variables that have nothing to do with acne. New acne-specific assessments are being developed which show some promise (45,46), but these need to be assessed for reliability and validity with additional randomized, placebo-controlled clinical trials utilizing representative population-based samples rather than samples of convenience. It is important, however, to continue to monitor for psychiatric difficulties from acne because effective treatments are available.

Treatment options for depression and social phobia include psychotherapy, group therapy, and recreational therapy (47). When indicated, one of these treatments should be included as part of a comprehensive treatment program. Depression is also treated effectively with pharmacotherapy. While antianxiety medications are effective for social phobia, cognitive behavioral therapy and systematic desensitization with exposure should also be considered.

PRIMARY PSYCHIATRIC DISORDERS INVOLVING A FOCUS ON ACNE

Acne can be the focus of even relatively mild psychiatric disorders. Teenagers may cite acne as an excuse to avoid social and occupational challenges that are inherent in the process of individual psychosocial development. Unfortunately, not all emotional issues that center around acne are mild.

Acne excoriée is an example of a more serious interplay between a primary psychiatric disorder and acne (48,49). The frequent end result is severe disfigurement from scarring. It is important to recognize that the diagnosis of acne excoriée refers only to the behavioral manifestation of picking acne lesions. The primary psychiatric disturbance may be a simple habit or something more serious. An example is obsessive-compulsive disorder (OCD), in which an urge to pick at acne cannot be resisted. Acne excoriée may represent a manifestation of delusion or depression for a minority of patients.

OCD patients can be distinguished from those with delusions by their retention of insight. OCD patients are usually aware that they should avoid their picking and that their behavior will cause damage to their skin. However, in trying to inhibit their destructive behavior, they instead experience a steady increase in a "compulsive urge," which typically makes them restless and "ill at ease" the longer they resist picking. Eventually, their motivation to stop their behavior is overwhelmed by the intensity of their urge to pick.

Anti-OCD medications such as fluoxetine (Prozac®) and paroxetine (Paxil®) can decrease obsessive thoughts and compulsive urges along with behavioral and psychotherapeutic interventions (50). If depression is the main psychopathology underlying acne excoriée, psychotherapy in addition to pharmacotherapy may provide significant relief. In mixed depression-OCD cases, antidepressants with anti-OCD properties (usually SSRIs) are preferred. The medication should not be regarded as a magic pill, however. Only if the individuals are motivated will the medication help control the compulsion by depressing the obsessive urge. Delusional patients, on the other hand, by definition cannot be persuaded away from their delusional idea. Fixed somatic delusional disorders are categorized under the term monosymptomatic hypochondriacal psychosis (MHP). For example, patients may express a rigid belief that a certain "object" must be extracted from the skin for acne to resolve. Delusional patients seen in dermatological practice are more likely to be convinced that they have living things in their skin, such as worms or insects (51), but they can also develop fixations regarding the presence of an inanimate object in the skin. Acne excoriée secondary to delusion is similar to delusions of parasitosis, in that patients harbor a fixed, delusional idea regarding a specific aspect of their health. The mainstay of treatment for these psychotic disorders involves pimozide(Orap®) (52) or other antipsychotic agents.

OTHER PSYCHIATRIC DISORDERS ASSOCIATED WITH ACNE

A discussion of all the psychiatric disorders that may have a relationship with acne is beyond the scope of this chapter, but one example—eating disorders—illustrates how other psychiatric disorders may be correlated with acne (13). The association is probably both psychological and physiological. Since both acne and eating disorder patients have trouble with body image, either can exacerbate or precipitate the other. It has been shown that improvement in eating disorder–related symptoms correlates with improvement in acne (53). Improvement in acne is also related to increased satisfaction with overall body weight and shape (38). Physiologically, decreased androgen levels are characteristic of anorexia nervosa and starvation. Because androgens are also known to be involved in the pathogenesis of acne, it is possible that some acne patients restrict their diets to reduce the amount of androgens in their body (54).

CONCLUSION

In summary, the interaction of acne and psychiatric processes takes place on many different levels. Delineating the specific type is important treatment appropriate for the underlying psychopathology.

REFERENCES

1. Koo JYM, Smith LL. Psychologic aspects of acne. Pediatr Dermatol 1991; 8(3):185–188.
2. Sulzberger MB, Zaidens SH. Psychogenic factors in dermatologic disorders. Med Clin North Am 1948; 32:669–685.
3. Griesemer RD. Emotionally triggered disease in a dermatologic practice. Psychiatr Ann 1978; 8:407–412.
4. Lorenz TH, Graham DT, Wolf S. The relation of life stress and emotions to human sebum secretion and to the mechanism of acne vulgaris. J Lab Clin Med 1953; 41:11–28.
5. Levi L. Endocrine reactions during emotional stress. In: Levi L, ed. Emotional Stress. New York: Grune & Stratton, 1967; 61–86.
6. Cunliffe WJ, Holland DB, Clark SM, et al. Comedogenesis: new aetiological, clinical, and therapeutic strategies. Br. J Dermatol 2000; 14:1084–1091.
7. Stratakis CA, Mastorakos G, Mitsiades NS, et al. Skin manifestations of Cushing disease in children and adolescents before and after the resolution of hypercortisolemia. Pediatr Dermatol 1998; 15:253–258.
8. Scholl GM, Wu CH, Leyden J. Androgen excess in women with acne. Obstet Gynecol 1984; 64:683–688.
9. Gupta MA, Gupta AK. Depression and suicidal ideation in dermatology patients with acne, alopecia areata, atopic dermatitis and psoriasis. Br J Dermatol 1998; 139:846–850.
10. Moussavian H. Improvement of acne in depressed patients treated with paroxetine. J Am Acad Child Adolesc Psychiatry 2001; 40(5):505–506.
11. Hughes H, Brown BW, Lawlis GF, Fulton JE. Treatment of acne vulgaris by biofeedback relaxation and cognitive imagery. J Psychosom Res 1983; 27(3):185–191.

12. Shenefelt PD. Hypnosis in dermatology. Arch Dermatol 2000; 136:393–399.
13. Hollander MB. Excoriated acne controlled by post-hypnotic suggestion. Am J Clin Hypn 1959; 1:122–123.
14. Mallon E, Newton JN, Klassen A, et al. The quality of life in acne: a comparison with general medical conditions using generic questionnaires. Br J Dermatol 1999; 140:672–676.
15. Gupta MA, Gupta AK. Psychological comorbidity in acne. Clin Dermatol 2001; 19:360–363.
16. Medansky RS, Handler RM, Medansky DL. Self-evaluation of acne and emotion: a pilot study. Psychosomatics 1981; 22(5):379–383.
17. Garrie SA, Garrie EV. Anxiety and skin disease. Cutis 1978; 22:205–208.
18. van der Meeren HL, Van der Schaar WW, Van den Hurk CM. The psychological impact of severe acne. Cutis 1985; 36(1):84–86.
19. Wu SF, Kinder BN, Trunnell TN, Fulton JE. Role of anxiety and anger in acne patients: a relationship with the severity of the disorder. J Am Acad Dermatol 1988; 18(2):325–333.
20. Smithard A, Glazebrook C, Williams HC. Acne prevalence, knowledge about acne and psychological morbidity in mid-adolescence: a community-based study. Br J Dermatol 2001; 145:274–279.
21. Khan MZ, Naeem A, Mufti KA. Prevalence of mental health problems in acne patients. J Ayub Med Coll Abbottabad 2001; 13:7–8.
22. Cotterill JA, Cunliffe WJ. Suicide in dermatological patients. Br J Dermatol 1997; 137:246–250.
23. American Psychiatric Association. Diagnostic and Statistical Manual of Mental Disorders. 4th ed. Washington, DC: American Psychiatric Publishing, 1994, 335–336.
24. Goldman HH, ed. Review of general psychiatry. East Norwalk, CT: Lange, 1984:497.
25. Hazen PG, Carney JF, Walker AE, et al. Depression—a side effect of 13-*cis*-retinoic acid therapy. J Am Acad Dermatol 1983; 9:278–279.
26. Scheinman PL, Peck GL, Rubinow DR, et al. Acute depression from isotretinoin. J Am Acad Dermatol 1990; 22:1112–1114.
27. Lamberg L. Acne drug depression warnings highlight need for expert care. JAMA 1998; 279:1057.
28. Jick SS, Kremers HM, Vasilakis-Scaramozza C. Isotretinoin use and risk of depression, psychotic symptoms, suicide, and attempted suicide. Arch Dermatol 2000; 136:1231–1236.
29. Panconesi E, Cossidente A, Giorgini S, et al. A psychosomatic approach to dermatologic cosmetology. Int J Dermatol 1983; 22:449–454.
30. Jowett S, Ryan T. Skin disease and handicap: an analysis of the impact of skin conditions. Soc Sci Med 1985; 20(4):425–429.
31. Motley RJ, Finlay AY. How much disability is caused by acne? Clin Exp Dermatol 1989; 14:194–198.
32. Shuster S, Fisher GH, Harris E, et al. The effect of skin disease on self-image. Br J Dermatol 1978; 99:18–19.

33. Cunliffe WJ. Acne and unemployment. Br J Dermatol 1986; 115:386.
34. Lasek RJ, Chren MM. Acne vulgaris and the quality of life of adult dermatology patients. Arch Dermatol 1998; 134:454–458.
35. Newton JN, Mallon E, Klassen A, et al. The effectiveness of acne treatment: an assessment by patients of the outcome of therapy. Br J Dermatol 1997; 137:563–567.
36. Seaton ED, Baxter KF, Cunliffe WJ. Familial dysmorphophobia. Br J Dermatol 2001; 144:439–440.
37. Hull SM, Cunliffe WJ, Hughes BR. Treatment of the depressed and dysmorphophobic acne patient. Clin Exp Dermatol 1991; 16:210–211.
38. Koo J. The psychosocial impact of acne: patients' perceptions. J Am Acad Dermatol 1995; 32:S26–30.
39. Cunliffe WJ, Hull SM, Hughes BR. The benefit of isotretinoin in the severely depressed/dysmorphophobic patient. Second International Congress on Psychiatry and Dermatology, University of Leeds (abstr), 1989.
40. Rubinow DR, Peck GL, Squillace KM, Gantt GG. Reduced anxiety and depression in cystic acne patients after successful treatment with oral isotretinoin. J Am Acad Dermatol 1987; 17(1):25–32.
41. Gupta MA, Gupta AK, Schork NJ, et al. Psychiatric aspects of the treatment of mild to moderate facial acne: some preliminary observations. Int J Dermatol 1990; 29:719–721.
42. Mulder MMS, Sigurdsson V, Zuuren EJ. Psychosocial impact of acne vulgaris: evaluation of the relation between a change in clinical acne severity and psychosocial state. Dermatology 2001; 203:124–130.
43. Rubinow DR, Peck GL, Squillace KM, et al. Reduced anxiety and depression in cystic acne patient after successful treatment with isotretinoin. J Am Acad Dermatol 1987; 17:25–32.
44. Krowchuk DP, Stancin T, Keskinen R, et al. The psychosocial effects of acne on adolescents. Pediatr Dermatol 1991; 8:332–338.
45. Martin AR, Lookingbill DP, Botek A, et al. Health-related quality of life among patients with facial acne—assessment of a new acne-specific questionnaire. Clin Exp Dermatol 2001; 26:380–385.
46. Gupta MA, Johnson AM, Gupta AK. The development of an Acne Quality of Life scale: reliability, validity and relation to subjective acne severity in mild to moderate acne vulgaris. Acta Derm Venereol (Stockh) 1998; 78:451–456.
47. Greist JH. Treatment of obsessive compulsive disorder: psychotherapies, drugs, and other somatic treatment. J Clin Psychiatry 1990; 51(8 suppl):44–50.
48. Kent A, Drummond LM. Acne excoriée—a case report of treatment using habit reversal. Clin Exp Dermatol 1989; 14:163–164.
49. Sneddon J, Sneddon I. Acne excoriée: a protective device. Clin Exp Dermatol 1983; 8:65–68.
50. Kearney CA, Silverman WK. Treatment of an adolescent with obsessive-compulsive disorder by alternating response prevention and cognitive therapy: an empirical analysis. J Behav Ther Exp Psychiatry 1990; 21(1):39–47.
51. Hopkinson G. Delusion of infestation. Acta Psychiatr Scand 1970; 46:111–119.

52. Riding J, Munro A. Pimozide in the treatment of monosymptomatic hypochondriacal psychosis. Acta Psychiatr Scand 1975; 52:223–230.
53. Gupta MA, Gupta AK, Ellis CN, Voorhees JJ. Bulimia nervosa and acne may be related: a case report. Can J Psychiatry 1992; 37:58–61.
54. Pochi PE, Downing DT, Strauss JS. Sebaceous gland response in man to prolonged total caloric deprivation. J Invest Dermatol 1970; 55:303–309.
55. Goulden V, Clark SM, Cunliffe WJ. Post-adolescent acne: a review of clinical features. Br J Dermatol 1997; 136(1):66–70.

23

Psychiatric Issues in Vitiligo

Ernest Lee and John Y. M. Koo
University of California, San Francisco
San Francisco, California, U.S.A.

INTRODUCTION

It has long been postulated that the pathogenesis of many skin disorders may have a psychological component, and the psychological consequences of disfiguring skin disease have been well documented. The interplay between vitiligo and psychiatry occurs on at least two levels. Psychiatric issues can exacerbate and affect the natural course of vitiligo, and vitiligo in turn has psychological consequences for many patients (Fig. 1).

NORMAL PIGMENTATION OF THE SKIN

Melanocytes derive from melanoblasts that migrate from the neural crest and the outer layer of the optic cup during the first 2 months of fetal development (1). In the skin, melanocytes are associated with the hair follicle and in some mammals, including humans, are also found in the basal layer of the interfollicular epidermis (2). They are also found in mucous membranes, the central nervous system (leptomeninges), the eye (uveal tract, pigment epithelium of retina), the inner ear, the oral cavity, and cochlea.

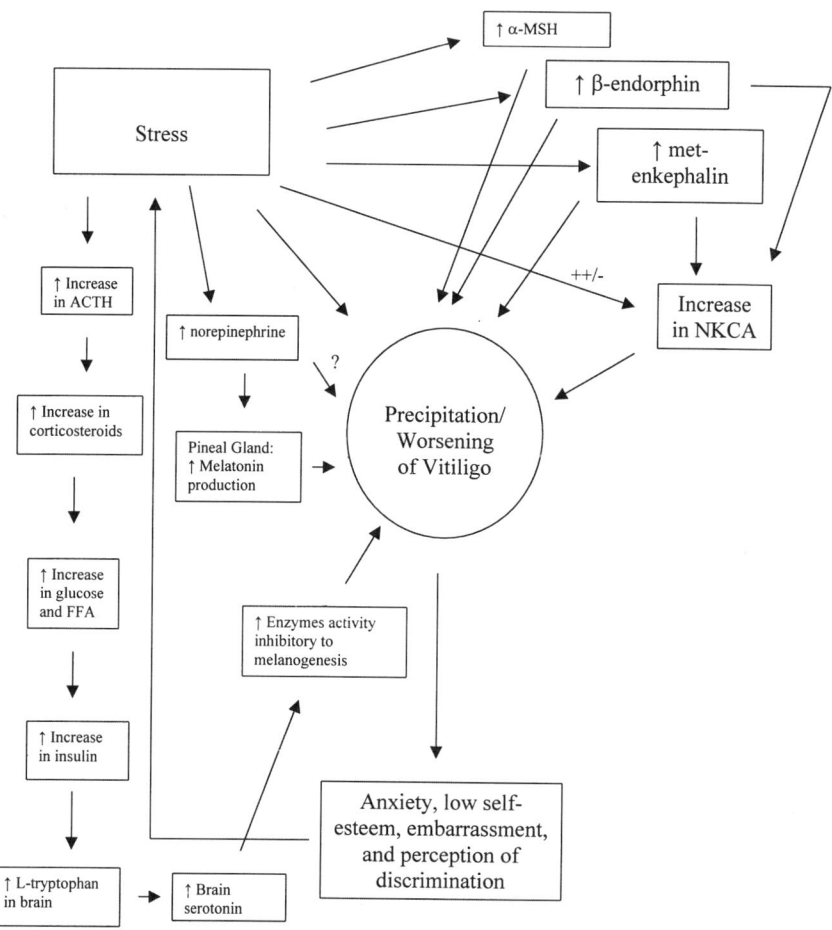

FIGURE 1 Hypothetical relationship of stress and vitiligo. NKCA: natural killer cell activity; α-MSH: alpha-melanocyte–stimulating hormone; FFA: free fatty acids.

However, only melanocytes of the epidermis and hair follicle are capable of forming melanin throughout life and of inserting their melanosomes into adjacent cells (3). Melanin is produced from tyrosine, a derivative of the essential amino acid derivative phenylalanine.

PSYCHOLOGICAL FACTORS IN THE DEVELOPMENT AND NATURAL HISTORY OF VITILIGO

Data Supporting Stress as a Significant Etiological Factor in Vitiligo

The relationship between stressful life events and skin disease has been carefully studied (4). In vitiligo, patients often associate the onset of their disease with emotional or physical stress (5). Nordlund and Lerner found that in 20% of cases, vitiligo is precipitated by severe sunburn or emotional stress (6). Others put the number as high as 50% (7). Griesemer (8) recorded the incidence of emotional triggering of dermatoses in 4576 patients during 1 year and, for the subset of patients with vitiligo, found that one third of vitiligo cases were reportedly induced by stress. The average latency period between the onset of emotional stress and a noticeable change in skin pigmentation was 2–3 weeks. Research suggests that vitiligo patients have endured a significantly higher number of stressful events in their life compared to patients with skin disease not thought to be associated with stress (e.g., epidermolysis bullosa) giving some support to the possibility of a psychological dimension to its etiology (9).

Current Theories Regarding the Etiology of Vitiligo

There are three theories concerning the etiology of vitiligo. The autoimmune hypothesis developed from the association between autoimmune diseases and vitiligo. Naughton's group has been instrumental in demonstrating that antibodies against melanocyte surface antigens exist and that the extent of depigmentation in vitiligo is correlated with the incidence and level of antibodies against melanocytes (10–12). The autocytotoxic theory suggests that increased melanocyte activity leads to its own demise by producing too many cytotoxic precursors to melanin synthesis leading to melanocytic cell death (13). The neural supposition, initiated by Lerner over 40 years ago (14), states that a neurochemical mediator (such as epinephrine, norepinephrine, or acetylcholine from nerve endings) destroys melanocytes or inhibits melanin production. This applies primarily to segmental vitiligo. There is also a composite theory, which brings elements of these three together.

The Human Body's Physiological Response to Stress

When human bodies are subjected to a stressful condition, a host of stress-related neurotransmitters, including endogenous opioids (mainly enkephalin and endorphin), corticotropin-releasing factor (CRF), adrenocorticotropic hormone (ACTH), and catecholamines are released (15). These responses in turn have effects on immune function and production of other hormone peptides. How does stress specifically affect vitiligo? Stress and the neurotransmitters released during stress could work through any of the above-mentioned mechanisms. Its effect on immune function could lead to autoimmune destruction of melanocytes, the increased production of melatonin may produce an autocytotoxic impact, and the increase in catecholamines could inhibit melanin production neurochemically.

Possible Psychophysiological Model of Vitiligo

The mechanism by which stress affects vitiligo could be either physiological, psychological, or a combination of the two. Stress has several physiological consequences. These include:

1. Direct effects on the immune response (16,17), including modulating natural killer cell activity (NKCA) (18). NKCA is a spontaneous cytotoxic function that is known to be crucial in the immediate host defense against viral and other infections and in natural resistance toward malignant cells (19). A consequent hypothesis is that stress affects vitiligo though the immune system by upregulating immune mechanisms targeted against the melanocyte or melanin. In a study by Mozzanica et al., NKCA was higher in vitiligo patients than in controls but had similar circadian rhythms (20). However, the extent of the difference was higher in patients with stable disease versus those with active vitiligo. These results imply that NKCA may be chronically active in vitiligo but involved in the "maintenance" rather than the "initiation" of the disease. It is important to note, however, that others have shown that NKCA and lymphokine-activated killer cell cytotoxicity are normal in patients with progressive vitiligo (21).

2. Increased production of opioid peptides such as β-endorphin, met-enkephalin, and α-melanocyte-stimulating hormone (α-MSH). The increase in α-MSH during times of stress comes from the pituitary gland (22) in humans (23) as well as rats (24). All these peptides act as immunomodulators, indicating that they may also affect vitiligo by upregulating the immune system surveillance of melanocytic antigens. In the Mozzanica et al. study (20), with regards to the neurohormones, daily met-enkephalin and β-endorphin oscillations in vitiligo patients were not circadian, whereas they were circadian in patients without vitiligo. β-

Endorphin plasma levels were higher in stable vitiligo patients than in controls, but only in the nadir phase (6:00 p.m.). There were, however, no differences in β-endorphin plasma levels between active vitiligo patients and normal subjects. Met-enkephalin plasma levels were generally higher in vitiligo patients, particularly ones with active disease, than in controls. In contrast, Katsambas et al. (25) reported that mean β-endorphin serum levels in patients in the early years of vitiligo were statistically significantly elevated compared to those in patients with chronic vitiligo and those in controls. It is probable that emotional stress during the early time of disease leads to increased opioid system activity and hence the elevated β-endorphin levels. As the vitiligo stabilizes, the β-endorphin levels decrease because of its depletion through nerve endings and/or increased metabolism of the peptide.

Most recently, investigators found that both β-endorphin plasma levels in 23 cases of progressive vitiligo and 17 cases of stable vitiligo were significantly higher than in normal controls (26). In addition, the overall levels of β-endorphin in skin tissue fluids from the lesions of patients with vitiligo were increased in comparison with uninvolved skin. As one can see, there are conflicting results in terms of whether β-endorphin is elevated more in stable or in progressive cases of vitiligo or if in fact there is no difference between the two disease states.

The Mozzanica study showed no differences in α-MSH levels or rhythm between controls and vitiligo patients. However, even if α-MSH was found to be elevated in vitiligo patients, it probably acts through a different mechanism from the other opioids. Pawelek et al. demonstrated increased melanocyte susceptibility to autocytotoxic cell death from accumulation of precursor molecules of melanin synthesis (e.g., dopachrome) with exposure to melanotropin, i.e., MSH (27).

3. Indirect effects on NKCA through β-endorphin and met-enkephalin (28–30). Many studies have been performed in order to assess the influence of opioid peptides on the activity of natural killer cells. While most of the studies have shown a clear stimulatory effect exerted by opioids on this immune function (31), a few studies suggest an inhibitory effect. Nonspecific responses, such as those mediated by polymorphonuclear (PMN) cells, natural killer cells, and macrophages are generally stimulated by opioids; whereas antigen-driven immune responses, such as those mediated by T cells, are generally inhibited by

opioids. The conflicting results may be due to differences in the concentration of opioid peptides utilized, subjects from whom the cells were obtained, and the cell populations utilized. The mechanism by which these endogenous opioids generally increase NKCA is not entirely clear, but a possibility involves calmodulin activation (32).

A possible mechanism of stress induction of vitiligo is that stress increases β-endorphin and met-enkephalin levels, stimulating NKCA as well as macrophage and polymorphonucleocyte (PMN) activity. This increase in activity is maintained in chronic vitiligo by the continued production of β-endorphin. The resulting increase in immune surveillance may precipitate the destruction of melanocytes and hence a decrease in pigmentation, particularly if preformed antibodies against melanocytes are present.

Catecholamines are also elevated in stress. In a recent study by Cucchi et al. (33), 70 patients with vitiligo (49 in the active phase and 21 in the stable phase) were compared with 35 controls. Levels of norepinephrine (NE), epinephrine (E), normetanephrine (NMN), metanephrine (MN), homovanillic acid (HVA), and 5-hydroxyindolacetic acid (5-HIAA) were higher in patients compared to controls, indicating that vitiligo patients may be undergoing a stress response on a hormonal level with or without their sensing it. NMN, MN, and HVA are all metabolites of NE and E, while 5-HIAA is a major metabolite of serotonin, which is a precursor of melatonin. There were also significantly higher levels of NE, NMN, MHPG, and HVA in active phase patients than in stable phase patients. The patients with a more recent onset (< 1 year) progressive vitiligo showed significantly increased levels of E, NE, and MN in comparison with long-term sufferers. Other investigators have found slightly different results. Salzer and Schallreuter (34) conducted an investigation of 117 patients with vitiligo and found that plasma norepinephrine was significantly higher compared to controls, whereas epinephrine was within the normal range. It has also been found that in vitiligo there is overproduction of norepinephrine and concomitant increased density of β_2-adrenorecptors in differentiating keratinocytes (35). This increase in catecholamine levels may occur in response to initial stress and, in total, suggests that the stimulated activity of the monoaminergic systems is not essential for subsequent progression of the disease.

Catecholamines may have a more direct role in vitiligo onset (36) because these compounds can easily undergo oxidation by different oxidant systems, with the formation of quinines, semi-quinone radicals, and oxyradicals, which are toxic for melanocytes (similar to autocytotoxic theory) (37). In fact, in vitiliginous patients, several detoxifying enzymes show reduced activity (38). Catecholamines can also influence depigmentation indirectly. Slominski et al. showed the phenomenon of very early increased activation of melatonin receptors in vitiliginous melanocytes (39). Melatonin is synthesized in the pineal gland, the retina, and certain areas of the gastrointestinal tract, and its synthesis and secretion are stimulated primarily by catecholamines. Increased catecholamines from stress could hyperactivate these melatonin receptors. With hyperactivation of the melanocyte, toxic metabolites and free radicals from melanogenesis may begin to accumulate, resulting in damage to melanocytes in addition to changes in neighboring keratinocytes. The keratinocytes are affected by both the toxins released by nearby melanocytes and the transport of these products to the keratinocyte via melanosomes (40). Since melanocytes are sustained in large part by keratinocytes through basic fibroblastic growth factor (bFGF), a cycle of destruction is initiated: melanocyte destruction → keratinocyte alterations → lack of bFGF secretion → decreased proliferation and vitality of melanocytes (41). In genetically predisposed subjects, an alteration in cell surface proteins could occur with damage to the melanocyte. This could be followed by an autoimmune antibody and lymphocyte-mediated response that could lead to a significant and irreversible loss of melanocytes (40).

In addition, the immunomodulating properties of melatonin released during stress may contribute further to vitiligo through an autoimmune pathway. Two groups have shown that the effect of melatonin on immunity may be mediated by endogenous opioids, in particular β-endorphin (42,43). Maestroni and Conti showed that melatonin works via the endogenous opioid system on antigen-activated immunocompetent cells (44).

Stress may also affect vitiligo through other hormone pathways (45). Stressful situations cause an increase in ACTH levels, increasing the production of corticosteroids, mobilizing glucose and free fatty acids, and stimulating insulin secretion. Insulin directly stimulates L-tryptophan in the brain, leading to an increase in brain serotonin synthesis. Because melatonin is a serotonin metabolite, vitiligo could be precipitated (see above). Serotonin hyperactivation could also lead to increased activity of enzymes inhibitory to melanogenesis.

In summary, there are several promising leads in linking stress and the development/exacerbation of vitiligo. However, the presence of contradictory data requires that further investigations are needed to elucidate the psychoneuroendocrine aspects of vitiligo.

PSYCHOLOGICAL IMPACT OF VITILIGO

The psychological impact of vitiligo can be significant. Cosmetic disfigurement from this disease tends to disrupt and cause anxiety in the lives of those with lower ego strength, particularly younger patients. Feelings of stress, embarrassment, or self-consciousness when in casual contact with strangers, perception of discrimination, and low self-esteem can all be brought about by vitiligo and be significantly detrimental to patients, especially those with lesions in visible locations (46). Approximately one quarter of patients believe their disease has interfered with sexual relationships; males, unmarrieds, those with low self-esteem, and those who rate appearance as important to them are at increased risk for adjustment problems. The factors determining to what overall extent vitiligo affects a patient's life is not as closely correlated to the extent of involvement as it is to lower self-esteem, higher levels of perceived stigma and disability, and younger age (47). The psychological impact can be of paramount importance in deeply pigmented races, in whom the contrast between normal and affected skin is marked, and the disease can carry a serious social stigma.

In a U.S. comparison of 66 patients with vitiligo, an equal number of control subjects, as well as 25 psoriasis patients and 11 patients with other pigment skin disorders (hypo- or hypermelanosis) (48), the social stigma of vitiligo resulted in lower self-esteem than those without skin disease. There was also no difference between patients with vitiligo and patients with other pigment disorders with regards to psychosocial effect. However, vitiligo patients did exhibit better adjustment to their disorder and experienced less social discrimination than did psoriasis patients, though the two groups did not differ in regards to self-esteem. The comparison of psoriasis and vitiligo patients is interesting because both of these are very common diseases. While vitiligo is primarily a pigmentary disease, psoriasis has a more painful physical component to the disease. In two studies from India, the psychiatric morbidity from these two diseases showed conflicting results. In a study by Sharma et al. (49) the prevalence of psychiatric morbidity, as assessed by the General Health Questionnaire (GHQ-H), was found to be 53.3% and 16.22% in psoriasis and vitiligo patients, respectively. In contrast, another group of investigators (50) from India using the same questionnaire found psychiatric morbidity rates of 33.63% and 24.7% for vitiligo and psoriasis, respectively.

Because a person's appearance is a major determinate of attributed personality traits, vitiligo can have a major impact on personality (51). Many psychological studies indicate that appearance correlates with the personality traits that people attribute to strangers (52). Attractive persons of both sexes are presumed to have more socially desirable traits, to be kinder and more intelligent, to have greater internal control and competence, and to have made greater achievements (52). Many studies show that people respond differently to those who are physically handicapped, such as an amputee, compared with those who are visibly disfigured. Traits attributed to those who are visibly disfigured are more frequently negative in character (53). For example, studies have demonstrated that people are less likely to help a facially disfigured person that a nondisfigured person (54). Therefore, it is understandable that patients who have extensive disfigurement from vitiligo may encounter many difficulties, not only in terms of emotional equilibrium, but also as a victim of negative perceptions from others.

While the psychosocial impact of vitiligo can be quite severe, treatment of the disease can lead to an improved quality of life for patients. In an open, uncontrolled trial of 51 children (20 males, 31 females) with generalized vitiligo, treatment with narrow-band (TL-01) UVB radiation therapy twice weekly resulted in more than 75% overall repigmentation in 53% of patients and stabilization of disease in 80% (55). Quality of life was compared using a Children's Dermatology Life Quality Index (CDLQI), before and after therapy. A lower CDLQI score indicated a higher quality of life. In the patient group that had < 25% repigmentation, the CDLQI scores were not significantly decreased after therapy ($p = 0.09$). However, in patients with > 25% repigmentation, the difference in CDLQI scores, before and after therapy, was significant; the greater the repigmentation, the more significant the decrease in the CDLQI scores, signifying improved psychological equilibrium.

CONCLUSION

Stress appears to exacerbate vitiligo in various ways, including 1) changing immune function, 2) increasing production of opioid peptides, 3) increasing catecholamine release, and 4) affecting other hormone pathways. Vitiligo in turn causes disfigurement, leading to 1) an increase in anxiety, 2) a lowering of self-esteem, and 3) increasing psychiatric morbidity.

The role of stress in the development/maintenance of vitiligo has important implications for future advances in therapy. Neuropeptides and their agonists/antagonists are already being pursued as potential therapies in other dermatological diseases such as psoriasis and Raynaud's disease (56). If stress exacerbates/precipitates vitiligo through a neuropeptide pathway(s), antagonists(e.g., naloxone)/antibodies for those mediators or drugs that reduce the levels of those mediators can be potential therapeutic agents. For conditions associated with increased β-endorphins, such as personality disorders and self-injurious behavior (57), antagonists of β-endorphin have already been used.

Any clinical intervention that reduces the extent and visibility of depigmentation will be of psychological benefit. However, with a disease such as vitiligo, which is not only incurable, but can also be progressive, it is important to recognize and deal with the social and psychological consequences of the condition. This applies not only to physicians but to other healthcare workers as well (58). With the known connection between stress and vitiligo, psychological interventions such as training in relaxation skills and other psychotherapeutic interventions may be helpful, as has been demonstrated in other psychophysiological disorders such as psoriasis (59,60). In fact there is preliminary evidence that cognitive-behavioral therapy may have a positive effect on the progression of vitiligo itself (61). Occasionally, patients with vitiligo have improved using hypnotic suggestion as complementary therapy (62,63). When vitiligo patients are able to adjust to the reality of their disfigurement, they will be less distressed by others' reactions and more able to form new relationships (64). In summary, vitiligo is a condition that is best approached from both psychological and physiological perspectives, much like many other psychophysiological disorders.

REFERENCES

1. Fitzpatrick T, Szabo G. The melanocyte: cytology and cytochemistry. J Invest Dermatol 1959;32:197–209.
2. Tsatmali M, Ancans J, Thody AJ. Melanocyte function and its control by melanocortin peptides. J Histochem Cytochem 2002;50:125–133.
3. Sams WM. Structure and Function of the Skin. In Sams WM, Lynch PJ, eds. Principles and Practice of Dermatology. 2nd ed. Churchill Livingstone Inc., 1996, New York.
4. Picardi A, Abeni D. Stressful life events and skin diseases: disentangling evidence from myth. Psychother Psychosom 2001;70(3):118–136.
5. Kovacs SO. Vitiligo. J Am Acad Dermatol 1998;38:647–666.
6. Nordlund JJ, Lerner AB. Vitiligo: it is important. Arch Dermatol 1982;118:5–8.
7. Agarwal G. Vitiligo: an under-estimated problem. Fam Pract 1998; 15:S19–23.
8. Griesemer RD. Emotionally triggered disease in a dermatological practice. Psychiatr Ann 1978; 8:49–56.
9. Papadopoulos L, Bor R, Legg C, et al. Impact of life events on the onset of vitiligo in adults: preliminary evidence for a psychological dimension in aetiology. Clin Exp Dermatol 1998; 23:243–248.
10. Naughton G, Eisinger M, Bystryn J. Antibodies to normal human melanocytes in vitiligo. J Exp Med 1983; 158:246–251.

11. Naughton G, Eisinger M, Bystryn J. Detection of antibodies to melanocytes in vitiligo by specific immunoprecipitation. J Invest Dermatol 1983; 81:540–542.

12. Naughton G, Reggiardo D, Bystryn J. Correlation between vitiligo antibodies and extent of depigmentation in vitiligo. J Am Acad Dermatol 1986; 15:978–981.

13. Lerner A. On the etiology of vitiligo and gray hair. Am J Med 1971; 51:141–147.

14. Lerner A. Vitiligo. J Invest Dermatol 1959; 32:285–310.

15. Drolet G, Dumont EC, Gosselin I, et al. Role of endogenous opioid system in the regulation of the stress response. Prog Neuro-Psychopharmacol Biol Psychiatry 2001; 25:729–741.

16. Dantzer R, Kelley KW. Stress and immunity: an integrated view of relationships between the brain and the immune system. Life Sci 1989; 44:1995–2008.

17. Khansari DN, Murgo AJ, Faith RE. Effect of stress on the immune system (review). Immunol Today 1990; 11:170–175.

18. Schlesinger M, Yodfat Y. Effect of psychosocial stress and natural killer cell activity. Cancer Detect Prev 1988; 12:9–14.

19. Herberman RB, Djeu J, Kay HD, et al. Natural killer cells: characteristics and regulation of activity. Immunol Rev 1979; 44:43–70.

20. Mozzanica N, Villa M, Foppa S, et al. Plasma α-melanocyte-simulating hormone, β-endorphin, met-enkephalin, and natural killer cell activity in vitiligo. J Am Acad Dermatol 1992; 26:693–700.

21. Durham-Pierre DG, Walters CS, Halder RM, et al. Natural killer cell and lymphokine-activated killer cell activity against melanocytes in vitiligo. J Am Acad Dermatol 1995; 33:26–30.

22. Lindley SE, Lookingland KJ, Moore KE. Dopaminergic and beta-adrenergic receptor control of alpha-melanocyte stimulating hormone secretion during stress. Neuroendocrinology 1990; 52:46–51.

23. Slavnov VN, Luchitski EV, Oleinik VA, et al. The secretion of alpha-melanotrophin in disease of the hypothalamas-hypophysis adrenal cortex system. Probl Endokrinol (Mosk) 1990; 36:40–43. (In Russian, abstract in English.)

24. Cannon JG, Tatro JB, Reichlin S, et al. Alpha-melanocyte stimulating hormone inhibits immunostimulatory and inflammatory actions of interleukin-1. J Immunol 1986; 137:2232–2238.

25. Katsambas AD, Schulpis KH, Antoniou C, et al. Beta endorphin serum levels in patients with vitiligo. J Eur Acad Dermatol Venereol 1994; 3:22–26.

26. Tu C-X, Zhao D-M, Lin X-R. Levels of β-endorphin in the plasma and skin tissue fluids of patients with vitiligo. J Dermatol Sci 2001; 26:62–66.

27. Pawelek J, Korner A, Bergstrom A, et al. New regulators of melanin biosynthesis and the autodestruction of melanoma cells. Nature 1980; 286:617–619.

28. Shavit Y, Lewis J, Terman G, et al. Opioid peptides mediate the suppressive effect of stress on natural killer cell cytotoxiciy. Science 1984; 223:188–193.

29. Plotnikoff N, Good RA, Faith RE, Murgo AJ. Enkephalins and Endorphins: Stress and the Immune System. New York: Plenum Press, 1986.

30. Jeijnen CJ, Zijlstra J, Kavelaars A, et al. Modulation of the immune response by POMC-derived peptides. Brain Behav Immun 1987; 1:284–291.

31. Kay N, Allen J, Morley JE. Endorphins stimulate normal human peripheral blood lymphocyte natural killer activity. Life Sci 1984; 35:53–59.

32. Baram D, Simantov R. Enkephalins and opiate antagonists control calmodulin distribution in neuroblastoma-glioma cells. J Neurochem 1983; 40:55–63.

33. Cucchi ML, Frattini P, Santagostino G, Orecchia G. Higher plasma catecholamine and metabolite levels in the early phase of nonsegmental vitiligo. Pigment Cell Res 2000; 13:28–32.

34. Salzer BA, Schallreuter KU. Investigation of the personality structure in patients with vitiligo and a possible association with impaired catecholamine metabolism. Dermatology 1995; 190:109–115.

35. Schallreuter KU, Wood JM, Pittelkow MR, Steinkraus V. High expression of beta-2 adrenoreceptors in vitiligo. Arch Dermatol Res 1993; 285:215–220.

36. Shelley WB, Ohman S. Epinephrine induction of white hair in AC1-rats. J Invest Dermatol 1969; 53:155–158.

37. Morrone A, Picardo M, DeLuca C, et al. Catecholamines and vitiligo. Pigment Cell Res 1992; 5:65–69.

38. LePoole C, Das KP. Microscopic changes in vitiligo. Clin Dermatol 1997; 15:863–873.

39. Slominski A, Paus R, Bormiski A. Hypothesis: possible role for the melatonin receptor in vitiligo: discussion paper. J Roy Soc Med 1989; 82:539–541.

40. Fabbri P. Immunodermatologia. Brescia: ISED, 1993:337–363.

41. Halaban R, Langdon R, Birchall N. Basic fibroblast growth factor from human keratinocytes is a natural mitogen for melanocytes. J Cell Biol 1988; 107:1611–1619.

42. Lakin ML, Miller CH, Stott Ml, et al. Involvement of the pineal gland and melatonin in murine analgesia. Life Sci 1981; 19:2543–2547.

43. Lissoni P, Esposti D, Esposti G, et al. A clinical study on the relationship between the pineal gland and the opioid system. J Neural Trans 1986; 65:63–73.

44. Maestroni GJM, Conti A. β-Endorphin and dynorphin mimic the circadian immunoenhancing and antistress effects of melatonin. Int J Immunopharmacol 1989; 11:333–340.

45. Le Poole C, Das PK, van der Wijngaard RM, et al. Review of the etiopathomechanism of vitiligo: a convergence theory. Exp Dermatol 1993; 2:145–153.

46. Porter JR, Beuf AH, Lerner AB, et al. The effect of vitiligo on sexual relationships. J Am Acad Dermatol 1990; 22:221–222.

47. Kent G, Al' Abadie M. Psychologic effects of vitiligo: a critical incident analysis. J Am Acad Dermatol 1996; 35:895–898.

48. Porter JR, Beuf AH, Lerner A, Nordlund J. Psychosocial effect of vitiligo: a comparison of vitiligo patients with "normal" control subjects, with psoriasis

patients, and with patients with other pigmentary disorders. J Am Acad Dermatol 1986; 15:220–224.

49. Sharma N, Koranne RV, Singh RK. Psychiatric morbidity in psoriasis and vitiligo: a comparative study. J Dermatol 2001; 28(8):419–423.

50. Matto SK, Handa S, Kaur I, Gupta N, Malhotra R. Psychiatric morbidity in vitiligo and psoriasis: a comparative study from India. J Dermatol 2001; 28:424–432.

51. Porter J, Beuf A, Nordlund J, et al. Psychological reaction to chronic skin disorders. Gen Hosp Psych 1979; 1:73–77.

52. Dion K, Bersheid E, Walster E. What is beautiful is good. J Pers Soc Psychol 1972; 24:215–220.

53. Siller J, Ferguson L, Vann D, Holland B. Structure of attitudes toward the physically disabled: the disability factor scale: amputation, blindness, cosmetic conditions. Proceedings of 76th Annual Convention of American Psychological Association, San Francisco, 1968, pp. 651–652.

54. Piliavin IM, Piliavin JA, Rodin J. Costs, diffusion, and the stigmatized victim. J Pers Soc Psychol 1975; 32:429–438.

55. Njoo MD, Bos JD, Westerhof W. Treatment of generalized vitiligo in children with narrow-band (TL-01) UVB radiation therapy. J Am Acad Dermatol 2000; 42:245–253.

56. Gomez-Bezares P, Vazquez-Doval FJ. Neuropeptides in dermatologic therapy. Rev Neurol 1997; 25(3):S320–324.

57. Konicki PE, Schulz SC. Rationale for clinical trials of opiate antagonists in treating patients with personality disorders and self-injurious behavior. Psychopharmacol Bull 1989; 25:556–563.

58. Mason PJ. Vitiligo: the psychosocial effects. Medsurg Nurs 1997; 6:216–218.

59. Winchell S, Watts R. Relaxation therapies in the treatment of psoriasis and possible pathophysiological mechanisms. J Am Acad Dermatol 1988; 18:101–104.

60. Price M, Mottahedin I, Mayo P. Can psychotherapy help patients with psoriasis? Clin Exp Dermatol 1991; 16:114–117.

61. Papadopoulos L, Bor R, Legg C. Coping with the disfiguring effects of vitiligo: a preliminary investigation into the effects of cognitive-behavioral therapy. Br J Med Psychol 1999; 72:385–396.

62. Scott MJ. Hypnosis in Skin and Allergic Diseases. Springfield, IL: Charles C Thomas, 1960.

63. Tobia L. L'ipnosi in dermatologia. Minerva Med. 1982; 73:531–537.

64. Patridge J. Changing Faces. The Challenge of Facial Disfigurement. London: Changing Faces, 1994.

24

Psychological Impact of Aging and the Skin

Madhulika A. Gupta
University of Western Ontario
London, Ontario, Canada

Aditya K. Gupta
University of Toronto
Toronto, Ontario, Canada

INTRODUCTION

The integumentary changes associated with aging are typically one of the first external indicators of the overall aging of the body in the otherwise healthy individual. Most of the clinical changes associated with aging, such as wrinkling, pigmentary changes, roughness, laxity, and telangiectasia, are due to photodamage. The skin as a powerful organ of communication represents various socially important attributes such as social status, wealth, and sexuality, in addition to age (1–4). Aging not only represents tangible change, it also necessitates adaption to change. Therefore, among most individuals, aging of the skin can result in an adjustment reaction as they adjust to the bodily changes associated with mid- and later life and affect, to varying degrees, their interpersonal interactions both socially and vocationally. Over the last several decades the social and cultural meanings of growing old have changed (5). The idea of old age has started to acquire increasingly negative connotations (5), and old age is widely viewed as a specific medical and social problem that has to be addressed by professionals. The view that chronological age itself does not signal the beginning of old age (5) has also become increasingly prevalent, with a high value placed by society on the maintenance of a youthful appearance and the reversal of some of the aging-related bodily changes. These factors have culminated in a range of psychological reactions to aging of the skin.

AGING SKIN AND INTERPERSONAL INTERACTIONS

Physical appearance, especially the appearance of the face, plays a major role in human transactions (3,4), and youthful skin contributes significantly to an individual's physical attractiveness. A youthful appearance has been shown to be associated with both increased self-esteem and improved social relations (6). In one study (7), 20 observers representing both sexes rated photographs of 48 white women (age range 54–96 yr) for physical attractiveness. Two essentially nonoverlapping groups of 16 women each who were on the opposite ends of the attractiveness spectrum were selected from the 48 subjects (7). The attractiveness ratings were strongly affected by cutaneous signs typically associated with aging (wrinkling, sagging, sallowing, etc.) by both the male and female judges (4,7). Furthermore, the group of women rated as good-looking by the observers also reported greater satisfaction with their lives and described themselves as more socially outgoing (3,7), further supporting the view that an attractive appearance has a positive influence upon social functioning. In a study of 20 patients with clinically mild to moderately aged skin secondary to photodamage (8) who had entered a clinical trial to evaluate the efficacy of topical tretinoin for the treatment of photodamaged skin, it was observed that at baseline the study volunteers had high scores on Interpersonal Sensitivity and Phobic Anxiety subscales of the Brief Symptom Inventory (BSI) (9). High scores on these subscales suggest that these subjects with photodamaged skin were experiencing uneasiness during their interpersonal interactions. The Interpersonal Sensitivity (BSI) (9) subscale measures a lack of ease during interpersonal interactions, and the Phobic Anxiety (BSI) (9) subscale provides an index of a persistent fear response to certain situations, including social situations, that leads to avoidance of the situations that provoke anxiety. After 24 weeks of therapy, both the Interpersonal Sensitivity (BSI) and Phobic Anxiety (BSI) scores decreased significantly ($p < 0.05$) in the topical tretinoin but not the control group (receiving the inactive vehicle) (8). These findings were confirmed in another study (10) involving 40 additional subjects with moderate to severe photodamage among whom a significant decrease in Phobic Anxiety (BSI) (8) ($p < 0.05$) was observed after 24 weeks of therapy with topical tretinoin, with an increase ($p < 0.05$) in this symptom dimension in the group receiving the inactive vehicle (10). These findings indicate that aging-related changes affecting the skin cause increased social anxiety in some subjects, and this anxiety decreases with treatment of some of the cutaneous changes of photodamage. Increased ease during interpersonal interactions usually translates into increased socialization and possibly increased physical activity. These lifestyle-related factors may have a protective effect upon the overall physical health of older adults, especially those with chronic health problems (11). These findings support the view that patients with cutaneous aging and/or photodamage should be informed about the therapies that can ameliorate some of the cutaneous changes and the use of such interventions should not be considered to be simply an expression of vanity (6).

The aging of the appearance can elicit certain reactions from caregivers and employers which can affect the individual's quality of life and psychological well-being. Aging skin does not generally have a direct impact upon the physical functioning of an individual (4). However, when the individual depends on others to carry out his or her physical activities, an aging appearance can have an important effect on the type of care the individual receives (4). In such instances the psychology of the caregiver becomes an important factor for the patient. For example, it has been observed that caregivers in nursing homes and hospitals sometimes emotionally disengage from a patient when their grooming habits and hygiene and/or appearance begin to deteriorate or when the patient appears aged (12). Alternately, an improved appearance secondary to improved hair care and cosmetics has been associated with increased interest by the caregiver and even taken as evidence by the caregiver that the patient's physical state is improving (12). It is likely that the older individual in the community who uses community resources to be able to maintain an independent lifestyle also experiences similar reactions (4).

Physical appearance plays an important role in the business world, and professional image consultants help both men and women project confidence and authority through their appearance and their clothing (12). Society tends to equate both beauty and productivity with youth (13), a factor contributing to the age discrimination faced by older individuals. This is especially relevant for women (13,14), because the "double standard of aging" (15) continues to be an important factor in the workplace. It has been observed, however, that an increasing number of men are also seeking a youthful appearance with the use of haircoloring, topical skin exfoliators, and cosmetic surgery (13). In contrast to older men, older women tend to face problems in the workplace to a greater degree and at an earlier age (4,13,16). In a study involving 8 women (ranging in age from the late 20s to the 60s) photographs "before" and "after" cosmetic makeovers were attached to resumés and submitted to personnel interviewers in 120 major private employment agencies and large corporations (4,12). The physical appearance of the applicant was observed to play an important role in the hiring process in all skill levels with greatest differences noted on jobs requiring the lowest skill level where a better appearance (i.e., associated with the photograph "after" the cosmetic makeover) yielded a 8–20% higher salary for the applicant.

AGING SKIN AND THE PSYCHOLOGICAL STATE

An aging appearance can have a significant psychological impact on the individual (4). Pearlman (17) describes a transitional developmental phase, sometimes reaching the proportions of a developmental crisis, that she has termed "late mid-life astonishment" (17). She describes a psychological reaction to a sudden awareness of the acceleration and stigmatization of aging which may manifest as amazement, despair, a disruption of one's sense of self or identity, feelings of heightened vulnerability, shame, depression, and severe loss of self-esteem (4,17). Other cofactors such as declining health and menopause can further lead to a sense of diminished physical and/or sexual attractiveness (4,17). Pearlman observes that in late mid-life it is no longer possible to "pass" as younger than one's chronological age, and this factor makes the psychological adjustment to aging more difficult (4). This may be one reason why studies involving treatment of photodamaged skin with topical tretinoin (8,10) and cosmetic makeovers to cover the cutaneous changes associated with aging (3,7), have been shown to be associated with an increased sense of well-being (3,7), increased ease during interpersonal interactions (3,7,8,10), and decreased anxiety (8,10).

Patients with severely narcissistic personalities may develop a major adjustment disorder in reaction to the cutaneous signs of aging (2,4). Among such narcissistic individuals who have a desperate need to be admired, having a youthful appearance is often a precondition for self-acceptance and trusting that they will be accepted by others and an aging appearance can result in a significant emotional crisis (2,4), including a severe depressive reaction. The incidence of some psychiatric emergencies such as suicide increases with age (18). Suicide rate peaks among men after age 45 years and among women after age 65 years (18). After age 75 years the suicide rate rises in both sexes (18), and older persons attempt suicide less often but are more successful in committing suicide (18). It is conceivable that some of the psychosocial reactions to aging appearance such as social isolation, decreased self-esteem, and depression also make some individuals more vulnerable to psychiatric emergencies such as suicide.

A psychological dimension that plays a critical role in the degree to which an individual is affected by cutaneous aging is the individual's internal locus of control or the degree to which an individual sees life's outcomes as being dependent upon his or her own abilities and efforts (4). It has been observed that patients who were concerned about their photodamaged skin and volunteered for studies (10) evaluating the efficacy of topical tretinoin also had obsessive-compulsive traits as measured by high Obsessive-Compulsiveness on the Brief Symptom Inventory (BSI) (9). Obsessive-compulsiveness is associated with perfectionistic personality traits, a tendency to be excessively self-critical, and an inordinate need to be in control of one's life (9). These personality traits probably predisposed these subjects to seek treatment for their wrinkles (10). After 24 weeks of therapy with topical tretinoin, the subjects reported a decrease in the Obsessive-Compulsiveness (BSI) scores, but those receiving the inactive vehicle reported an increase in this symptom dimension (10). These findings also suggest that external life events that adversely affect an individual's internal locus of control and make them feel more vulnerable may heighten their concern about their aging appearance and predispose them to seek treatment for their aging skin (2).

AGING SKIN AND BODY IMAGE

The impact of aging skin on body image, which is defined as the mental representation of the body and its organs, may generalize to concerns about overall body image not related directly to the skin (4). In a study of 71 men and 102 women who were all nonclinical subjects attending a shopping mall (19), it was observed that concerns about the effect of aging on the appearance correlated directly $(r = 0.4; p < 0.05)$ with the Drive for Thinness subscale of the Eating Disorder Inventory (EDI) (20) even after the possible effects of body mass index (weight in kilograms divided by height in square meters) and chronological age were partialed out statistically. This correlation was significant among both men and women. The Drive for Thinness subscale of the EDI measures an excessive preoccupation with dieting and exercise and an ardent desire to lose weight (20). Furthermore, among the women the belief that having young-looking skin is a prerequisite to good looks correlated directly with Drive for Thinness (EDI) (20) $(r = 0.3; p < 0.01)$ and Body Dissatisfaction (EDI) (20)

$(r = 0.4; p < 0.01)$ after the effects of age and body mass index were partialed out statistically. The Body Dissatisfaction subscale of the EDI (20) measures dissatisfaction with body shape and weight and measures the concern that certain body regions such as the abdomen, hips, and thighs are too fat. This finding was replicated among another randomly selected sample of nonclinical subjects (21). Furthermore, in a prospective, controlled study (21) of patients undergoing treatment for photodamaged skin with topical tretinoin or the inactive vehicle (the control group), it was observed that patients receiving the active treatment with topical tretinoin and not the control group reported a significant decline $(p < 0.01)$ in both Drive for Thinness (EDI) and Body Dissatisfaction (EDI) after 24 weeks (21). These findings highlight the significant impact of photodamaged skin on satisfaction with the overall body image, including aspects of body image not necessarily related to aging (2).

A youthful look is typically associated with a slim and well-toned physique, and some individuals may become obsessively preoccupied with diet and exercise as they develop the cutaneous stigmata of aging (2). In the small subgroup of individuals who have other risk factors for the development of an eating disorder, the fear of aging precipitated by the cutaneous changes of aging can culminate in anorexia nervosa (2,22). Eating disorders such as anorexia nervosa and bulimia nervosa are associated with distortion of body image perception, which mainly manifests as a fear of fatness and drive for thinness. In some eating-disordered patients the body image concerns generalize to other aspects of the appearance in addition to body weight, including concerns about the cutaneous body image. As a result, among some eating-disordered patients, concerns about cutaneous aging may be grossly inconsistent with the norms for their age group (23). In a study examining concerns about various aspects of skin appearance among 30-year-old eating-disordered patients $(n = 32)$ and randomly selected, age-matched nonclinical controls $(n = 34)$, it was observed that 81% of the eating-disordered patient sample versus 56% of the controls reported dissatisfaction with the appearance of their skin in the cross-sectional survey $(p = 0.03)$ (23). The cutaneous attributes of concern that were rated more frequently by the eating-disordered patients were those also associated with aging and photodamage, e.g., "darkness" under the eyes, freckles, fine wrinkles, and patchy hyperpigmentation, in addition to dryness and roughness of the skin (possible cutaneous features of eating disorders). One of the central psychological conflicts in eating disorders, which has a peak incidence during the teenage years, involves difficulties in dealing with the developmental tasks of adolescence and young adulthood, especially social tasks. The extreme starvation and secondary amenorrhea in anorexia nervosa is often an attempt to regress the pubertal or postpubertal body to a prepubertal stage. It is possible that greater concerns about aging skin in the eating-disordered sample is an index of the overall difficulties in coping with "growing up and growing old." Some patients with eating disorders may therefore present to the dermatologist with complaints about cutaneous stigmata of aging, and their concerns are likely to be grossly out of proportion to the objective clinical dermatological findings.

The cutaneous changes associated with aging can be minimized by avoiding photodamage. In an attempt to achieve a socially desirable body image consisting of a "healthy and tanned look," a significant minority of American youth between the ages of 11–18 years use indoor tanning sunlamps (24), thereby increasing the risk of photodamage. Among some of these teenagers the acute desire for approval by the peer group by projection of the tanned appearance overrides concerns about the long-term effects of photodamage, including premature aging of the skin.

SUMMARY

In contrast to most dermatological conditions, aging and/or photodamaged skin lies within the spectrum of normal human experience. Therefore, there is most likely a wide variation in the degree to which an individual will cutaneous aging to be a dermatological problem. In the process of promoting good skin care, the dermatologist should not place undue emphasis on some of the normal aspects of aging, which can further add to the negative view of aging that is already prevalent. Some of the major psychosocial factors that are associated with aging skin include the effect of an aging appearance upon interpersonal interactions, which can lead to social anxiety, social isolation, or a more serious emotional crisis in severely narcissistic individuals who have a desperate need to be admired and for whom having a youthful appearance is often a precondition for self-acceptance. Aging of the appearance can adversely affect the quality of life. Caregivers sometimes emotionally disengage from an individual who appears less attractive due to aging. This may adversely affect the quality of support and care the individual receives in the community. Older individuals, especially women, may face age-related discrimination in the workplace.

Excessive concerns about an aging appearance may be associated with body image disorders. Some individuals may engage in extreme dieting and/or exercise in an attempt to acquire a youthful, trim, and well-toned body. In some individuals, this can culminate in an eating disorder. Furthermore, eating-disordered patients who typically have difficulties coping with the tasks and changes associated with adulthood may become excessively preoccupied with cutaneous stigmata of aging that are grossly inconsistent with the clinical dermatological evaluation. Before treating such patients dermatologically, it is important to recognize that they have an underlying body image disorder and are likely to have unrealistic expectations of what treatment has to offer.

REFERENCES

1. Kligman AM. Psychological aspects of skin disorders in the elderly. Cutis 1989; 43:489–501.
2. Gupta MA. The aging face: a psychocutaneous perspective. Facial Plastic Surg 1995; 11:86–90.
3. Kligman AM, Graham JA. The psychology of appearance in the elderly. Dermatol Clin 1986; 4:501–507.
4. Gupta MA. Aging skin and quality of life. In: Rajagopalan R, Sheretz EF, Anderson RT, eds. Care Management of Skin Diseases: Life Quality and Economic Impact. New York: Marcel Dekker, 1998:245–251.
5. Hirshbein LD. Popular views of old age in America, 1900–1950. J Am Geriatr Soc 2001; 49:1555–1560.
6. Kligman AM, Koblenzer C. Demographics and psychological implications for the aging population. Dermatol Clin 1997; 15:549–553.
7. Graham JA, Kligman AM. Physical attractiveness, cosmetic use and self-perception in the elderly. Int J Cosmet Sci 1985; 7:85–97.
8. Gupta MA, Goldfarb MT, Schork NJ, Weiss JS, Gupta AK, Ellis CN, Voorhees JJ. Treatment of mildly to moderately photoaged skin with topical tretinoin has a favorable psychosocial effect: a prospective study. J Am Acad Dermatol 1991; 24:780–781.
9. Derogatis LR, Spencer PM. The Brief Symptom Inventory (BSI), Administration, Scoring and Procedures Manual—I. Baltimore: Clinical Psychometric Research, Johns Hopkins University 1982.
10. Gupta MA, Schork NJ, Ellis CN. Psychosocial correlates of the treatment of photodamaged skin with topical retinoic acid: a prospective controlled study. J Am Acad Dermatol 1994; 30:969–972.
11. Seeman T, Chen X. Risk and protective factors for physical functioning in older adults with and without chronic conditions: MacArthur Studies of Successful Aging. J Gerontol B Psychol Sci Soc Sci 2002; 57:S135–144.
12. Waters J. Cosmetics and the job market. In: Graham JA, Kligman AM, eds. The Psychology of Cosmetic Treatments. New York: Praeger, 1986:113–124.
13. Rodeheaver D. Labor market progeria. Gender & Aging, Generations 1990, Summer:53–58.
14. Banister EM. Women's midlife confusion: "Why am I feeling this way?" Issues Ment Health Nurs 2000; 21:745–764.
15. Sontag S. The double standard of aging. In: Williams J, ed. Psychology of Women. New York: Academic Press, 1979:462–478.

16. Hutchens RM. "Do job opportunities decline with age?" Ind Labor Relations Rev 1988; 42:89–99.

17. Pearlman SF. Late mid-life astonishment: disruptions to identity and self-esteem. Women Ther 1993; 14:1–12.

18. Sadock BJ, Sadock VA. Suicide, violence and other psychiatry emergencies. In: Kaplan & Sadock's Pocket Handbook of Clinical Psychiatry. 3rd ed. Philadelphia: Lippincott Williams & Wilkins; 261–274, 2001.

19. Gupta MA, Schork NJ. Aging-related concerns and body image: possible future implications for eating disorders. Int J Eating Disord 1993; 14:481–486.

20. Garner DM, Olmstead MP. Eating Disorder Inventory Manual. Lutz, FL: Psychological Assessment Resources, 1984.

21. Gupta MA. Concern about aging and a drive for thinness: a factor in the biopsychosocial model of eating disorders? Int J Eating Disord 1995; 18:351–357.

22. Gupta MA. Fear of aging: a precipitating factor in late onset anorexia nervosa. Int J Eating Disord 1990; 9:221–224.

23. Gupta MA, Gupta AK. Dissatisfaction with skin appearance among patients with eating disorders and non-clinical controls. Br J Dermatol 2001; 145:110–113.

24. Cokkinides VE, Weinstock MA, O'Connell MC, Thun MJ. Use of indoor tanning sunlamps by US youth, ages 11–18 years, and by their parent or guardian caregivers: prevalence and correlates. Pediatrics 2002; 109:1124–1130.

25

Skin Disease and Sexuality

Volker Niemeier and Uwe Gieler

Justus-Liebig University
Giessen, Germany

Well into the twentieth century, open discussions of sexuality were practically taboo. Opportunities to talk about sexuality with a doctor frequently arose only in connection with diseases that had a shameful character. The reprehensible character of venereal disease was automatically extended to sexuality. Recently, however, in addition to the pathological aspects, the physiological—and erotic—aspects of the skin have been examined and studied (1).

Beautiful skin is erotic and attractive and elicits a desire in the observer to touch it, while ugly skin often causes feelings of disgust, aversion, and repugnance (2). Skin is the organ that initiates sexual contact in erotic foreplay and, in touching and looking, contributes to stimulation and continuance of sexual desire (3).

From a psychoanalytical point of view, the skin—in addition to its many other functions—has the function of intersensorality, i.e., the interweaving of a wide variety of sensory impressions and the function of sexual excitability and of the libido. Nursing and feeding are associated with sensuous skin contact. Later, erogenous zones develop in the skin (1).

In addition to the nervous system and other sensory organs, the skin is the organ of communication between an individual and the environment. The first impressions created by a person's outward appearance are decisive for how that person is received by others (4).

Disorders of sexuality among the general population have not become less frequent, even since the "sexual liberation" of the 1970s. Although psychogenic sexual disorders are common among the general population (5), among sexual problems skin patients have rarely been systematically examined in the Anglo-American area. It has long been known that the estimation of the frequency of sexual disorders partly depends on the attitude of the treating physician. Doctors who initiate discussions of sexual problems with their patients estimate the percentage of patients with such disorders to be higher than doctors who never or only rarely ask about sexual complaints (6).

Fantasies about skin disease, shared by patients and onlookers alike, relate to guilt, control of bodily boundaries, and perfectionist yearnings. Some issues involved in these fantasies include distorted beliefs about contagion, dirt, and sexuality (7).

Bosse and Hünecke (8) used a questionnaire to ask 119 acne and 346 psoriasis patients about the everyday situations in which they fear psychosocial rejection from persons with healthy skin. They demonstrated that the fear exists particularly in the areas of "erotic-sexual rejection," "close living," "personal relationships," "café table contact," and "aesthetics." In addition, persons with healthy skin were asked about their difficulties in dealing with persons with skin diseases. The evaluation showed that the psychosocial rejection experienced subjectively by skin disease patients stems from those with healthy skin. With respect to everyday situations, only men with healthy skin saw no problem in the erotic-sexual area in dealing with women with diseased skin (8). Patients with serious acne should expect discrimination from their fellow workers. The skin-diseased person reacts to his environment with emotional inhibition, so that interpersonal communication is impaired by the skin disease (9–11).

The negative social impact of skin diseases is also expressed in the attitude of persons with healthy skin. Disgust is a frequent reaction to skin diseases. Hornstein et al. determined that two thirds of persons with healthy skin are reluctant to visit a dermatology clinic (12). Often, a parallel is drawn between skin diseases and venereal diseases. The cause of skin disease is frequently cited as "lack of hygiene" and "promiscuity." The danger of contagion, even just from shaking hands, was considered important by half of those questioned (12).

Early investigators addressed the interaction between skin disease, scratching, and sexuality. Stokes (13) saw the imperative urge to scratch as a masturbation equivalent in the framework of sexual conflicts, but this can be proven only in the context of depth-psychological heuristics in individual cases. In a study of patients with psychogenic pruritus, Musaph concluded that itching may be a sign of suppressed anxiety, rage, or sexual excitement (14).

In a study of 20 male patients with herpes genitalis recidivans, the investigators found that the emotional situation that preceded the onset or recurrence of the disease was characterized by two specific mechanisms: a physically or morally "impure" experience or a conscious or unconscious attempt to flee from sexual contact that was inwardly undesired or impermissible. Since the emotional factors cited are similar to those responsible for impotence, it is hypothesized that herpes genitalis recidivans, psychologically speaking, is a variant of impotence, having the somatic basis for a loss of sexual function (15).

Vulvar disorders (bacterial and fungal vulvitis, dermatitis, inflammatory dermatoses, secondary drug reactions, viral infections, vulvar tumors) can be extremely anxiety provoking, especially in adolescent females who are dealing with issues surrounding self-image, physical maturation, and sexuality (16).

In sexually transmitted infection, particularly in terms of teenage sexuality, physicians are often unaware of the limitations of the protection provided by condoms against sexually-transmitted infections. Condoms offer inadequate protection against three of the most common sexually transmitted infections: human papillomavirus, type 2 herpesvirus, and chlamydia (17). We mention in passing here the problems arising from HIV positivity and AIDS—various skin changes often accompany the start of the manifest disease. From an epidemiological perspective and in the context of developments in the medical treatment of AIDS, it is important to address the sexuality of HIV-infected people (18). Sex is different for seropositive persons than for people who are seronegative. Among seropositives, sex is also related to dilemmas involving disclosure of serostatus to potential sex partners and the motivation to protect one's partners as well as oneself against sexually transmitted disease (STD) and suprainfection.

Furthermore, having to cope with a serious disease induces negative mood states and may compromise sexual functioning. Other stigmatizing diseases often lead to pronounced impairment of sexuality, with pair conflicts not infrequently at the root (19). Burn patients, in particular, may later develop problematical sexual disorders (20). Koblenzer emphasized the consequences of aging, which also includes the area of sexuality (21).

Clinical experience shows that attention is usually paid to the sexual aspect of the skin only in venereal diseases or when the sexual organs themselves are involved. Even in such cases, medical interest is concentrated primarily on the skin lesions or infection pathways and less on the effects on the patient's sex life. In recent years, only a few studies have addressed the effects of chronic skin diseases on sexual behavior (22,23).

In order to determine the effect of chronic skin disorders on sexuality, a cross-sectional study was carried out in the Dermatological Outpatient Clinic of Leiden University Hospital. Fifty-two patients with psoriasis and 25 patients with atopic dermatitis filled out a questionnaire including items on sexual responsiveness and satisfaction. The response rate was 84%. One third of the patients, especially those with psoriasis, had problems with dating and starting sexual relationships and were embarrassed in these relationships. The sexual responsiveness of both male and female patients was below that of the normal population. Women appeared to have more problems in this area then men. Their sexual satisfaction was lower than in the average Dutch population, whereas in men this trend was found to be reversed. Sexual responsiveness did not correlate with the extent of the skin disease or location around genital areas, but was associated with self-esteem. Groups that are especially affected are females and young psoriatics who have their first sexual relationship (23).

According to Paulus, touching results in a loss of personal distance. The space surrounding the individual is experienced as a personal space, belonging to the individual (24). When this border is violated, the proximity of the other may appear threatening. In psychodynamic theory, it is assumed that atopic dermatitis (AD) and psoriasis vulgaris may also serve to create interpersonal distance towards others and thus unconsciously to avoid physical contact (25).

From psychosocial research it is well known that qualities like "friendly," "socially skilled," and "intelligent" are attributed more often to physically attractive strangers than to physically unattractive strangers (26). The importance of physical attractiveness to the exchange of physical contact was demonstrated in earlier studies (27). Subjects who considered themselves physically attractive received more attention than those who considered themselves normally or less attractive (27).

Niemeier et al. (22) investigated whether disfiguring skin diseases influence the sex life of the patient as well as which aspects of sex life are altered compared to patients with healthy skins. Patients with psoriasis vulgaris and AD were enrolled, since both diseases are characterized by frequently generalized and disfiguring symptoms and are among the most frequent skin diseases confronted by dermatologists.

Fifty-three patients with psoriasis, 24 patients with AD, and 52 controls with healthy skin were compared with regard to their sexual behavior. Questionnaires on sexuality and partnership were used. Patients with skin diseases had significantly impaired sex lives compared to those with healthy skin. There was a highly significant reduction in the exchange of tenderness in patients of both sexes and in the capacity for orgasm in female patients. On the other hand, no significant difference was found in the frequency of intercourse. Patients with psoriasis felt more impaired than those with AD. Ninety-three percent of psoriatics and 96% of patients with AD had not been asked about their sexual life by their attending doctor. These results indicate that the disfiguring skin disease is associated with avoidance of body contact. The reason why the psoriasis patients examined showed a greater deficit in the exchange of caresses than the AD patients can be attributed to the more disfiguring, more stigmatizing symptoms of psoriasis. Patients with AD suffer more and have greater emotional stress than psoriasis patients, but patients with psoriasis still feel more stigmatized (28).

It was demonstrated with respect to inhibitedness versus uninhibitedness in sexual contact that psoriasis patients view themselves as significantly more inhibited than control persons, possibly as a result of the serious disfiguring aspects, while there were no statistically significant differences between control persons and patients with AD.

It is remarkable that there is no difference in coitus frequency between the test groups. Apparently there is only slight limitation at the level of pure drive satisfaction, since there is also no significant difference in the three groups with respect to age at first sexual intercourse. Three fourths of the patients also deny that they have less frequent intercourse because of their skin disease. Persons with skin diseases may attempt to compensate for their lack of physical contact on a genital-sexual level. Desire for skin contact and caresses may at the same time be experienced as threatening, as endangering the personal boundaries and may possibly be sexualized as a result and satisfied at a genital-sexual level (29). How coitus is experienced by those afflicted, whether it is desired or whether it is seen as "fulfillment of duty" in the sense of a purely mechanical sexuality, cannot be answered based on the questionnaires used.

There was no evidence of a reduction in the quality of genital sexuality in the replies to the question concerning the frequency of orgasm. While orgasm capability was not reported as reduced in skin-diseased men, skin-diseased women reported that they experience significantly fewer orgasms during intercourse than women with healthy skin. The difference between men and women may be explained by the greater susceptibility to disruption in female orgasm. While impaired excitability and orgasm are in the forefront of functional sexual disorders among women, the men complain predominantly of problems with erection (30). Stigmatization may partly explain why women with skin diseases have fewer orgasms. In addition, there is a deflation of the erotic stimulating self-image, which contributes to difficulties with continuance of desire during sexual intercourse (31).

Feeling stigmatized is a central experience of patients with AD and psoriasis. This was estimated using the Questionnaire on Experience with Skin Complaints (QES) in three groups of patients: 76 with AD and 81 and 217 with psoriasis. The comparison of subgroups with different affected regions revealed that the genital region is especially relevant for the stigmatization experience in these patients (32).

Since 93% of psoriasis patients and 96% of patients with AD had obviously never been asked about their sexuality by their personal physicians, disorders in this area and secondary effects of the disease may also not have been recognized (22). Despite the problems in addressing this intimate area, the specialist in skin and venereal diseases should be a competent discussion partner for questions about the disease and its consequences for the patient's sex life. It is essential to develop a trusting relationship between the doctor and the patient. Usually a doctor's question about sexuality is the first approach to such a discussion. If sexual difficulties are reported, it is important that they be taken seriously. It is helpful to ask concrete questions: "I can imagine that your skin disease also affects your sex life?" or "Perhaps you would like to tell me when you last slept together, what was good about it and when did the problems arise?" Open and unemotional language, clear and down to earth, has been found useful. For the patient, encouraging nonverbal signals from the doctor (facial expressions, gestures, eye contact) are also helpful. Frequently, the topic of sexuality is burdened with shame (33). It may be necessary to address the patient's feeling of embarrassment. It is helpful when the doctor can talk about sexual matters without prejudice. After a confidential discussion, the doctor should decide whether referral to a sexual therapist or andrologist is indicated.

Annon (34) has devised a graded consultation model for patients with sexual disorders from a behavior-therapeutic approach: the PLISSIT Model (Permission–Limited Information–Specific Suggestions–Intensive Therapy). This is a graded model that may be applied in the psychosomatic care of patients with sexual disorders as well as in other areas. Depending on the (psycho) therapy motivation and introspection capability of the patient and the doctor's assessment of the need for additional psychosocial care, the patient is treated with adjuvant psychosocial interventions at various intensity levels. It is often sufficient to let the patient know that the doctor understands the patient's difficulties (permission). Depending on the assessment, a more intensive therapy can be offered gradually up to referral to a psychotherapist or sexual therapist (intensive therapy).

REFERENCES

1. Anzieu D. Le Penser. Du Moi-peau au Moi-pensant. Paris: Dunod, 1994.
2. Pasini W. Sexologic problems in dermatology. Clin Dermatol 2:59–65, 1984.
3. Musaph H. Skin, touch and sex. In: Money J and Musaph H, eds. Handbook of Sexology. Elsevier-North Holland Biomedical Press, 1157–1165, 1977.
4. Jürgens H. Der Mensch und seine Umwelt. Die menschliche Körperform im sozialen Umfeld. Ärztl Kosmetol 8:61–75, 1978.
5. Spector JP, Carrey MP. Incidence and prevalence of the sexual dysfunctions: a critical review of the empirical literature. Arch Sex Behav 19:389–408, 1990.
6. Pacharzina K. Der Arzt und die Sexualität seines Patienten. Ergebnisse einer Studie an 100 Ärzten für Allgemeinmedizin. In: V Sigusch, ed. Sexualität und medizin. Kiepenheuer and Witsch: Köhr, 17–40, 1979.
7. Ginsburg IH. The psychosocial impact of skin disease. An overview. Dermatol Clin 14(3):473–484, 1996.
8. Bosse K, Hünecke P. Psychodynamik und Soziodynamik bei Hautkranken. Göttingen: Verlag Vandenhoek & Ruprecht, 1976.
9. Gloor M, Eichler C, Wiebelt H, Moser G. Soziologische Untersuchung bei der Acne vulgaris. Z Hautkr 53(23):871–880, 1979.
10. Koo J. The psychosocial impact of acne: patients' perceptions. J Am Acad Dermatol 32(5 pt 3):S26–30, 1995.
11. Niemeier V, Kupfer J, Demmelbauer-Ebner M, Stangier U, Effendy I, Gieler U. Coping with acne vulgaris. Dermatology 196: 108–115, 1998.
12. Hornstein O, Brückner G, Graf U. Über die soziale Bewertung von Hautkrankheiten in der Bevölkerung. Methodik und Ergebnisse einer orientierenden Befragung. Hautarzt 24:230–235, 1973.
13. Stokes JH. The effect on the skin of emotional and nervous states. Arch Dermatol 22:803–810, 1930.
14. Musaph H. Psychodynamics in itching states. Int J Psycho-Anal 49:336–339, 1968.
15. Dimitrov CT. Psychische Faktoren bei Herpes Simplex Recidivans Genitalis. Z Psychosom Mcd Psychoanal 19(3):279 287, 1973.
16. Fivozinsky KB, Laufer MR. Vulvar disorders in adolescents. Adolesc Med 10(2):305–319, 1999.
17. McIlhaney JS Jr. Sexually transmitted infection and teenage sexuality. Am J Obset Gynecol 183(2): 334–339, 2000.
18. Schiltz MA, Sandfort TG. HIV-positive people, risk and sexual behaviour. Soc Sci Med 50 (11): 1571–1588, 2000.
19. Niemeier V, Mayser P, Weyers W, Schill WB. Lepromatöse Lepra. Therapiemöglichkeiten bei Glucose-6-Phosphat-Dehydrogenasemangel [Lepro-

matous Leprosy—Therapeutic Possibilities in Patients with Glucose-6-Phosphate-Dehydrogenase Deficiency]. Z Hautkr 71(6): 625–629 1996.
20. Bogaerts F, Boeckx W. Burns and sexuality. J Burn Care Rehabil 13(1):39–43 1992.
21. Koblenzer CS. Psychologic aspects of aging and the skin. Clin Dermatol 14(2):171–177, 1996.
22. Niemeier V, Winkelsesser T, Gieler U. Hautkrankheit und Sexualität [Skin disease and sexuality. An empirical study of sex behavior on patients with psoriasis vulgaris and neurodermatitis in comparison with skin-healthy probands]. Hautarzt 48:629–633, 1997.
23. van Dorssen IE, Boom BW, Hengeveld MW. Experience of sexuality with psoriasis and constitutional eczema. Ned Tijdschr Geneeskd 136 (44):2175–2178, 1992.
24. Paulus P. Zur Erfahrung des eigenen Körpers Weinheim: Beltzverlag, 1982.
25. Gieler U, Detig-Kohler C. Nähe und Distanz bei Hautkranken. Psychotherapeut 39:1–5, 1994.
26. Feingold A. Good-looking people are not what we think. Psychol Bull 111:304–341, 1992.
27. Jourard S. An exploratory study of body accessibility. Br J Soc Clin Psychol 5:221–231, 1966.
28. Gieler U, Stangier U, Ehlers A. Der Marburger Neurodermitisfragebogen. In: Gieler U, Stangier U, Brähler E, eds. Jahrbuch der medizinischen Psychologie. Götlinger: Hogrefe Verlag für Psychologie, 115–134, 1992.
29. Pfitzner R. Die Psychodynamik der Psoriasis vulgaris im Rorschach-Test. Z Psychosom Med Psychoanal 22(2):190–197, 1977.
30. Bräutigam W, Clement U. Sexualmedizin im Grundriß. Stuttgart: Thieme Verlag, 1989.
31. Martini M, Cossidente C, Giorgini S, Melli MC, Sarti MG, Panconesi E. Haut, Kosmetik und Sexualität. Dynam Psychiatry 20:201–216, 1987.
32. Schmid-Ott G, Kuensebeck HW, Jaeger B, Werfel T, Frahm K, Ruitman J, Kapp A, Lamprecht F. Validity study for the stigmatization experience in atopic dermatitis and psoriatic patients. Acta Derm Venereol 79(6):443–447, 1999.
33. Wurmser L. The mask of shame [Die Maske der Scham]. Berlin; Heidelberg, NY: Springer, 1997.
34. Annon JS. The Behavioral Treatment of Sexual Problems. Vol. 1: Brief Therapy. Honolulu: Enabling Systems, 1974.

26

Psychiatric Issues in Cutaneous Surgery

Ernest Lee and John Y. M. Koo
University of California, San Francisco
San Francisco, California, U.S.A.

INTRODUCTION

The expansion of dermatology over the past decade has in large part been spearheaded by the growth in demand for cutaneous surgery. The growth of cutaneous surgery, specifically cosmetic surgery, likewise has been driven by society's greater emphasis on youthfulness, physical fitness, and acceptable standards of physical appearance (1). This recent explosion in the demand for aesthetic surgery has increased the importance of recognizing psychiatric issues that may present to the dermatologist.

When a cosmetic surgical procedure is performed, there are at least four possible scenarios, of which three are undesirable. The first situation involves the patient who is satisfied with the results. That patient obviously needs only routine follow-up. The second scenario is the unhappy patient who requests and obtains additional unnecessary procedures. Third, the patient sues the physician, claiming that the surgeon should have identified that this procedure was unnecessary and known that the operation should not have been performed (2). Lastly, in very rare instances completion of the surgery can precipitate psychosis. For example, a patient who has rhinoplasty performed may actually be "screening" and suppressing their psychiatric illness from the conscious awareness by focusing on their bodily defect. Once the procedure is finished, the patient no longer has a cosmetic issue to focus on and their psychosis overwhelms this mode of "coping." To avoid these pitfalls, it is necessary for the cutaneous surgeon to have some understanding of psychosurgical issues.

How can the dermatological/cosmetic surgeon identify the patient who is not a suitable candidate for surgery or at least not the surgery that the patient requests? Some of the characteristics of such patients include:

1. Complaints out of proportion to the actual physical defect
2. Idealization/devaluation/splitting of medical personnel suggestive of borderline personality disorder
3. Delusional thinking characteristic of some psychotic disorder
4. Signs and symptoms of depression (e.g., tearfulness, insomnia, decreased appetite, significant weight loss) where the patient may be "somatizing" his or her depression onto a cosmetic complaint
5. Signs and symptoms of anxiety
6. Multiple somatic complaints suggestive of somatization disorder

Once such a "problem" patient is identified, how does one broach this topic with the patient? Should the dermatological surgeon approach the issue with the patient, or is it better to refer to psychiatry or neurology? Is there any role for psychiatric medications? How does the physician work with psychiatrists or other mental health professionals regarding these cases? These are some of the questions this chapter will address in order to provide a framework of management for the cutaneous surgeon.

PSYCHIATRIC ISSUES

There are three critical psychiatric issues in the management of cutaneous surgery patients (3). The first situation involves the patient who has an alleged cosmetic defect that is nonexistent or minimal but who demands a cosmetic surgical procedure. The second scenario deals with a patient who experiences significant psychological problems because of disfigurement resulting from surgery. Such an instance would most likely occur in extensive cutaneous procedures such as the removal of a large neoplasm. The third arises when the patient has no desire to undergo the procedure for which he or she has been referred. This chapter will focus on these three scenarios, with an emphasis on understanding their psychiatric differential diagnosis and management, along with suggestions on how to best interact with these patients.

Patients Who Exaggerate Their Cosmetic Defects

When encountering a patient who demands a surgical procedure for the correction of a "cosmetic defect" that is minimal or nonexistent, the first step in managing such a case involves making an attempt to understand the nature of the underlying psychopathology. At least 10 disorders are seen among patients with psychiatric conditions that create an exaggerated perception of an alleged cosmetic defect (Table 1). Of these, 5 are most commonly encountered: monosymptomatic hypochondriacal psychosis (MHP), body dysmorphic disorder (BDD), somatization of depression, chronic anxiety disorder, and borderline personality disorder (BDD).

Monosymptomatic Hypochondriacal Psychosis

MHP refers to a group of disorders characterized by an encapsulated delusional belief system that is hypochondriacal (Table 2) (4). A delusional disorder is characterized by a false idea that is rigidly held by the individual but not shared by other people in the same cultural or social group. MHP is frequently a chronic condition but is easily distinguished from other forms of chronic psychosis, like schizophrenia, by its encapsulated nature. These patients may appear normal except when expressing concern about the hypochondriacal delusional idea. This is in contrast to schizophrenics, who develop other symptoms such as hallucinations, flat or inappropriate affect, deterioration in interpersonal relationships, grossly disorganized or catatonic behavior, and disorganized speech in addition to a delusional belief system (5).

TABLE 1   Common Psychiatric Conditions That Predispose Patients to Have An Exaggerated Perception of Cosmetic Deficiencies

Bipolar disorder
Body dysmorphic disorder
Borderline personality disorder
Chronic anxiety disorder
Dysmorphophobia
Gender identity disorder
Major depression with somatization
Monosymptomatic hypochondriacal psychosis
Schizoaffective disorder
Schizophrenia

TABLE 2   Features of Monosymptomatic Hypochondriacal Psychosis

Chronic in nature
Encapsulated delusional belief system
Hypochondriacal complaints
Patient is not grossly pathological in other respects

One type of MHP is dysmorphophobia, a condition in which the patient is occupied with an imaginary or exaggerated cosmetic defect (6). However, concern has been raised that this term is actually a misnomer for a large proportion of the patients who present with such a complaint that is actually delusional (7), not phobic. In phobias, patients usually recognize that their fear is irrational or exaggerated. However, in delusions, patients truly believe in their distorted perception and exhibit little insight into their problem. Since most of these patients truly believe in the unsightly nature of their physical appearance, the preferred term for this subset of delusional patients is "delusions of dysmorphosis."

The term MHP is most often used in Europe. In American psychiatric nosology, this group of disorders can be classified under delusional disorder, somatic subtype (8). In general dermatology, the other subsets of MHP include "delusions of bromosis" and "delusions of parasitosis." In delusions of bromosis, patients falsely believe they are emitting a bad odor that offends people and drives them away. In a cutaneous surgery practice, however, delusional concerns regarding the cosmetic appearance typically predominate (9). The management of "delusions of dysmorphosis" is discussed later.

Body Dysmorphic Disorder

In BDD, the patient has a preoccupation with an imagined defect in appearance. If a slight physical anomaly is present, the person's concern is grossly excessive. The preoccupation tends to cause clinically significant distress or impairment in social, occupational, or other important areas of functioning (10).

Distinction Between MHP and BDD

One may notice the similarity in definition between MHP and BDD. In fact, in the European literature, body dysmorphic disorder is synonymous with "dysmorphophobia," so it is important to distinguish between this condition and delusions of dysmorphosis (11). Much of the literature on this subject does not make a clear distinction between the two entities. BDD is a condition where the feeling of being deformed is an overvalued idea, whereas "delusions of dysmorphosis" is an isolated belief reaching delusional intensity. One can think of the entities as dysmorphic neuroses versus dysmorphic delusions (12). Although it may be difficult for even the most astute clinician to determine the delusional intensity of a belief in the dermatological setting (13), the distinction between overvalued idea and delusion is important both theoretically and because of treatment implications (14). For example, as will be discussed in more detail in the management section of this chapter, pimozide is effective for MHP but may not be the first-line agent for neurotically based dysmorphophobias where selective serotonin reuptake inhibitors (SSRIs) may be preferred.

By definition, patients cannot be persuaded away from their delusions, and the dermatologist will find that delusional patients insist on the presence of their deformity without possibility of rational discussion. BDD can be distinguished from MHP because the patient can acknowledge the possibility that the complaint may be exaggerated or that there may be no defect at all. In other words, the patient's belief system is not of delusional intensity. With their insight relatively retained, these patients may be reassured that their concerns are exaggerated and that surgical correction is neither advisable nor necessary.

Somatization of Depression

When suffering from major depressive episodes, patients may develop exaggerated physical complaints. This phenomenon is called somatization of depression (15). In this situation, the depressed patient comes to the physician with an exaggerated physical complaint without recognizing its relationship to the underlying depression. To make this diagnosis, it must be clear that the patient is suffering from a major depressive episode (16). The symptoms of a major depressive episode are listed in Table 3. Of course, not every patient will exhibit all of these psychological symptoms and physiological signs. Moreover, some patients may consciously or unconsciously deny some of the subjective symptoms, such as depressed mood. However, the diagnosis of major depression can be postulated if enough (five or more of nine over a 2-week period) symptoms and signs of depression can be detected during the evaluation. The management of depression is discussed in a later section of this chapter.

TABLE 3 Major Depressive Symptoms

Depressed mood
Markedly diminished interest or pleasure in activities
Significant weight loss when not dieting or weight gain or decrease or increase in appetite
Insomnia or hypersomnia
Psychomotor agitation or retardation
Fatigue or loss of energy
Feelings of worthlessness or excessive or inappropriate guilt
Diminished ability to think or concentrate
Recurrent thoughts of death, recurrent suicidal ideation, or suicide attempt

A diagnosis of major depressive episode can be made when five (or more) of the above symptoms have been present during the same 2-week period and represent a change from previous functioning; at least one of the symptoms is either 1) depressed mood or 2) loss of interest or pleasure.

Anxiety Disorder

Patients with chronic anxiety disorder frequently experience many physical complaints (Table 4) (17). These complaints can be either purely psychiatric or psychophysiological in nature. When the physical complaints merely represent a psychological fixation on the part of the anxious patient, there is no demonstrable physiological abnormality. In contrast, psychophysiological disturbances such as psoriasis or atopic dermatitis are exemplified by the presence of real physiological pathology that is exacerbated by anxiety. It has been speculated that patients experiencing chronic recurrent anxiety find the anxiety most unbearable when it is "free floating" and undefined in character. One way to make this amorphous anxiety more psychologically manageable is to "fixate" the anxiety into some concrete, visible physical complaint, including cosmetic complaints.

The physician should question these patients regarding any symptoms of generalized anxiety disorder to try to confirm or rule out the diagnosis of underlying anxiety disorder. As in the case of depression, the manifestations of underlying anxiety disorder can be either physiological or subjective. Frequently, there are both physiological and subjective signs and symptoms of anxiety disorders. Subjective symptoms of anxiety are manifested by a recurrent and chronic worry that is often excessive or unrealistic in nature. The physiological manifestations of anxiety may include motor tension such as trembling, twitching, muscle tension, restlessness, and a feeling of shakiness. Alternatively, hyperactivity of the autonomic nervous system may be observed. This consists of dyspnea, tachycardia, palpitations,

TABLE 4   Physiological Manifestations of Anxiety Disorders

Restlessness or feeling keyed up or on edge
Being easily fatigued
Difficulty concentrating or mind going blank
Irritability
Muscle tension
Sleep disturbance (difficulty falling or staying asleep, or restless unsatisfying
   sleep)
Trembling
Twitching
Feeling shaky
Aches/soreness
Cold, clammy hands
Dry mouth
Sweating
Nausea or diarrhea
Urinary frequency
Trouble swallowing or a "lump in the throat"
Exaggerated startle response

The diagnosis of generalized anxiety disorder can be made when anxiety and worry are associated with three or more of the first six listed symptoms, with at least some symptoms present for more days than not for the past 6 months.

sweating, clammy hands, dry mouth, dizziness, nausea, diarrhea, hot flashes, frequent urination, and trouble in swallowing. At times, the patient may also experience hyperreactivity (e.g., an exaggerated irritability or startle response). The physician can be quite confident that an underlying anxiety disorder is present if enough symptoms and signs are present (anxiety and worry associated with three or more of the first six symptoms listed in Table 4). The management of anxiety disorder is discussed later.

Borderline Personality Disorder

BPD is a commonly encountered chronic personality disturbance that most frequently affects young women (Table 5) (18). One of the central deficits in this disorder is a sense of identity that is poorly defined, precarious, and unstable in nature. The psychic manifestations can include chronic feelings of emptiness and boredom, impulsiveness, intense or inappropriate feelings of anger, and instability of affect. The patient may shift quickly from baseline mood to anxiety, depression, or irritability. This vague sense of self may lead to a pattern of intense and unstable interpersonal relationships

TABLE 5   Features of Borderline Personality Disorder

Most frequently affects young women
Unstable and intense interpersonal relationships
Instability of affect
Instability of self-image
Marked impulsivity beginning in early adulthood and present in a variety of
    contexts (spending, sex, substance abuse, reckless driving, binge eating)
Frantic efforts to avoid real or imagined abandonment
Extremes of idealization and devaluation
Recurrent suicidal behavior, gestures, or threats, or self-mutilating behavior
Marked reactivity of mood
Chronic feelings of emptiness
Inappropriate, intense anger, or difficulty controlling anger
Transient, stress-related paranoid ideation or severe dissociative symptoms

characterized by alternating extremes of idealization and devaluation of the people with whom emotional attachments have been made.

These patients also frequently experience difficulties with regard to body image. In this context, body image refers to patients' psychological and mental representation of their body. The patient's body image is known to diverge from their actual physical appearance in several psychiatric disorders (e.g., anorexia nervosa, bulimia). For example, anorectic patients typically engage in extreme forms of exercise and diet to lose weight, even though they are already emaciated (19–21). In their body image they see themselves as obese. In borderline personality disorder, there are also distortions of body image. In a study among 48 women in a psychiatric outpatient setting (22), the association between borderline personality and body image was examined. Using the borderline personality scale of the Personality Diagnostic Questionnaire-Revised (PDQ-R) (23), scores were significantly related to self-rated bodily attractiveness ($p < 0.05$), self-rated facial attractiveness ($p < 0.05$), and social avoidance due to body image concerns ($p < 0.05$) even after controlling for body mass index (BMI). These patients may try to define their amorphous sense of self by externalizing their core psychological problems and working on altering their physical appearance instead.

Patients with BPD can be classified into those with a low psychosocial functional level and those with a high psychosocial functional level. Low-functioning patients may chronically engage in promiscuous sex, chaotic relationships, binge eating, reckless spending, repeated suicidal gestures, or other self-mutilating behaviors. High-functioning patients may appear fairly normal, except for a pattern of intense and unstable interpersonal relationships, chronic feeling of emptiness, uncertainty regarding self-esteem and self-image, ill-defined long-term goals, and unstable or undefined preferred personal values where their values may be easily defined by the values of significant others. With experience, it is not difficult to identify patients with BPD by merely observing the way they look at or talk to the physician. They typically have an intense look, with a touch of adoration, and the content of their verbal expression idealizes the physician. BPD is most frequently seen in young women, and consequently male physicians are often the focus of attention of these patients. Needless to say, surgical correction of the imaginary or exaggerated cosmetic defects cannot repair their chronic sense of defective identity.

Alternative Psychiatric Diagnoses

Even though many patients with exaggerated complaints regarding real or imaginary cosmetic defects fall into one of the five psychiatric diagnoses previously described, other patients may fall into some other psychiatric diagnostic category, such as narcissistic personality disorder, schizophrenia, schizoaffective disorder, bipolar disorder, or gender identity disorder.

Narcissistic Personality Disorder

Narcissistic personality disorder is characterized by a pervasive pattern of grandiosity (in fantasy or behavior), need for admiration, and lack of empathy, beginning by early adulthood and present in a variety of contexts (24). This condition has been reported to be common in patients seeking cosmetic surgery (25). It would not be surprising that in attempting to achieve greater admiration for oneself, a patient may develop an exaggerated perception of a physical defect in her tireless effort to make herself even more "beautiful" and "superior."

Schizophrenia

In schizophrenia, it is not unusual for patients to develop bizarre delusions concerning their physical appearance. However, it is relatively easy to diagnose schizophrenic patients because of their multiple florid psychological impairments, including marked social or occupational dysfunction, hallucinations, affective flattening, alogia (restrictions in the fluency and productivity of thought and speech), avolition (restrictions in the initiation of goal-directed behavior), bizarre delusional belief system, and failure to establish interpersonal rapport with the physician (26). Therefore, request for inappropriate cosmetic procedures by schizophrenic patients is probably easiest for dermatological surgeons to identify and deny.

Schizoaffective Disorder

The essential feature of schizoaffective disorder is an uninterrupted period of illness during which, at some time, there is a major depressive, manic, or mixed episode concurrent with symptoms of schizophrenia (27). During that same period of illness, there have been delusions or hallucinations for at least 2 weeks in the absence of prominent mood symptoms. Also, the symptoms that meet criteria for a mood episode are present for a substantial portion of the total duration of the active and residual periods of the illness, and the disturbance is not due to a substance or medical condition. This disorder is relevant because during episodes with depression as a major component, patients may somatize depression in the form of an exaggerated physical defect.

Bipolar Disorder

Bipolar disorder is divided into two types: bipolar I disorder consisting of depression and mania, and bipolar II disorder consisting of depression and hypomania. The diagnosis can usually be established by asking the patient questions about experiencing symptoms that are the opposite of depression, i.e., mania or hypomania. These symptoms include grandiosity, inflated self-esteem, flight of ideas, racing thoughts, exaggerated self-confidence, psychomotor agitation, distractibility, pressured speech, sexual indiscretion, spending sprees, or involvement in unrealistic business ventures (28). This disorder is included for the same reason that schizoaffective disorders are discussed. During the episodes of depression, the patient may develop somatization of their disorder.

Gender Identity Disorder

Patients who suffer from gender identity disorder have a strong and persistent cross-gender identification (note merely a desire for any perceived cultural advantages of being the other sex) (29). In adolescents and adults, the disturbance is manifested by symptoms such as a stated desire to be the other sex, frequent passing as the other sex, desire to live or be treated as the other sex, or the conviction that he or she had the typical feelings and reactions of the other sex. These patients may request a variety of cosmetic surgical procedures. However, the underlying diagnosis becomes apparent when the nature of gender confusion is recognized as being "generalized," and the patient's request is only one small manifestation of this underlying confusion.

Is Psychopathology More Prevalent in Cosmetic Surgery Patients?

In a study by Vargel and Ulusahin (30), 20 cosmetic surgery patients and 20 control patients were evaluated for the presence of psychopathology. The control patients underwent minor noncosmetic surgical procedures to control for the possible psychological effects of the operation itself. Symptom Check List-90 Revised (SCL-90-R), Beck Depression Inventory (BDI), and the Multi-Dimensional Body Self Relations Questionnaire (MBSRQ) were administered to both groups. The SCL-90-R is a self-report checklist developed by Derogatis (31) as a screening test for psychiatric symptoms in outpatients, the BDI is a well-validated self-report inventory, and the MBSRQ is an instrument developed by Cash et al. (32) to evaluate the perceptual, behavioral, and attitudinal aspects of body image. The General Symptom Index (GSI) of the cosmetic operation candidates was higher than that of the control group, though the difference was not significant. Fifty percent of the cosmetic group and 40% of the control group GSI scores were over 1, indicating the presence of psychopathology. The mean GSI of the cosmetic group was also over 1, whereas the control group's mean GSI score was 0.89.

The mean BDI score of the cosmetic group was higher than that of the control group, but not at a statistically significant level. The depression rate according to BDI scores, on the other hand, was higher in the general surgery patients (50%) than in the cosmetic patients (35%), but again this difference was not statistically significant. Moderate depression (BDI = 13–24) was present in five (25%) of the cosmetic patients and 10 (50%) of the control group. Two subjects from the cosmetic group had severe depression (BDI scores 33 and 35). The BDI scores of these two subjects increased the mean of the cosmetic group's BDI score.

Neither MBSRQ total nor subscale average scores differed significantly between cosmetic and control groups. According to the body areas satisfaction subscale, 55% of the cosmetic and 50% of the control group were happy with their faces. Twenty-five percent of the cosmetic and 65% of the control group were happy with their body weights. Thirty percent of the cosmetic group were unhappy with their appearance, whereas none of the control group felt so. Feelings about other body parts did not vary between the two study groups. Of note, 4 (20%) of the cosmetic patients were diagnosed with body dysmorphic disorder.

In another recent study of cosmetic surgery patients, 103 patients from three hospitals in the Paris area were examined for depression, anxiety, and quality of life (QOL) (33). Evaluation was performed using a structured interview and three assessment scales: the MADRS (Montgomery and Asberg Depression Rating Scale), the SISST (Social Interaction Self Statement Test), and the EQ-5D (EuroQol), which measures quality of life. The MADRS index was higher in the cosmetic surgery group than in the control group ($p < 0.001$), signifying a greater degree of depression with 20% of cosmetic surgery patients having depression. From the SISST, the social anxiety of cosmetic patients was greater than that of the control group ($p < 0.001$), but more in regards to fear of speaking in public rather than a fear of social interaction. The EQ-5D visual analogue scale average was 77.39%, indicating that there was no significant difference between the two groups, but the descriptive EQ-5D revealed an overrepresentation of the anxiety/depression category ($p < 0.01$) in the cosmetic group. In addition, from the structured interview it was shown that 50% (52/103) of the cosmetic surgery patients had already been treated with psychotropic medications, of which 27% were an antidepressant.

In a recent study of psychiatric morbidity in cosmetic surgery candidates, 84 plastic surgery patients in western Australia were evaluated (34). Half were requesting surgery for cosmetic reasons, while the other half acted as controls (referrals to this clinic for medically oriented symptoms). Patients were administered the dysmorphic concern questionnaire (DCQ) and the General Health Questionnaire (GHQ). The DCQ is a self-report questionnaire validated as a reliable diagnostic instrument for BDD (35), while the GHQ is a 12-item measure of psychiatric symptoms (36). Patients presenting for cosmetic reasons were 13 times more likely to be female (95% CI 4.3–41), nine times more likely to have high DCQ scores (95% CI 3.3–24), and six times more likely to be GHQ cases (patients with some degree of psychiatric morbidity) (95% CI 2.1–17). In total, these results suggest that patients who present for cosmetic surgery have higher rates of dysmorphic concern and psychiatric morbidity than patients presenting for plastic surgery with medical justifications.

MANAGEMENT

General Concepts

Ideally, patients with psychopathology could simply be referred to a mental health professional. In reality, many of these patients refuse to recognize the psychological nature of their condition or refuse a referral to a mental health professional, even if they recognize their psychiatric disturbance. Thus, it is useful for the dermatological surgeon to have some knowledge about how to manage these patients and the forms of treatment available. The expectation is not that the dermatological surgeon will take total responsibility for treatment of the psychiatric disorder, but that he or she will recognize that even partial treatment may benefit the patient who might otherwise go untreated. Before discussing how to treat these psychiatric diseases, a framework for how to evaluate these patients is provided.

Approach to the Patient with an Exaggerated Cosmetic Concern

Philips suggested five useful questions to evaluate patients with body dysmorphic disorder (37). These can be used with any patient that has an exaggerated cosmetic concerns:

1. Do you worry about the appearance of your face or body?
2. If so, what is your concern? How bad do you think your face or body part appears?
3. How much time do you spend worrying about the appearance of your face or body part?
4. Have you done anything to hide the problem or rid yourself of the problem?
5. Does this concern with your appearance affect any aspect of your life (e.g., school, job, or social life)?

If in asking these questions, an underlying psychopathology is suspected, referral to a psychiatrist would be most helpful. As these patients may be reluctant to see a mental health professional, the referral can be explained to the patient as potentially beneficial in the following ways: 1) the symptoms of emotional distress can be treated, 2) the patient receives psychological help in adapting to a physical feature that is a particular problem for the patient, and 3) the patient will have a higher level of psychological support.

In the end, the decision as to whether or not to proceed with the cosmetic procedure lies with the dermatologist. The evaluation to obtain an answer to this question should include the following questions (38):

1. Who is our patient, and what are his or her personality traits, likes, and dislikes?
2. What are his or her goals for surgery, and can we accomplish these goals safely?

3. When is the best time to perform the surgery? Is he or she experiencing problems that might make surgery a bad option at this time?
4. Why does the patient want this procedure, and does he or she have realistic expectations and understand the limitations of the surgery?

If the dermatologist feels comfortable with the answers given to these questions, a satisfactory result is the most probable outcome.

Monosymptomatic Hypochondriacal Psychosis

By definition, patients with delusional beliefs cannot be persuaded to give up their delusions. In these cases, reassurances and explanations are unlikely to be adequate. The treatment of choice for encapsulated delusional disorders may be pimozide (Orap) (39), a diphenylbutylpiperidine derivative and the most potent oral antipsychotic medication available in the United States. Because of this potency, treatment with pimozide should be started at a lower dosage than other antipsychotic medications. The most conservative starting oral dosage is 1 mg daily. Pimozide can be given at bedtime if the patient experiences sedation. Conversely, the mediation can be taken in the morning if the patient experiences increased energy levels. The dosage may be increased every other day according to the patient's tolerance and therapeutic response (40). Because of pimozide's elimination half-life [55 hours (41)], the dosage can be increased at longer intervals (e.g., every 5–7 days). Most patients are adequately treated with dosages of less than 10 mg daily, and, if at all possible, this dosage should not be exceeded in dermatological usage since cardiac side effects may become more relevant at dosages above 10 mg/day (42). Usually, 4–6 mg or less per day is effective in decreasing the intensity of the somatic delusions (43).

The most frequent and potentially severe adverse effects of pimozide involve the central nervous system (CNS) (44). Extrapyramidal reactions may occur with pimozide, especially during the early phase of therapy. In most patients, these reactions consist of parkinsonian symptoms (e.g., tremor, rigidity, akinesia) that are mild to moderate in severity and usually reversible following discontinuation of the drug. Dystonic reactions (a more severe muscle stiffness and rigidity) and feelings of motor restlessness (i.e., akathisia) occur less frequently. Generally, the occurrence and severity of extrapyramidal reactions are dose related, since they occur at relatively high dosages and disappear or become less severe following a reduction in dosage. Extrapyramidal reactions have been reported to appear in about 10–15% of patients receiving dermatological dosages of pimozide (up to

10 mg/day). Administration of anticholinergic antiparkinsonian agents (e.g., benztropine, trihexyphenidyl) or diphenhydramine may be necessary to control parkinsonian extrapyramidal reactions (45). If persistent extrapyramidal reactions occur, pimozide therapy may have to be discontinued.

The most common dystonic reaction is torticollis, which is generally accompanied by orofacial symptoms and, in rare instances, oculogyric crisis, as well as spasms of the face, tongue, and jaw. Dyskinesias of the mouth and throat areas, trismus, dysarthria, muscle cramps, and athetoid movements may occur rarely. Akathisia occurs relatively frequently in patients receiving pimozide, but can usually be managed by reducing the dosage of pimozide or by concomitant administration of an anticholinergic antiparkinsonian agent, diphenhydramine, a benzodiazepine, or propranolol.

Pimozide-induced neuroleptic malignant syndrome (NMS) has not been reported except for one case. Nomifensine (75 mg/d), an antidepressant inhibiting the reuptake of norepinephrine and dopamine, and pimozide (4 mg/d) were used to treat a 20-year-old patient hospitalized with depressive schizoidia (term not defined by authors) (46). Four days later, he showed a clinical picture the authors felt was consistent with NMS. No further details were provided.

There is also the theoretical risk of developing tardive dyskinesia with pimozide. This side effect is characterized by rhythmic involuntary movements of the face, mouth, tongue, or jaw, which may be accompanied by involuntary movements of the trunk or extremities. No cases of pimozide use for MHP causing tardive dyskinesia have been reported except for one questionable case. Lindskov and Baadsgaard (47) reported one patient with delusions of parasitosis treated with 6 months of pimozide (4 mg/d maximum dose) exhibiting slight twisting of her lips, present since the treatment. The original authors did not label this as tardive dyskinesia, but rather it was interpreted as such by another author in a separate publication (44). There is also an extremely rare phenomenon called withdrawal dyskinesia in which a patient who is tapered off a neuroleptic may start to have involuntary movements around the mouth. This dyskinesia is self-limited in duration. Its importance lies in the clinician's knowledge of this condition so she does not confuse it with tardive dyskinesia (48). It is not known if withdrawal dyskinesia occurs with pimozide.

Pimozide can also theoretically cause arrhythmias by prolonging the QT interval. Thus, it is recommended that patients have a pretreatment electrocardiogram to make sure that the patient does not have any underlying cardiac abnormalities if the dosage is greater than or equal to 10 mg/day (49). If the dosage is < 10 mg/day in a relatively young healthy patient with no history of cardiac arrhythmias, it is controversial if an EKG is warranted (42).

Body Dysmorphic Disorder

Because BDD is a broader term that includes, at one end of the spectrum, delusions of dysmorphosis, the distinction between delusional and nondelusional subtypes of BDD may be difficult for the dermatologist to separate out. Delusional BDD (i.e., delusions of dysmorphosis) is treated as MHP as discussed above. The treatment of nondelusional BDD often involves the use of SSRIs and cognitive-behavioral psychotherapy (50). Dosages of these SSRIs often need to be higher than those typically recommended for depression or eating disorders, i.e., up to 40–80 mg/day of fluoxetine (Prozac®) or 40–60 mg/d of paroxetine (Paxil®) (37).

Somatization of Depression

Therapy for somatization of depression is directed at treating the underlying depression. Treatments for depression include psychopharmacotherapy, individual psychotherapy, and group therapy. The patient who refuses to see a psychiatrist or other mental health professional or refuses to recognize the presence of depression may still be helped by antidepressant medications. However, it is useful to determine to what extent the depression stems from difficulties in the patient's life and to what extent it may be endogenous in origin. An extra effort should be made to refer the patient to a psychotherapeutic setting where counseling can be provided if some real life issue such as financial difficulty or stress at work precipitated or contributed to the episode of depression.

All drugs currently approved for treating depression are nearly equally effective, and no drug seems to work much more rapidly than another. A newly selected antidepressant, however, may fail to be effective 25% of the time. The best antidepressant to use in recurrent depression is the one that worked well in the past if the patient can tolerate the side effects. Because all antidepressants are equally effective, most physicians choose one based on its side-effect profile. If a patient's primary complaint is tiredness, an activating SSRI such as fluoxetine (Prozac) may be preferred, whereas if anxiety is a major component, a more sedating drug such as paroxetine (Paxil) may work best. Cancer patients who have anorexia and weight loss may do better receiving a tricyclic antidepressant (TCA) that is associated with increased appetite and weight gain. The most troubling side effects of tricyclic antidepressants are those due to excessive anticholinergic activity, namely dry mouth, blurred vision, constipation, memory disturbance, and urinary retention. These can be particularly troublesome for elderly patients who already have many of these problems.

Most physicians prefer to select a drug that is not lethal if taken in overdose because most patients who commit suicide by ingestion do not stockpile their medicine but take the last prescription given. The lethal dose for a tricyclic antidepressant such as amitriptyline (Elavil®) is 1.5 g or about 10 times the daily therapeutic dose.

The usual preferred first-line drug currently used is either an SSRI [fluoxetine, sertraline (Zoloft®), paroxetine, etc.] or one of the newer agents such as venlafaxine (Effexor®), nefazodone (Serzone®), or mirtazapine (Remeron®). The remaining drugs fall into the tricyclic or miscellaneous categories. The tricyclic agents were first on the market, and although as effective as other agents, they have more severe side effects and can be lethal in overdose. A final category are the monoamine oxidase inhibitors (MAOIs), but these are rarely used because of their severe side effects, the most serious of which is potentially fatal hypertensive crisis if taken with certain drugs or foods containing tyramine. Therefore, MAOIs are not discussed in detail in this chapter.

Chronic Anxiety Disorder

For many years, benzodiazepines have been the treatment of choice for patients with anxiety disorders. The benzodiazepines have a broad spectrum of effects, including sedation, muscle relaxation, anxiety reduction, and decreased physiological arousal (51). Individual benzodiazepines are differentiated by their potency and elimination half-life. These differences have important treatment implications. For a relatively short-acting drug such as alprazolam (Xanax®), with a half-life of 10–14 hours, dosing may be required three or four times a day to avoid interdose symptom recurrence. On the other hand, use of longer-acting clonazepam (Klonopin®), with a half-life of 20–50 hours, may minimize the risk of interdose symptom recurrence.

Several controlled studies have demonstrated the efficacy of different benzodiazepines (BZ), namely chlordiazepoxide (Librium®), alprazolam, and diazepam (Valium®), in the treatment of generalized anxiety disorder (52). Currently, clonazepam and alprazolam are used most often. Interestingly, studies indicate that benzodiazepines have the most pronounced effect on hypervigilance and somatic symptoms (e.g., fatigue, weakness, diaphoresis, insomnia, flushing, chills) of anxiety disorder but exhibit fewer effects on psychic symptoms such as dysphoria (i.e., depressed mood or feeling), interpersonal sensitivity, and obsession (53). Benzodiazepines are particularly effective in the acutely anxious patient because they exert their therapeutic effects quickly, often after a single dose. They have few drug interactions and are widely accepted by patients and generally well tolerated. Surprisingly, even though benzodiazepines like alprazoalm are widely abused, even as a street drug, some authors have suggested that the long-term treatment of anxiety disorder patients with this class of drugs is not associated with abuse or tolerance to anxiolytic effects (54).

A final daily dosage of alprazolam at 2–4 mg/d, diazepam at 15–20 mg/d, or clonazepam at 1–2 mg/d is usually sufficient for the majority of patients. However, these figures are for chronic psychiatric patients. Dermatology patients who are "therapeutic virgins" with regards to these agents often show optimal response at much lower doses. The author usually starts with a very low dose of alprazolam (half of a 0.25 mg tablet) p.o. QID prn acutely and rarely prescribes more than 0.25 mg p.o. QID prn. It is helpful for patients to take an initial dose at home in the evening to see how it affects them when treatment is initiated, especially with regard to the possible sedative effect. Unwanted adverse effects can be limited by gradual titration to an effective dose.

Daytime drowsiness is the main side effect of benzodiazepines, but this usually subsides after several days of treatment. Memory and mild cognitive impairments have been demonstrated but are generally not serious except in the elderly patient. During tapering of benzodiazepines, the reemergence of symptoms is common. With chronic anxiety disorder, it should be expected that symptoms may reappear during tapering after successful BZ treatment. Therefore, for the treatment of chronic anxiety disorder, nonaddictive, nonbenzodiazepine alternatives such as low-dose doxepin or paroxetine (Paxil) need to be considered. Distinguishing between reemergence of anxiety disorder (AD) and withdrawal symptoms can be difficult. This distinction can often be made by stopping the taper when symptoms emerge. It is most likely due to the recurrence of AD if symptoms persist for 3–4 weeks; if they improve, it is more likely due to withdrawal.

In summary, the available literature suggests that BZ are effective for the acute treatment of anxiety disorder. Even though BZ can be used for long-term control of anxiety, nonaddictive, nonbenzodiazepine alternatives are preferred for safety.

The other significant agent used for anxiety is the azapirone busiprone (BuSpar®), a serotoninergic 5-HT receptor partial agonist. The anxiolytic response is generally less pronounced than most BZ. However, it poses no apparent risk for abuse, physical dependence, or withdrawal, and it is not synergistic with alcohol or other sedatives. Its main disadvantage is its delayed onset of action. Buspirone must be administered for at least 2 weeks before a significant therapeutic effect occurs. Because the elimination half-life of buspirone ranges from 2 to 8 hours, a three times daily dosing schedule is generally required. Buspirone is usually given in dosages of 5–10 mg per dosing, but this must be individualized beginning with the lowest dosage and titrating upward until an optimal dosage is reached. Its side effect profile is quite benign but may include gastrointestinal system–related side effects (appetite disturbances and abdominal complaints). Low-dose tricyclics and other antidepressants, such as certain SSRIs, may also be effective in the treatment of generalized anxiety disorder.

Borderline Personality Disorder

The mainstay of treatment for this disorder remains long-term psychotherapy (55). It is important for the clinician to recognize certain aspects of the doctor-patient relationship so that interpersonal problems can be minimized. The physician needs to watch out for idealization, devaluation, and splitting by the patient.

Idealization is seeing others as all-powerful, ideal, or godlike. The most common situation involves a young female patient and a older male physician. This can be a problem for the surgeon if he makes an error in judgment by performing a procedure that is not medically justified because of seductive flattering by these types of patients.

Devaluation is the opposite of idealization and involves depreciating others. The BPD patient may devalue and be extremely angry with the physician the moment she does not obtain the care she expects. This leads to treating the physician as the worst doctor she has had and can catch the dermatological surgeon totally off-guard. As a consequence, the physician may respond with personal rage against the patient and not exercise proper legal and medial judgment.

Splitting is experiencing oneself and others as all good or all bad. This can result in confusion and antagonism among the physician and medical staff or between physicians. The process of splitting involves the patient giving different stories to different staff members, resulting in conflicts among them. It is critical that the staff meet periodically and exchange information to make sure that everyone is in agreement as to how to handle these patients.

Even though the dermatologist is not expected to engage in psychotherapy or pharmacotherapy, it is useful for the clinician to know about possible therapies used for this disorder to facilitate proper referral. Although medication has traditionally been limited in usefulness for this disorder, there may still be some role. Neuroleptics are the best studied of the psychotropic medications in BPD (56). The empiric literature supports the use of low-dose neuroleptics for the acute management of symptoms, with increased specificity in the treatment of schizotypal symptoms and psychoticism, anger, and hostility (57). A role for low-dose neuroleptics in continuation and maintenance therapies has yet to be established despite multiple controlled treatment trials. The Cornelius study (58) supports modest use against irritability and hostility, whereas the Montgomery study (59) is highly supportive of efficacy against parasuicidal behaviors. Compliance with continuation therapy is the essential condition for a successful trial. Many clinicians have used low-dose neuroleptics as maintenance prophylaxis against borderline patients' vulnerability to cognitive-perceptual distortions, disruptive anger, and impulsive aggression. The clinician must carefully weigh the risks of tardive dyskinesia against the benefits in each patient. If in the future, efficacy in BPD is established for the new atypical neuroleptics, concerns with tardive dyskinesia in continuation and maintenance therapies may be lessened. Antidepressants, anticonvulsants, lithium carbonate, and anxiolytic agents have all been used with only limited success in the treatment of this disorder.

Other Psychiatric Disorders

The management of other, less frequently encountered psychiatric disturbances such as schizophrenia, schizoaffective illness, and bipolar disorder is beyond the scope of this chapter and can likely be found in any standard psychiatric textbook.

Other Treatments

As medical knowledge expands, new treatments for these diseases undoubtedly will arise. Though we could not identify any literature indicating its use in place of cosmetic cutaneous surgery, hypnotherapy is an interesting future possibility for the treatment of the patient who exaggerates his or her cosmetic defect (60).

PSYCHIATRIC DISORDERS RESULTING FROM DISFIGUREMENT

The importance of beauty and the emphasis that society places on it cannot be underestimated (61). In social interaction, a person's physical appearance is the personal characteristic most accessible and obvious to others (62). We live in a society that values youth and beauty. It is not surprising then that patients who undergo significant cutaneous surgery may have trouble adjusting to their "new look" and as a result develop psychiatric problems. While this does rarely occur, it should be remembered that most patients adjust well to the consequences of their procedure.

Many psychological studies indicate that strangers assume beauty to be associated with more socially desirable personality traits (63). The more attractive individual also tends to attain higher social status (64). It is understandable, then, that trauma patients or those who have extensive disfigurement from skin cancer surgery may encounter many difficulties, not only in terms of personal emotional distress, but also as victims of negative perceptions from others.

Patients who have a disfigurement are at greater risk of developing psychiatric problems. In a prospective study of 45 burn patients, Madianos and colleagues (65) found psychological impairment in 40–45% of patients right after their burn and at follow-up assessments. Fukunishi (66) found that, at least in female patients, posttraumatic stress disorder (PTSD) was more common after cosmetic disfigurement. Stoddard et al. (67) found that in children and adolescents with severe burns, unrecognized depression was common during their lifetimes. Traumatic injury/disfigurement patients also bring unique psychiatric issues that the cosmetic surgeon should be made aware of (68). These include PTSD, phobias, flashbacks, depressed mood, fear of reinjury, anticipated peer group rejection, and negative body image. It is important to recognize the psychiatric consequences of surgical disfigurement, since many of these patients can be encouraged to seek professional help. Unlike chronic psychiatric patients, many of these individuals had reasonable presurgical psychological adaptation levels, and if they can be helped through their current crisis through referral to mental health professionals, they can become quite functional again.

Social Phobia

For many individuals, aesthetic disfigurement can cause a significant amount of social stress. This anxiety often manifests itself in situations requiring interaction with others. When this anxiety reaches pathological proportions, the consequences can be debilitating for some. Social phobia, also known as social anxiety disorder, is a marked and persistent fear of one or more social or performance situations in which the person is exposed to unfamiliar people or to possible scrutiny by others. The individual fears that he or she will act in a way (or show anxiety symptoms) that will be humiliating or embarrassing (69). Exposure to the feared social situation almost invariably provokes anxiety, which may take the form of a panic attack.

Generally speaking, three types of treatment are available for social phobia. The first is systematic desensitization and exposure. The patient gradually learns not to fear the social situation by being presented with increasingly anxiety-provoking social situations, first in imagery and later in real life. At each stage of exposure, care is taken to make sure the patient's anxiety level does not go out of control. In a related treatment known as "flooding" or "implosion," the patient is rapidly exposed to an enormous volume of phobic material to try to overwhelm the phobic response. Another treatment available is cognitive behavioral therapy. The therapist actively tries to change the patient's thinking habits by challenging existing semiautomatic and automatic thought patterns. The last therapy available is medications. Beta-blockers may be effective in treating performance-anxiety symptoms. Drugs used in generalized social phobias include SSRIs [in doses similar to those used in depression (70)] or a monoamine oxidase inhibitor (MAOI), such as phenelzine (Nardil®).

Patients Who Refuse Treatment

What are the justifiable reasons for seeking the services of a cosmetic/ dermatological surgeon? The most obvious scenario is the patient with a blatant cosmetic defect resulting from trauma, genetics, or birth defects. It is important for the surgeon to determine whether this deformity is in fact grossly disfiguring to the observer, including the surgeon and the patient and the values of the society and culture in which he or she lives. Dr. Jefferson tells the story of such a candidate (71):

> I am reminded of a patient referred by a dermatologist for psychiatric evaluation because she refused treatment of a keloid on her neck. She had been referred to the dermatologist by her family practitioner who felt the keloid unsightly. The dermatologist agreed and recommended removal which the patient refused. Irritated by her decision, she was referred to me. During the evaluation it became apparent that the dermatologist and family practitioner were far more conflicted about the presence of the keloid than the patient. She had made a more than satisfactory adjustment to its presence, over the 40 years of her life. It had not interfered in her social life or employment and indeed, was not as unsightly to this examiner as it was to the physicians responsible for her care. She had no desire to undergo the procedure which, had it occurred may have set in motion the forces that would have created more problems than those it attempted to solve.

In a situation such as this, it is obvious that the cutaneous surgeon should not place his own values ahead of that of the patient.

The Dissatisfied Patient

Psychological issues are not only important preoperatively, but post-operatively as well. A certain percentage of cosmetic surgery patients will be dissatisfied with an operation that did not turn out well. In addition, some patients will be also be dissatisfied despite excellent results from a purely technical point of view (72).

The approach to the former should begin with addressing the suboptimal result frankly and openly (73). Then a plan should be articulated and, with the patient's approval, a correction or revision should be performed. In regards to the latter patient, retrospective analysis usually reveals some facet of psychopathology that was missed or a perceived betrayal of the patient's expectations. Given the difficulty of such patients, the dermatological surgeon will need to spend a significant amount of time with these patients discussing the problem and providing encouragement. In some cases, the patient will eventually respond favorably with increasing acceptance of the result; in other instances, the patient may become discouraged and depressed. It is critical for the dermatologist to watch for this and enlist the assistance of the patient's other physicians and a psychiatric consultation as needed.

Special Considerations in the Adolescent Patient

While appearance-enhancing cosmetic surgery for adults is generally accepted, its appropriateness for younger adolescents is still questioned. In a study centered in the Netherlands by Simis et al., a group of 184 adolescent plastic surgery patients (corrective for aesthetic deformities, $n = 100$; reconstructive for congenital or acquired deformities, $n = 84$) and a control group of 83 adolescents selected at random from three municipalities (corrective $n = 67$; reconstructive, $n = 16$) were studied for the effects of appearance-related surgery on psychosocial functioning (74). These patients, 12–22 years old, were studied at two time points, with a 6-month interval. The plastic surgery patients were studied presurgically and postoperatively. Structured telephone interviews and postal questionnaires were used to determine adolescent's rating of their appearance, bodily satisfaction and attitudes, and appearance-related burdens. All patients reported a significant decrease in burdens (with regards to topics such as "making friends," "romantic relationships," and "future plans") after surgery compared with the control group, indicating a much more prominent improvement in the patient sample compared with the developmental changes that may be expected to occur in adolescence. The corrective patient group reported the least burdens after the operation.

While adolescent patients are unique because of their constantly changing and developing sense of self, adolescents can also reap the benefits of cosmetic surgery. Cosmetic surgery appears to improve bodily satisfaction and relieve many appearance-related burdens.

DISCUSSION

A 1998 study by Sarwer et al. found that cosmetic surgery patients did not demonstrate greater dissatisfaction with their overall appearance compared to the normal values of the measures used in this investigation (75). A more recent study by Sarwer et al. (76) suggests that cosmetic surgery patients seek surgery not because of global dissatisfaction with the entire body, but rather because of heightened dissatisfaction with the specific body feature considered for surgery. Following cosmetic surgery, women reported significant improvements in the level of body image satisfaction with specific features altered by surgery, but no significant changes in overall body image satisfaction. For example, a patient who has a rhinoplasty will have improvement in her image of her nose with successful surgery, but overall she will not feel more satisfied with her total body appearance. Patients did report a significant improvement in self-rated attractiveness following cosmetic surgery, as assessed by a single question in the patient information questionnaire. Patients' scores on the Appearance Evaluation subscale of the Multi-Dimensional Body-Self Relations Questionnaire, which measures a global evaluation of one's appearance, also increased, but not at a statistically significant level. No improvements were noted in the degree of investment with their overall appearance. There was also no increase in satisfaction or investment with their physical fitness or health. It appears that cosmetic surgery has positive effects on an individual's thoughts and feelings about the specific feature altered by surgery, but these effects may not generalize to the overall body image.

While there are many potential psychiatric pitfalls in cosmetic procedures, surgery can have a positive impact on the patient's psyche. The core value of the cosmetic procedure appears to be derived from the patient's opinion and reaction to the result and not from the objective beauty of the visible change (73).

CONCLUSION

In the practice of cosmetic/dermatological surgery, many different psychiatric issues may arise. The greatest of these is the management of patients with exaggerated or nonexistent cosmetic complaints. In addition, there can be psychiatric consequences of traumatically or surgically induced disfigurement. Lastly, the physician may recommend a procedure not desired by the patient. Some treatments have been described, but cutaneous surgeons cannot be expected to treat psychiatric problems on a regular basis. If the patient refuses a referral to a psychiatrist for care, one-time consultation from a psychiatrist or another mental health professional would still be helpful. Even limited advice from a mental health provider can be helpful for the clinician in effectively handling psychological problems at hand.

REFERENCES

1. Reich J. The interface of plastic surgery and psychiatry. Clin Plast Surg 1982; 9:367–377.
2. Kaplan R. What should plastic surgeons do when obsessed patients can't stop? New York Obsrver. July 31, 2000.
3. Koo JYM. Psychiatric aspects of cutaneous surgery. In: Wheeland RG, ed. Cutaneous Surgery. Philadelphia: WB Saunders, 1994:935–942.
4. Bishop ER. Monosymptomatic hypochondriacal syndromes in dermatology. J Am Acad Dermatol 1983; 9:152–158.
5. DSM-IV: Diagnostic and Statistical Manual of Mental Disorders. Washington, DC: American Psychiatric Association, 1994:291–292.
6. Birtchnell SA. Dysmorphophobia: a centenary discussion. Br J Psychiatry 1988; 153(suppl 2):41–43.
7. Thomas CS. Dysmorphophobia: a question of definition. Br J Psychiatry 1984; 144:513–516.
8. DSM-IV: Diagnostic and Statistical Manual of Mental Disorders. Washington, DC: American Psychiatric Association, 1994:309–310.
9. Woods LW. Psychiatry, body image, and cosmetic surgery. Appl Therapeut 1968; 10:451–454.
10. DSM-IV: Diagnostic and Statistical Manual of Mental Disorders. Washington, DC: American Psychiatric Association, 1994:481.
11. Philips KA. Body dysmorphic disorder: the distress of imagined ugliness. Am J Psychiatry 1991; 148:1138–1149.
12. Schachter M. Dysmorphic neurosis (ugliness complexes) and delusions or delusional conviction of ugliness. Ann Med Psychol 1971; 129:723–745.
13. Braddock L. Dysmorphophobia in adolescence: a case report. Br J Psychiatry 1982; 140:199–201.
14. Munro A. Monosymptomatic hypochondriacal psychosis. Br J Hosp Med 1980; 24:34–38.
15. Sadock BJ, Sadock VA. Kaplan & Sadock's Comprehensive Textbook of Psychiatry. 7th ed. Lippincott, Williams & Wilkins, Baltimore, 2000:584.
16. DSM-IV: Diagnostic and Statistical Manual of Mental Disorders. Washington, DC: American Psychiatric Association, 1994, 335–336.

17. DSM-IV: Diagnostic and Statistical Manual of Mental Disorders. Washington, DC: American Psychiatric Association, 1994, 444–448.

18. DSM-IV: Diagnostic and Statistical Manual of Mental Disorders. Washington, DC: American Psychiatric Association, 1994, 672–673.

19. Franzen U, Florin I, Schneider S, Meier M. Distorted body image in bulimic women. J Psychosom Res 1988; 32:445–450.

20. Heilbrun AB, Witt N. Distorted body image as a risk factor in anorexia nervosa: replication and clarification. Psychol Rep 1990; 66:407–416.

21. Heilbrun AB, Friedberg L. Distorted body image in normal college women: possible implications for the development of anorexia nervosa. J Clin Psychol 1990; 46(4):398–401.

22. Sansone RA, Wiederman MW, Monteith D. Obesity, borderline personality symptomatology, and body image among women in a psychiatric outpatient setting. Int J Eat Disord 2001; 29:76–79.

23. Hyler SE, Rieder RO. Personality Diagnostic Questionnaire-Revised (PDG-R). New York: New York State Psychiatric Institute, 1987.

24. DSM-IV: Diagnostic and Statistical Manual of Mental Disorders. Washington, DC: American Psychiatric Association, 1994, 658–661.

25. Napoleon A. The presentation of personalitites in plastic sugery. Ann Plast Surg 1993; 31:193–208.

26. DSM-IV: Diagnostic and Statistical Manual of Mental Disorders. Washington, DC: American Psychiatric Association, 1994:279–292.

27. DSM-IV: Diagnostic and Statistical Manual of Mental Disorders. Washington, DC: American Psychiatric Association, 1994, 300–304.

28. DSM-IV: Diagnostic and Statistical Manual of Mental Disorders. Washington, DC: American Psychiatric Association, 1994, 214–218.

29. DSM-IV: Diagnostic and Statistical Manual of Mental Disorders. Washington, DC: American Psychiatric Association, 1994, 321.

30. Vargel S, Ulusahin A. Psychopathology and body image in cosmetic surgery patients. Aesth Plast Surg. 2001; 25:474–478.

31. Derogatis LR. SCL-90: administration, scoring, and procedure manual-I for the revised version. Baltimore: Johns Hopkins University, School of Medicine, Clinical Psychometrics Unit: 1977.

32. Cash TF, Winstead BA, Janda LH. Body image survey report: the great American shape-up. Psychol Today 1986; 20:30–44.

33. Meningaud JP. Benadiba L, Servant JM, et al. Depression, anxiety, and quality of life among scheduled cosmetic surgery patients: multicentre prospective study. J Craniomaxillofac Surg 2001; 29(3):177–180.

34. Kisely S, Morkell D, Allbrook B, et al. Factors associated with dysmorphic concern and psychiatric morbidity in plastic surgery outpatients. Aust NZ J Psychiatry 2002; 36(1):121–126.

35. Jorgensen L, Castle D, Roberts C, et al. A clinical validation of the Dysmorphic Concern Questionnaire. Aust NZ J Psychiatry 2001; 35(1):124–128.

36. Goldber DP, Williams P. A users' guide to the general health questionnaire. Windsor: NFER-Nelson, 1988.

37. Slaughter JR, Sun AM. In pursuit of perfection: a primary care physician's guide to body dysmorphic disorder. Am Fam Physician 1999; 60:1738–1742.
38. Rohrich RJ. The Who, What, when, and why of cosmetic surgey: Do our patients need a preoperative psychiatric evaluation? Plast Reconstr Surg 2000; 106(7):1605–1607.
39. Riding J, Munro A. Pimozide in the treatment of monosymptomatic hypochondriacal psychosis. Acta Psychiatr Scand 1975; 52:23–30.
40. Stat! Ref. AHFS Drug Information. p 4.
41. McCreadie RG, Heykants JJP, Chalmers, et al. Plasma pimozide profiles in chronic schizophrenics [letter]. Br J Clin Pharmacol 1979; 7:533–534.
42. Shatzberg AF, Cole JO, Degattista C. Antipsychotic drugs. In: Manual of Clinical Psychopharmacology. 3rd ed. Washington, D.C.: American Psychiatric Publishing, 1997:154–155.
43. Koo JYM, Pham CT. Psychodermatology: practical guidelines on pharmacotherapy. Arch Dermatol 1992; 128:381–386.
44. Driscoll MS, Rothe MJ, Grant-Kels JM, et al. Delusional parasitosis: a dermatologic, psychiatric, and pharmacologic approach. J Am Acad Dermatol 1993; 29:1023–1033.
45. Fernandez A. Pimozide in delusional dysmorphosis. Can J Psychiatr 1988; 33:425–426.
46. Ansseau M, Diricq S, Grisar T, et al. Biochemical and neuroendocrine approaches to a malignant syndrome of neuroleptics. Acta Psychiatr Belg 1980; 80:600–606.
47. Lindskov R, Baadsgaard O. Delusions of infestation treated with pimozide: a follow-up study. Acta Derm Venereol 1985; 65:267–270.
48. Koo J, Gambla C. Delusions of parasitosis and other forms of monosymptomatic hypochondriacal psychosis. Dermatol Clin 1996; 14:429–438.
49. Koo JYM, Strauss GD. Psychopharmacologic treatment of psychocutaneous disorders: a practical guideline. Semin Dermatol 1987; 6:83–93.
50. Rohrich R. Streamlining cosmetic surgery patient selection: Just say no! Plast Reconstr Surg 1999; 104:220–221.
51. Tasman A. Psychiatry. Philadelphia: WB Saunders, 1997:1110–1115.
52. Brawman-Mintzer O, Lydiard RB. Psychopharmacology of anxiety disorders. Psychiatr Clin North Am 1994; 1:51–79.
53. Hoehn-Saric R, McLeod DR, Zimmerli WD. Differential effects of alprazolam and imipramine in generalized anxiety disorder: Somatic versus psychic symptoms. J Clin Psychiatry 1988; 49:293–301.
54. Romach M, Busto U, Somer G, ct al. Clinical aspects of chronic use of alprazolam and lorazepam. Am J Psychiatry 1995; 152:1161–1167.
55. Chessick RD. Intensive psychotherapy of a borderline patient. Arch Gen Psychol 1982; 39:413–419.
56. Soloff PH. Psychopharmacology of borderline personality disorder. Psychiatr Clin North Am 2000; 23(1):169–192.
57. Brinkley J, Beitman D, Friedel R. Low dose neuroleptic regimens in the treatment of borderline patients. Arch Gen Psychiatry 36:319–326, 1979.

58. Cornelius JR, Soloff PH, Perel JM, et al. Continuation pharmacotherapy of borderline personality disorder with haloperidol and phenelzine. Am J Psychiatry 150:1843–1848, 1993.

59. Montgomery SA, Montgomery D. Pharmacologic prevention of suicidal behavior. J Affect Disord 4:291–298, 1982.

60. Shenefelt PD. Hypnosis in dermatology. Arch Dermatol 2000; 136:393–399.

61. Alam M, Dover JS. On beauty. evolution, psychosocial considerations, and surgical enhancement. Arch Dermatol 2001; 137:795–807.

62. Hautmann G, Panconesi E. Vitiligo: a psychologically influenced and influencing disease. Clin Dermatol 1997; 15:879–890.

63. Dion K, Bersheid E, Walster E. What is beautiful is good. J Pers Soc Psychol 1972; 24:285–290.

64. Anderson C, John OP, Keltner D, Kring AM. Who attains social status? Effects of personality and physical attractiveness in social groups. J Pers Soc Psychol 2001; 81:116–132.

65. Madianos MG, Papaghelis M, Ioannovich J, Dafni R. Psychiatric disorders in burn patients: a follow-up study. Psychother Psychosom 2001; 70:30–37.

66. Fukunishi I. Relationship of cosmetic disfigurement to the severity of posttraumatic stress disorder in burn injury or digital amputation. Psychother Psychosom 1999; 68:82–86.

67. Stoddard FJ, Stroud L, Murphy JM. Depression in children after recovery from severe burns. J Burn Care Rehabil 1992; 13:340–347.

68. Rusch MD, Gould LJ, Dzwierzynski WW, et al. Psychological impact of traumatic injuries: what the surgeon can do. Plast Recon Surg 2002; 109:18–24.

69. DSM-IV: Diagnostic and Statistical Manual of Mental Disorders. Washington, DC: American Psychiatric Association, 1994, 411–417.

70. Baldwin D, Bobes J, Stein DJ, et al. Paroxetine in social phobia/social anxiety disorder: randomised, double-blind, placebo-controlled study. Paroxetine Study Group. Br J Psychiatry 1999; 175:120–126.

71. Jefferson RS. The psychiatric assessment of candidates for cosmetic surgery. J Nat Med Assoc 1976; 68:411–419.

72. Gifford S. Cosmetic surgery and personality change: a review and some clinical observations. In: The Unfavorable Result in Plastic Surgery. Goldwyn RM, ed. Boston: Little, Brown, 1972:11–33.

73. McGrath MH, Mukerji S. Plastic surgery and the teenage patient. J Pediatr Adolese Gynecol 2000; 13:105–118.

74. Simis KJ, Hovius SER, de Beaufort ID. After plastic surgery: adolescent-reported appearance ratings and appearance-related burdens in patient and general population groups. Plast Reconstr Surg 2002; 109:9–17.

75. Sarwer DB, Wadden TA, Pertschuk MJ, et al. Body image dissatisfaction and body dysmorphic disorder in 100 cosmetic surgery patients. Plast Reconstr Surg 1998; 101:1644–1649.

76. Sarwer DB, Wadden TA, Whitaker LA. An investigation of changes in body image following cosmetic surgery. Plast Reconstr Surg 2002; 109:363–369.

27

Nonpharmacological Treatments in Psychodermatology

Richard D. Fried

Yardley, Pennsylvania, U.S.A.

INTRODUCTION

Nonpharmacological psychocutaneous treatments encompass a wide variety of structured and unstructured interventions, which may lead to amelioration of skin function. Nonpharmacological studies understandably lack the appeal of "drug studies" to the scientist. Drug studies allow for elucidation of chemical structures, pharmacological mechanisms of action, receptor specificity, etc. These are all relatively concrete constructs that allow the researcher to explain the observed defects. In contrast, nonpharmacological interventions are often more difficult to quantify and mechanisms of action more nebulous. Studies are often small, poorly controlled, and anecdotal and thus lack sufficient adherence to scientific method and statistical rigor to allow for definitive claims of efficacy. Further, the small numbers of patients in these studies do not adequately allow for the many biases influencing therapeutic outcome, e.g., investigator-patient individual characteristics, natural course of disease, and seasonal issues.

Recognizing the above caveats, there is little question that factors other than pharmacological agents affect psychocutaneous function. Recent studies (1) have shown that psychological stress directly perturbs epidermal permeability barrier homeostasis. Stress has also been shown to delay wound healing with a direct effect on interleukins (2), while other studies (3) have shown that acute immobilization stress triggers skin mast cell degranulation. Other studies have shown that stress and other emotional factors clearly lead to worsening of many common dermatosis including rosacea, psoriasis, eczema, acne, herpes simplex virus (HSV), and hyperhidrosis (4). Nonpharmacological interventions are generally stress-reducing adjuncts to traditional therapy which have been shown to enhance the efficacy of standard dermatological therapies. They can lead to a reduction in drug dosage, duration, or exposure to potentially toxic agents or modalities (5). The addition of a nonpharmacological intervention by definition offers and engages the patient in a broader care model. The concept of "total care" was championed by the late Eugene Farber (6,7).

Overall, studies do not suggest that nonpharmacological psychocutaneous interventions are disease specific. Rather, the observed benefits appear to be the result of global stress reduction, enhanced sense of control over the illness, and normalization of psychoneuroendocrine function. Thus, the organization of this chapter will be a brief review of efficacy studies of five categories of nonpharmacological interventions followed by several case illustrations. A legitimate criticism of the observed benefits of psychocutaneous interventions of all types is the contention that these modalities simply increase the patients' sense of subjective control over their illness. Thus, their enhanced sense of control leads to diminished anxiety and improved compliance with traditional regimens. I believe the data support a more direct influence on neuropeptides, mast cells, cutaneous, vasculature, etc. In fact, it is probably a combination of direct psychophysiological effects and enhanced compliance that accounts for the efficacy of these techniques. Some patients achieve greater benefits from psychocutaneous interventions than others. Unfortunately, there are not yet adequate selection criteria to define which patients will most benefit from nonpharmacological intervention. It can be stated with reasonable certainty that incorporation of these techniques into clinical practice adheres to the dictum of "do no harm" and most likely results in improvement in the patient's overall quality of life.

Nonpharmacological psychocutaneous interventions may be considered as legitimate adjunctive treatment for any of the following disorders: psoriasis, atopic dermatitis (including dyshidrotic eczema, rosacea, acne, acne excoriée, urticaria, hyperhidrosis, trichotillomania, chronic telogen effluvium, neurotic excoriations, dysesthetic syndromes including postherpetic neuralgia, chronic pruritus, scalp dysesthesia, glossodynia, vulvodynia, and body dysmorphic disorder (4,8–19).

BIOFEEDBACK THERAPY

Biofeedback is a noninvasive conditioning technique, which has wide applications in modern medicine. Electromyograph (EMG, muscle tension) and blood flow (temperature) training are the most commonly used modalities. The objective physiological data generated from biofeedback training are useful for research and clinical efficacy studies. The machinery provides excellent face validity for patients, providing objective visual and auditory feedback paralleling desired improvements in muscle tension and blood flow. Patients are often enthusiastic about this modality since the monitoring and feedback displays suggest that they are receiving "high-tech" intervention. In addition to reducing muscle tension and improving blood flow, an overall relaxation response is achieved with biofeedback training. Increased distal temperature and decreased muscle tension are the desired objective endpoints, while subjective endpoints include enhanced feelings of relaxation, well-being, symptom reduction, and increased patient sense of bodily control. Biofeedback has been studied for the treatment of acne, eczema (atopic dermatitis), urticaria, pain syndromes, and psoriasis (20–22,25).

Biofeedback training encompasses a wide variety of progressive muscle-relaxing techniques, autogenic training, imagery techniques, and straightforward conditioning techniques. No method has consistently demonstrated superior efficacy, and choices are usually made based on therapist and patient preference. Biofeedback training is best accomplished by a psychologist or BCIA (Biofeedback Certification Institute of America)-certified therapist. Training sessions are usually 45–60 minutes in length; and 8–20 sessions are usually required based upon patient progress. Patient homework in the form of charting and home practice is considered essential to therapeutic success.

RELAXATION TRAINING

Relaxation training can be accomplished by numerous techniques, all chiefly directed at minimizing sympathetic reactivity and enhancing parasympathetic function. Included in this group of procedures are progressive muscle relaxation, autogenic training, guided imagery, transcendental and other meditation techniques, and other relaxation directed programs (breathing techniques, self-talk, etc.). Relaxation training has been used as adjunctive therapy to treat acne, eczema, urticaria, psoriasis, hyperhidrosis, acne excoriée, and neurotic excoriations (23,24,26–28,39).

HYPNOSIS

The hypnotic phenomenon has been used since ancient times to assist in healing. Hypnotic trance can be defined as a heightened state of focus that can be helpful in reducing unpleasant sensations, i.e., pain, pruritus, dysesthesias, while simultaneously inducing favorable physiological changes. This receptive state of heightened suggestibility has been used to target behaviors (scratching, picking), emotional states, physical symptoms, and specific skin reactions. Hypnosis has been studied as monotherapy or complementary therapy for the treatment of acne excoriée, alopecia areata, atopic dermatitis, congenital ichthyosiform erythroderma, dyshidrotic eczema, erythromelalgia, glossodynia, lichen planus, neurodermatitis, nummular eczema, postherpetic neuralgia, pruritus, psoriasis, rosacea, trichotillomania, urticaria, verruca, and vitiligo (29–33,43,44). Documented physiological changes include favorable alteration in blood pressure, heart rate, muscle tension, blood flow, galvanic skin response, electroencephalographic output, T-cell function, and histamine release.

PSYCHOTHERAPY

Many psychotherapeutic approaches ranging from orthodox psychoanalysis to behavioral conditioning techniques have been employed in the treatment of psychocutaneous skin disease (34–37). Cognitive behavioral psychotherapy, behavior modification, insight-oriented psychotherapy, and supportive psychotherapy are psychotherapeutic interventions.

Efficacy studies have never clearly demonstrated superiority of any given therapeutic orientation or technique. It has been suggested that therapist preference and personal characteristics, along with a positive therapist patient alliance, add more prognostic value than specific techniques utilized. Effective psychotherapy should be directed at modifying disabling emotions and behaviors that interfere with psychosocial and vocational functioning and are suspected of maintaining or exacerbating the skin disease. Patients who are afflicted with chronic or disfiguring skin diseases may be in need of longer-term supportive or insight-oriented psychotherapy. The focus is frequently on gaining acceptance of the unpleasant realities of their disease and helping them to develop coping strategies to enable the patient to meet the demands, intrusions, and limitations imposed by their skin disease. Both individual and group psychotherapy may be encompassed under the general heading of psychotherapy. We may further broaden the conceptualization to include brief psychotherapeutic interventions (far less than the stated 45-minute hour) implemented by physician, psychologist, social worker, and office ancillary staff. The effects on the individual can be dramatic, improving not only skin function but overall survival (38,40,41).

PSYCHOEDUCATION AND SUPPORT

Several studies suggest that programs providing patients with detailed information about their skin disease, including etiology, therapeutic options, and prognosis, can be helpful in enhancing compliance with treatment regimen, as well as improving the emotional state of the patient (24,27,42).

Psychoeducation directed at educating the patient with regard to common emotional reactions to their skin disease can be helpful in reducing the patient's sense of isolation and confusion. Support groups, which are composed of individuals similarly affected, appear to provide companionship, consultation, and useful treatment and lifestyle suggestions. They have not only been suggested to improve the mood states and psychosocial status of the patient but may actually affect prognosis and perhaps survival. Spiegel et al. showed improved survival in patients with metastatic breast cancer (38), while Fawzy et al. showed similar findings for malignant melanoma (41).

CASE ILLUSTRATIONS

The following are some selected case illustrations in which nonpharmacological psychocutaneous techniques have been incorporated into the treatment regimens for common skin diseases. It must be recognized that there are no defined "standards" of care or defined treatment algorhythms which enable the clinician to select the most appropriate nonpharmacological intervention. Decisions should be made based on therapists' expertise and preference, patient expectation and desire, and availability of resources. Flexibility and creativity are essential ingredients in psychocutaneous treatment protocols as they are in any effective therapeutic intervention. These case illustrations represent only a sampling of the potential applications of the techniques thus far described.

Psoriasis

Ronald G. has had psoriasis for 11 years. He is a 27-year-old white man who returned to his dermatologist for treatment complaining of his "typical psoriasis flare." He had been in remission for the last 6 months without any significant skin lesions and now complains of a 3-week history of enlarging, hypertropic scaly plaques on the scalp, elbows, knees, buttocks, and hands. The micaceous scale that covered his plaques flaked almost continuously, and his lesions on the elbows and knees occasionally bled. His bedsheets were covered with scale and dry blood each morning. Uncharacteristically for the patient, two 3 cm erythematous plaques were prominently visible on his forehead. He noted extreme levels of pruritus that intensified his subjective discomfort, worsened the psoriasis, and markedly impaired his work and sleep patterns. The patient stated somberly that his psoriasis appears to worsen each year, and he stated "I will never have a normal life." On further questioning, he related moderate feelings of depression, characterized by mild anhedonia, lethargy, self-deprecating ideation, and feelings of futility. Suicidal and homicidal ideation and intent were denied. He related that he had had a recent romantic relationship with an older woman, which was terminated by her soon after his recent flare. Erectile dysfunction had been a prevalent and distressing feature in the sparse number of romantic relationships he has had since developing psoriasis. The small lesions on the glans penis served as a constant reminder of his ongoing illness.

Ronald G.'s case illustrates the broad-reaching emotional and functional effects which are only infrequently verbalized by patients with psoriasis. Treatment was initiated with topical corticosteroids, Dovonex, and antihistamines. He also began a 12-week biofeedback treatment program in which EMG training on the sternocleidomastoid and trapezius muscles was initiated. Autogenic imagery training accompanied his biofeedback, and imagery focused on slowing of the hyperproliferative rate of his keratinocytes. The slowing was accomplished using guided imagery: a warm Caribbean sun gently soothing and slowing his racing skin cells. Short-term cognitive behavioral psychotherapy proved effective in ameliorating his self-deprecating ideation and associated depressive symptoms. Evidence of a mild body dysmorphic disorder was apparent with the discovery that the patient believed that his penis had become smaller and disfigured with each subsequent psoriasis flare. Cognitive behavioral psychotherapy and physician support together with steady improvement in his psoriasis resulted in substantial improvement in his distorted body image. A psychoeducational support group also appeared to facilitate his recovery and improved his interpersonal skills. With this combined approach, his psoriasis cleared more quickly than in previous years, and it was obvious that his compliance with standard medication regimens was better. He no longer experienced the application of his psoriasis medications as a futile and anxiety-provoking chore. Rather, he reported that he experienced reduced anxiety and an enhanced sense of control with each application of medication. His erectile dysfunction resolved over the 3 months following the initiation of therapy, and at the termination of treatment he had entered an apparently healthy relationship with a woman and reported mutually satisfying emotional and sexual encounters.

Ronald G.'s case illustrates the potential effectiveness of a multimodal psychocutaneous intervention as adjunctive or complementary treatment. While his dermatologist continued his traditional treatments, the adjuctive psychocutaneous interventions were performed by a psychologist (cognitive-behavioral psychotherapy), a certified biofeedback therapist (biofeedback training), and a medical assistant supervising the support group.

Eczema

Robert G.'s mother was unable to contain her obvious frustration. She appeared exhausted. "You have to make him better. I can't stand it anymore!" She returned for her tenth visit over the last 4 months. Her 2-year-old son had severe atopic dermatitis and squirmed restlessly in her lap, scratching his severely excoriated skin. He had hypertropic, lichenified plaques on his arms and legs, and open impetiginized lesions were prominent on his trunk and scalp. Mrs. G. became tearful as she described his constant irritability, fitful restless sleep patterns, and insatiable demand for attention. She described a scenario in which she had become so exhausted that she was no longer able to rouse herself from bed to go to Robert's room numerous times each night. Therefore, she resorted to having him sleep between her and her husband. Through her tears, she explained "I have no life, I have no marriage, I hate him!"

Although this may sound extreme to the nondermatologist reader, it is a situation that is frequently encountered in dermatological practice. It certainly illustrates the complex and far-reaching effects of skin disease in young children. The demands and sequelae of chronic skin disease can easily overwhelm the emotional resources of even the best parent and disrupt all aspects of the family and marital system. The stress experienced by the family unit can result in exacerbation of the child's symptoms. This reciprocal interaction often results in greater irritability and demands for attention on the part of the child. A destructive cycle evolves which can lead to further stress and deterioration of the family-marital unit. The skin disease becomes an affliction borne by the entire family. Both individual and family intervention can be extremely beneficial for all affected individuals.

Despite the intense emotional and functional disruption caused by Robert's eczema, both Robert and his family did well. Although initially rejected by his parents, desparation led to reluctant acceptance and referral was made for family therapy. Mrs. G. was exhausted and appropriately experiencing feelings of rage toward her son. His skin disease and constant demands had disrupted all spheres of her functional world. She felt a subjective sense of inadequacy and failure as a mother that was dramatically worsened by her guilt elicited in response to her negative feelings and thoughts about her son. Her therapy was directed toward helping Mrs. G. accept the appropriateness and normalcy of her mixed feelings and helping her to provide concrete coping strategies and behavioral techniques to restore control and balance to her home. Because Robert's eczema is likely to persist for many years to come, longer-term planning and acceptance were important ingredients of the therapeutic process. Restoration of marital function and recruitment of her husband into the child care process were considered important ingredients. Her husband had both emotionally and physically removed himself from the family situation, partly based on his own rage toward both Mrs. G. and Robert and in part in response to his own feelings of helplessness and inadequacy. Robert's presence in the parental bed had made intimacy between Mr. and Mrs. G. impossible. Mr. G. refused to help in the care and management of Robert as a passive-aggressive expression of his anger toward Mrs. G., who "allowed Robert to intrude into their marital bed." Gradually, the marital relationship was restored, Robert was moved back to his room, firmer limits were set, and the intense stress in the family unit lessened. In response, Robert's sleep improved, his skin improved, and his eczema, while not clear, became manageable. Indeed, infantile and childhood eczema is often extremely sensitive to stress, parental stress, fatigue, and guilt-driven overindulgence.

Acne and Acne Excoriée

Anna S. sat nervously on the examination table. Examination revealed numerous new deeply excoriated aciniform lesions, many with fresh hemorrhagic crusts. She became tearful as she explained her fiancé's ridicule and stated that he had taken to calling her "scarface." Anna's acne excoriée had predated her present relationship, but had markedly intensified as conflicts and stresses leading up to her upcoming wedding intensified. She noted that she picked in response to "tense feelings and anger" and experienced transient reduction in anxiety while picking. Unfortunately, the visible lesions that resulted from her picking led to intensification of her anxiety and feelings of hopelessness. While Anna vehemently denied any suicidal or homicidal ideation or intent, she did state through her tears that "this was ruining my life."

Referral was made to a "skin emotion specialist" (a mental health professional knowledgeable about skin disease), and thereby the efforts of the dermatologist and mental health professional were coordinated. A combination of cognitive behavioral psychotherapy, behavioral techniques, including response prevention incorporating alternative behaviors, and biofeedback therapy were simultaneously initiated. Oral antibiotics and Zoloft 50 mg HS were prescribed by the dermatologist.

Anna gradually achieved control over her picking behavior and over a period of 8 weeks developed several alternative behaviors, which were moderately effective in reducing anxiety. She did go on to marry her fiancé, who was brought into therapy near termination. His role in maintaining her anxiety and self-injurious behaviors was explored. Anna still persists with occasional self-excoriation but has achieved much greater control and often employs her alternative behaviors, which are nonscarring in nature (finger rubbing, leg rubbing, deep breaths, etc.).

Adult Eczema

Robin S. had had eczema since early childhood; now, at age 24, she sat in the examination room, shaking her head slowly from side to side, stating "I thought I would outgrow this. I can't believe it is back." Her diffusely dry skin was evident on her arms and legs, but most striking were the thick dark plaques on her posterior cervical neck, antecubital and popliteal fossas. She stated that her itching was intolerable and that her level of anxiety and agitation had become so intense that performing her tasks as a CPA had become impossible. She complained that her time in bed at night had become a tortuous ordeal of persistent scratching, rubbing, and frustration.

This case illustrates several points. The first is the unpredictable and capricious nature of eczema. While many patients have predictable seasonal and emotional precipitants, many others find that their disease flares randomly and unpredictably. The second important point is that the pruritus associated with eczema can be both subjectively intolerable and functionally incapacitating. A vicious cycle exists between scratching and disruption of the skin, each intensifying the severity of the other.

Robin S. was treated with a regimen of topical tacrolimus, oral antihistamines, and liberal use of emollients. In addition, progressive muscle relaxation with guided imagery proved helpful in decreasing her anxiety and itching. It must be again reiterated that anxiety and pruritus reciprocally potentiate one another. She responded well, and no additional psychocutaneous interventions were necessary. Other interventions that have demonstrated efficacy as adjuncts to standard treatments would have included biofeedback, stress management, psychoeducational groups, and individual and group psychotherapy.

Urticaria

Roberta H. was angry. With infuriating predictability, her hives began to migrate from her central chest to the sides of her neck, cheeks, and arms. The burning, heat, and intense erythema were accompanied by intolerable itching, which compelled her to dig her fingernails deep into the involved areas of her skin. It was only a matter of minutes before this high-level advertising executive was to stand before a group of 100 and present her creative and well-thought-out advertising campaign. She knew that whatever creative genius she brought before this group would be over-shadowed by the visible blotches of disfigurement that encroached her neck and arms.

This case illustrates the intense embarrassment and physical discomfort that often accompanies urticaria. The etiology of urticaria can be varied, and all patients with persistent urticaria should be thoroughly evaluated for the myriad of underlying medical conditions that can contribute to their occurrence. Assuming that modifiable triggers and serious medical maladies have been eliminated, psychocutaneous techniques can be helpful in controlling these patients. Urticaria, akin to flushing and hyperhidrosis, often becomes amplified in a psychocutaneous cascading fashion. Specifically, it becomes intensified by cognitive and emotional factors that lead to greater sympathetic reactivity. It must be recognized that the onset of urticaria is frequently idiopathic without identifiable psychosocial stress or emotional reactivity. Further, recurrences often follow an unpredictable course. Despite this, psychocutaneous techniques have been suggested to be helpful in controlling their occurrence and severity. This patient was managed with a multimodal approach. She was treated with standard multiple agent antihistamine therapy and also began biofeedback training and cognitive behavioral psychotherapy. She gradually reduced her level of rage and intense anxiety that were elicited in response to her urticaria. She began to accept it as an unpleasant nuisance of life rather than a tragic occurrence. She was also taught specific self-talk and relaxation techniques that allowed her to intervene at the earliest occurrence of her urticaria. The interventions were designed to blunt her sympathetic response to the urticaria that resulted in an exacerbating neuroadrenergic cascade. She gradually found that the duration and severity of her urticarial episodes markedly diminished. At the end of therapy, the frequency of her urticaria had diminished from several times per day to several times per week. While the treatment protocol was not curative, it certainly improved the quality of her life and her subjective emotional state.

Pruritus

Sam H. scratched vigorously at his forearms as he recounted his lengthy saga. He described chronic full body itching of 2 years duration which had proven unresponsive to multiple interventions. He had seen numerous medical specialists, including his general internist, gastroenterologist, rheumatologist, endocrinologist, oncologist, pulmonologist, four dermatologists, and a psychiatrist. Each specialist performed a plethora of both noninvasive and invasive tests. Not surprisingly, each managed to find at most a minor malady which "could be contributing" to his pruritus. However, no diagnosis or intervention provided him with anything more than transient relief from his symptoms. He recounted a rather impressive medical history, including colon cancer, chronic obstructive pulmonary disease, coronary artery disease, type II diabetes, osteoarthritis, and generalized anxiety disorder. The list of medications was long and each was reported in the *Physicians' Desk Reference* (PDR) to cause pruritus in a small number of patients. Most of his medications were considered "essential" and cessation could prove problematic.

Physical examination revealed diffusely xerotic skin with scattered excoriations. Scattered discrete eczematous plaques were evident on the lower back and distal lower extremities. Significant pigmentary alteration was noted in areas of chronic excoriation. Examination failed to reveal any primary lesions suggestive of a primary skin disease, nor was there any evidence of malignancy, infection, or infestation. There was no rash consistent with a "classic drug eruption," and complete review of his laboratory data suggested no obvious organic basis for his itching. Review of systems was essentially negative for symptoms of underlying malignancy, but the possibility of an as yet undeclared malignant, collagen vascular, or neuropathic process remained prominent in the differential. When allowed to speak freely, the patient expressed a variety of emotional reactions, chiefly involving anger and fear. The patient was extremely angry at the medical profession because of its inability to provide a definitive answer and, more importantly, any degree of symptom amelioration. He was angry at his pruritus and how it had essentially robbed him of his daytime pleasures and nocturnal relaxation. He was extremely fearful that his itching represented a serious underlying malady, and in the course of his medical workup numerous ominous possibilities were entertained by various physicians, including malignancy, collagen vascular disease, infectious disease including HIV, hepatic, renal, and other disease.

Oral antihistamines and antidepressant medications were mandatory as part of the initial intervention. Patients such as Sam H. are invariably sleep deprived and anxiety ridden, and reactive depression is almost a certainty. Initial therapy must be directed toward reducing anxiety and increasing nighttime sedation to allow for some restoration of sleep. In addition, psychoeducation and relaxation training proved very helpful in reducing his level of anxiety and agitation and provided a great deal of "hand holding" that he needed. Another important aspect of treatment in these patients is reducing the self-inflicted components of skin disruption. The constant scratching and rubbing lead to further disruption of the integument and intensification of symptoms. Many such patients excoriate so frequently and furiously that the disrupted integument is vulnerable to additional irritation and impetiginization, leading to greater sensory disturbance. Finally, in the older patient, xerosis is frequently present and can contribute to itching. Thus, alternative methods to decrease pruritus, i.e., cold packs, topical doxepin, topical lidocaine (qualities small enough to avoid lidocaine toxicity from percutaneous absorption), and alternative behaviors as well as liberal use of emollients, are essential.

Sam H. did quite well with this multimodal approach and experienced a dramatic reduction in his itching. During anxiety-ridden times, his itching did intensify, but with much less severity and without the extreme anger and fearfulness. PRN use of benzodiazepine anxiolytics, daily buspirone and a serotonin selective reuptake inhibitor were helpful. A crucial caveat in this patient population is the necessity for the clinician to maintain vigilance for the possibility of an underlying organic or malignant process. Pruritus is well known to be a harbinger of underlying but as yet undeclared malignancy. Specifically, gastrointestinal malignancies, blood dyscrasias, Hodgkin's disease, polycythemia vera, and carcinoid syndrome are a few to be considered. Finally, HIV and CNS organic processes (Alzheimer's, multiple sclerosis, etc.) should always be considered with chronic pruritus.

The preceding case illustrations present only a minute sampling of the conditions amenable to psychocutaneous intervention, and the techniques described are certainly few in number. A myriad of possible psychological techniques are at the disposal of the experienced and creative clinician.

CONCLUSION

Psychocutaneous medicine has indeed come of age and is being incorporated into mainstream medical practice. Patients presenting to our offices today are more sophisticated and frequently dissatisfied with traditional medical therapies. They are actively seeking alternative approaches and adjuncts to standard treatments. In contrast to many other "alternativeholistic" treatments offered through nonmedical venues, we can assure our patients that there are controlled studies that support the efficacy of psychocutaneous techniques in improving many dermatological conditions. Psoriasis, rosacea, herpes simplex, body dysmorphic disorder, acne, eczema, urticaria, neurotic excoriations, acne excoriée, trichotillomania, dysesthetic syndromes, and delusions parasitosis are included in this incomplete list.

It is helpful for both the patient and therapist to define concrete and realistic goals for psychocutaneous intervention. Concrete observable or measurable goals can help the patient and clinician to gauge therapeutic progress and success. Specifically, goals can include reduction in pruritus (rating severity from 1 to 10), decreased scratching activity, decreased plaque extent or thickness, decreased number of urticarial plaques, decreased flushing, decreased anxiety, decreased anger, decreased social embarrassment, decreased social withdrawal and improved sleep. More global goals can include improved sense of well being, increased sense of control and enhanced acceptance of some of the inevitable aspects of a given skin disease. "Cure" should never be a goal because most disorders amenable to psychocutaneous techniques are the chronic nature, thus cure as an end point would only lead to disappointment.

I encourage the dermatologist reader to align themselves with what I call the "skin emotion specialist." This may be a psychiatrist, psychologist, social worker, biofeedback therapist, or other mental health or behavioral specialist. Patients are more likely to accept a referral to a "skin emotion specialist" since this destigmatizes psychological interventions. Incorporating these techniques and specialists into your clinical practice will expand your therapeutic horizons and improve the quality of life of many of the patients afflicted with chronic skin disease. A final caveat must be offered when attempting to make prognostic statements regarding the likelihood of therapeutic success. While all patients can potentially benefit from psychocutaneous interventions, those with severe psychopathology and poor pre-treatment functional status are likely to be more difficult to treat and achieve less optimal outcomes. Patients with personality disorders such as borderline, narcissistic, and schizotypal as well as patients with any active psychotic process certainly present a more resistant and difficult population with whom therapeutic success is less likely. However, these are also patients who are often in the greatest subjective distress and certainly can profit from any of the above interventions. According to W. Mitchell Sams, Jr., "although the physician is a scientist and clinician, he or she is and must be something more. A doctor is a caretaker and the patient's person—a professional advisor, guiding the patient through some of life's most difficult journeys. Only the clergy share this responsibility with us." This commitment is and hopefully will always be the guiding force in the provision of comprehensive and compatient patient care.

REFERENCES

1. Amit Garg BA, et al. Physiological stress perturbs epidermal permeability barrier homeostasis; implications for the pathogenesis of stress-associated skin disorders. Arch Dermatol 2001; 137:53–59.
2. Gleser R, et al. Arch Gen Psychiatry 1999; 56(5):450–456.
3. Singh Singh LK, Pang X, Alexacos N, Letourneau R, Theoharides TC. Acute immobilization stress trigger skin mast cell degranulation via corticotropin releasing hormone, neurotensin, and substance P: a link to neurogenic skin disorders. Brain Behav Immun 1999; 13(3):225–239.
4. Koo JYM, Do JH, Lee CS. Psychodermatology, periodic synopsis. J Am Acad Dermatol 2002; 43(5):848–853.
5. Kirby B, Richards JL, McElhone K, et al. Br J Dermatol 2000; 143(suppl 57): 15–16.
6. Farber EM, Raychaudhuri SP. Concept of total care: a third dimension in the treatment of psoriasis. Cutis 1997; 59:35–38.
7. Fried RG. Stress and the skin: Is holistic dermatology the solution? 1998; Skin Aging, 52–58.
8. Gupta AK. Psychodermatology: an update. J Am Acad Dermatol 1997; 34:130–146.
9. Koo JYM. Psychodermatology. Dermatol Clin 1996; 14(3).
10. Cotterill Ja. Psychophysiological aspects of eczema. Semin Dermatol 1990; 9:216–219.
11. Gastron L, Crombez JC, Lassonde M, Bernier-Buzzanga J, Hodgins S. Psychological stress and psoriasis; experimental prospective correlational studies. Acta Derm Venereol Suppl 1991; 156:37–43.
12. Iyer S, Washenik K, Shupack J. Can psychological stress affect psoriasis? Possible mechanisms. J Clin Dermatol 1998; 1:21–28.
13. Koo JYM, Smith L. Psychologic aspects of acne. Pediatr Dermatol 1991; 8:185–188.
14. White A, Horne DJ, Varigos GA. Psychological profile atopic eczema patient. Australas J Dermatol 1990; 31:13–16.
15. Fried RG. Evaluation and treatment of "psychogenic" pruritus and self excoriation. J Am Acad Dermatol 1994; 30:993–999.
16. Eli IE, Bhat R, Littner MM, Kleinhauz M. Detection of psychopathologic trends in glossodynia pateints. Psychosom Med 1994; 56:389–394.
17. Rojo L, Silbestre SJ, Vagan JV, DeVicente T. Psychiatric morbidity in burning mouth syndrome. Psychiatric interview versus depression and anxiety scales. Oral Surg Oral Med Oral Pathol 1993; 75:308–311.
18. Edwards, L Vulvadynia
19. Phillips KA. Body dysmorphic disorder: the distress of imagined ugliness. Am J Psychiatry 1991; 148:1138–1149.
20. Haynes SN, Wilson CC, Jaffe PG, Britton BT. Biofeedback treatment of atopic dermatitis. Biofeedback Self Reg 1979; 4:195–209.

21. Hughes H, Brown BW, Lawlis JF, Fulton GE. Treatment of acne vulgaris by biofeedback, relaxation and cognitive imagery. J Psychosom Res 1983; 27:185–191.

22. Manuso JSJ. The use of biofeedback hand warming training in the eczematous dermatitis of the hands: a case study. J Behav Ther Exp Psychiatry 1977; 8:445–446.

23. Cotterill JA. Psychophysiological aspects of eczema. Semin Derm 1990; 9:216–219.

24. Bilkis MR, Mark KA. Mind–body medicine: practical applications in dermatology. Arch Dermatol 1998; 134:1437–1441.

25. Hughes HH, England R, Goldsmith DA. Biofeedback and psychotherapeutic treatment of psoriasis: a brief report. Psychol Rep 1981; 48:99–102.

26. Winchell SA, Watts RA. Relaxation therapy in the treatment of psoriasis and possible pathophysiologic mechanisms. J Am Acad Dermatol 1988; 18:101–104.

27. Spiegel D. Healing words: emotional expression and disease outcome. JAMA 1999; 281:1328–1329.

28. Faulstitch ME, Williamson DA. An overview of atopic dermatitis toward a biobehavioral integration. J Psychosom Res 1985; 29:645–654.

29. Shenefelt PD. Hypnosis and dermatology. Arch Dermatol 2000; 136:393–399.

30. Spiegel H, Spiegel D. Trance and treatment: clinical uses of hypnosis. New York: Basic Books, 1978:35–78.

31. Spanos NP, Williams V, Gwynn MI. Effects of hypnotic, placebo, and salicylic acid treatments on wart regression. Psychosom Med 1990; 52:109–114.

32. Ewin DM. Hypnotherapy for warts (verruca vulgaris): 41 consecutive cases with 33 cures. Am J Clin Hypn 1992; 35:110.

33. Noll RB. Hypnotherapy for warts in children and adolescents. J Dev Behv Pediatr 1994; 15:170–173.

34. Koblenzer CS. Psychocutaneous Disease. 1987; Grune & Stratton Orlando FL.

35. Koblenzer CS. Cutaneous manifestations of psychiatric disease that commonly present to the dermatologist: diagnosis and treatment. Int J Psychiatry Med, 1992; 22:47–63.

36. Brown HE, Bettley FR. Psychiatric treatment of eczema: a controlled trial. Br Med J 1971; 2:729–734.

37. Koo Jym, Gabla C. Cutaneous sensory disorder. Dermatol Clin 1996; 14:497–502.

38. Spiegel D, Bloom JR, Kraemer HC, Gottheil E. Effect of psychosocial treatment on survival of patients with metastatic breast cancer. Lancet 1989; ii:888–891.

39. Kabat-Zinn J, Wheeler E, Light T, et al. Influence of a mindfulness meditation-based stress reduction intervention on rates of skin clearing in patients with moderate to severe psoriasis undergoing phototherapy (UVB) and photo-chemotherapy (PUVA). Psychosom Med 1998; 6:635–632.

40. Spiegel D, Sephton SE, Terr AL, Stites DP. Effects of psychosocial treatment in prolonging cancer survival may be mediated by auroaimmuameuroimmune pathways. Ann NY Acad Sci 1998; 840:674–683.
41. Fawzy FI, Fawzy NW, Hyun CS, et al. Malignant melanoma. Effects of an early structured psychiatric intervention, coping and effective state on recurrence and survival six years later. Arch Gen Psychiatry 1993; 50:681–689.
42. Roberts AH, Kewman DG, Mercier L, Hovell M. The power of non-specific effects in healing: implications for psychosocial and biological treatments. Clin Psychol Rev 1993; 12:375–391.
43. Stewart, AC, Thomas SE. Hypnotherapy as a treatment for atopic dermatitis in adults and children. Br J Dermatol 1995; 132:778–783.
44. Schertzer CL, Lookingbill DP. Effects of relaxation therapy and hypnotizability in chronic urticaria. Arch Dermatol 1987; 123:913–916.
45. Spiegel D. Healing words, emotional expression and disease outcome. JAMA 1999; 281:1328–1329.

28

The Use of Psychotropic Medications in Dermatology

Chai Sue Lee

Henry Ford Hospital
Detroit, Michigan, U.S.A.

John Y. M. Koo

University of California, San Francisco
San Francisco, California, U.S.A.

INTRODUCTION

Although the idea of using psychotropic medications may seem foreign to many dermatologists since dermatology as a specialty has had very limited exposure to psychopharmacotherapy, our opinion is that psychodermatological patients who refuse to be treated by a psychiatrist can still be greatly helped by a dermatologist who has an adequate knowledge base and the experience to prescribe psychotropic medications, especially when the alternative is for these problems to be left unattended.

There are certain situations in which it is not in the best interest of the patient for a dermatologist to attempt treatment alone. Some examples include suicidal or homicidal cases, if the dermatologist decides that the psychopathology involved is clearly beyond his or her capacity to analyze or treat, if the psychopathology is escalating despite the dermatologist's best efforts, and if the patient shows no improvement despite the dermatologist's best efforts to address the psychosocial aspect of the case. Fortunately, a large segment of psychodermatological cases are not so seriously mentally disturbed that they cannot be helped safely and effectively in a nonpsychiatric setting.

Because so many different types of conditions lie between the fields of psychiatry and dermatology, it is helpful to have classification systems that will help the clinician understand what he or she is dealing with. In Chapter 1, two clinically useful ways to classify psychodermatological cases were discussed in detail: first, by the category of psychodermatological condition, and second, by the nature of the underlying psychopathological condition. It is important to make the distinction between these categories and the underlying nature of the psychopathological condition because these distinctions help guide physicians to select the optimal approach to patients. Moreover, if a dermatologist seriously considers the challenge of treating these patients with psychopharmacological agents, the selection of appropriate agents is generally dictated by the nature of the underlying psychopathologies that need to be treated. The pharmacological treatment for the major types of psychopathological conditions encountered in a dermatology practice (anxiety, depression, delusion, and obsession-compulsion) are discussed in this chapter. The drugs discussed in this chapter pertinent to each of these diagnostic categories are listed in Table 1. A dermatologist can enhance his therapeutic armamentarium by becoming familiar with the use of selected psychotropic medications in each class of medications.

PHARMACOTHERAPY OF ANXIETY DISORDER IN DERMATOLOGY

In general, psychodermatological cases involving anxiety can be divided into two groups: acute versus chronic anxiety. The acute and time-limited episodes of anxiety usually involve a specific situational stress, such as increasing demands at work, interpersonal difficulties, or a financial crisis. Unlike patients with chronic anxiety, many of these patients with acute situational anxiety have a good premorbid functional level in society and adequate coping skills. They usually recover from the crisis after a few weeks. However, this period of stress can be long enough to exacerbate their skin disorder. The use of an antianxiety medication (Table 2) may be indicated short term to avert a flare of their psychodermatological condition, especially if the nonpharmacological measures are either not

TABLE 1 Psychotropic Agents

Generic name	Trade name
Anxiolytic medications	
Alprazolam	Xanax
Buspirone	BuSpar
Antidepressant medications	
Doxepin	Sinequan
Fluoxetine	Prozac
Paroxetine	Paxil
Sertraline	Zoloft
Citalopram	Celexa
Venlafaxine	Effexor
Nefazodone	Serzone
Bupropion	Wellbutrin
Antipsychotic medications	
Pimozide	Orap
Risperidone	Risperdal
Olanzapine	Zyprexa
Quetiapine	Seroquel
Anti–obsessive-compulsive medications	
Fluoxetine	Prozac
Paroxetine	Paxil
Sertraline	Zoloft
Fluvoxamine	Luvox
Citalopram	Celexa

Source: Ref. 48.

TABLE 2 Pharmacological Profile of Anxiolytic Medications

Drug	Brand name	Drug category	Preparations	Recommended dosage
Alprazolam	Xanax	Benzodiazepine	Tablet: 0.25, 0.5, 1, 2 mg	0.25–0.5 mg qd-qid prn
Buspirone	BuSpar	Nonbenzodiazepine	Table t: 5, 10 mg Dividose tablet: 15, 30 mg (scored to be easily bisected or trisected)	Begin with 15 mg "dividose" daily (7.5 mg po bid), usual effective dose 30 mg/day, max 60 mg/day

Source: Adapted from The 2002 Tarascon Pocket Pharmacopoeia.

TABLE 3 Key Pharmacological Concepts—Anxiolytic Medications

Drug	Absorption and bioavailability			Elimination		
	Peak levels	Bioavailable	Protein binding	Half-life	Metabolism	Excretion
Alprazolam	1–2 hr	—	80%	12–15 hr	Hepatic, active metabolite is alpha-hydroxy-alprazolam	Primarily renal
Buspirone	40–90 min	90%	86%	2–3 hr	Hepatic CYP3A4, active metabolite is 1-pyrimidinylpiperazine	Renal 29–63%, fecal 18–38%

Source: Ref. 48.

feasible or not adequate to control the patient's anxiety. Table 3 lists key pharmacological concepts for anxiolytic medications.

For the treatment of acute and self-limited stress, an antianxiety agent with a quick onset of action is indicated. Benzodiazepines take effect immediately and can almost always relieve anxiety if given in adequate doses. Alprazolam (Xanax) is a prototypical quick-acting benzodiazepine that is used to treat anxiety. Usually a half or a whole 0.5 mg tablet four times daily on an "as-needed" basis provides quick relief of acute anxiety for most patients. Because of the potential risk of addiction with long-term use, the physician should try to limit the duration of the treatment to no more than 3–4 weeks. When the therapeutic course is complete, alprazolam should be tapered rather than stopped "cold turkey" to prevent withdrawal. For short-term usage, sedation is usually the only adverse effect encountered, and this can easily be controlled by dosage adjustment.

Buspirone (BuSpar) may be a safer choice for long-term use for the treatment of anxiety because it is nonsedating and is not addicting. The major drawback of this medication is that its onset of action may be delayed for 2–4 weeks so that it cannot be used on an as needed basis. Therefore, buspirone is not useful for the treatment of acute anxiety because the therapeutic effect may not become evident until after the stressful event has resolved. The usual dosage of buspirone ranges from 7.5 to 30 mg twice daily. Buspirone is generally well tolerated. Most patients experience no side effects. Patients who have been previously treated with benzodiazepines or who have a history of substance abuse appear to have a decreased response to buspirone because it lacks the euphoria, sedation, and immediate action these patients may have come to expect with anxiety relief.

Antidepressants like paroxetine (Paxil) and extended-release venlafaxine (Effexor XR) are also used for the treatment of chronic anxiety. Rocca et al. (1) compared paroxetine, imipramine, and a standard benzodiazepine in the treatment of generalized anxiety disorder (GAD) in an open-label study. During the first 2 weeks of the study, the group receiving the benzodiazepine showed the greatest improvement; however, from the fourth week forward, the paroxetine and imipramine groups demonstrated superior improvement. Venlafaxine XR 225 mg/day was significantly more effective than placebo as measured on the Hamilton Rating Scale for Anxiety and the Clinical Global Impressions-Severity in an 8-week randomized, placebo-controlled study in 377 patients who met criteria for GAD without comorbid depression (2). Entsuah et al. (3) found 75 and 150 mg/day of venlafaxine XR to be significantly better than placebo or buspirone 30 mg/day on the Hospital Anxiety and Depression Scale, a patient-rated scale.

PHARMACOTHERAPY OF DEPRESSION IN DERMATOLOGY

There are many antidepressant agents to choose from. All antidepressants have been shown to have equivalent efficacy, with 60–80% of patients responding adequately. However, there is no sure way of predicting which patients will respond to a specific antidepressant based on clinical presentation. The selective serotonin-reuptake inhibitors (SSRIs) are commonly used as first-line agents for depression because they are generally better tolerated than the other antidepressants such as tricyclic antidepressants (TCAs) or monoamine oxidase inhibitors (MAOIs). Probably the only TCA still worth considering as a possible first-line antidepressant in dermatology is doxepin because of its combined antipruritic and antidepressant effects.

SSRI Antidepressants

The SSRIs include fluoxetine (Prozac), paroxetine (Paxil), sertraline (Zoloft), fluvoxamine (Luvox), and citalopram (Celexa). Fluvoxamine is FDA approved for obsessive-compulsive disorder in children and adults but is just as effective as the other SSRIs for depression. However, many drug interactions with cytochrome P450–metabolized medications have been reported with fluvoxamine. Therefore, it is not commonly used to treat depression because the other SSRIs are just as effective. The dosing guidelines of SSRIs and their key pharmacological concepts are listed in Tables 4 and 5. Table 6 lists drug interactions for SSRI antidepressants.

The side-effect profiles of the SSRIs are more alike than different. Gastrointestinal effects, such as nausea and diarrhea, are the most common side effects. Giving the medication with food often alleviates the nausea. Nausea usually improves after several days. Insomnia may occur with any of

TABLE 4 Pharmacological Profile of SSRIs

Drug	Brand name	FDA-approved indications	Preparations	Recommended dosage
Fluoxetine	Prozac	Depression and OCD	Capsule: 10, 20, 40 mg Tablet: 10, 20 mg Solution: 20 mg/5 mL	Begin with 20 mg qam, increase dose by 20 mg/day each month in partial responders, usual effective dose 20–40 mg/day, max 80 mg/day
Paroxetine	Paxil	Depression and OCD	Tablet: 10, 20, 30, 40 mg Solution: 10 mg/5 mL	Depression: begin with 20 mg qam, increase dose by 10–20 mg/day each month in partial responders, usual effective dose 20–50 mg/day, max 50 mg/day OCD: begin with 10–20 mg/day, usual effective dose 10–60 mg/day, max 60 mg/day
Sertraline	Zoloft	Depression and OCD	Tablet: 25, 50, 100 mg Solution: 20 mg/mL	Begin with 50 mg qd, increase dose by 50 mg/day each month in partial responders, usual effective dose 50–200 mg/day, max 200 mg/day
Fluvoxamine	Luvox	OCD	Tablet: 25, 50, 100 mg	Begin with 50 mg qhs, usual effective dose 100–300 mg/day divided bid, max 300 mg/day OCD in children age 8–17: begin with 25 mg qhs, usual effective dose 50–200 mg/day divided bid, max 200 mg/day
Citalopram	Celexa	Depression and OCD	Table t: 10, 20, 40 mg Solution: 10 mg/5 mL	Begin with 20 mg qd, max 60 mg/day

Source: Adapted from The 2002 Tarascon Pocket Pharmacopoeia.

TABLE 5 Key Pharmacological Concepts—Selective Serotonin Reuptake Inhibitors

Drug	Absorption and bioavailability			Elimination		
	Peak levels	Bioavailable	Protein binding	Half-life	Metabolism	Excretion
Fluoxetine	6–8 hr	N/A	94.5%	1–3 days after acute administration and 4–6 days after chronic administration; norfluoxetine 4–16 days	Hepatic	Renal
Paroxetine	5.2 hr	N/A	93–95%	21 hr	Hepatic	Renal 64%, fecal 36%
Sertraline	4.5–8.4 hr	N/A	98%	26 hr	Hepatic	Renal 40–45%, fecal 40–45%
Fluvoxamine	3–8 hr	53%	80%	15.6 hr	Hepatic	Renal 94%
Citalopram	4 hr	80%	80%	35 hr	Hepatic	Renal 20%

Source: Ref. 48.

the SSRIs, but it is more common with fluoxetine. The SSRI should be given in the morning if insomnia occurs. Sedation can occur with paroxetine or fluvoxamine. If sedation occurs, the medication should be given at bedtime. The SSRIs can be associated with sexual dysfunctions, most commonly involving difficulties with orgasm. When sexual side effects occur, switching to another class of antidepressants that causes less sexual dysfunctions than the SSRIs, such as nefazodone or bupropion, is recommended.

Like other antidepressant treatments, full clinical response to SSRIs is gradual. The onset of response to SSRIs usually begins about 2–3 weeks after the optimal therapeutic dosage is reached, and 4–6 weeks is required before the full therapeutic effect is apparent. There is no linear relationship between SSRI dose and response. For partial responders, however, the dosage may be increased to maximize therapeutic effect. The lack of response to one SSRI or inability to tolerate one SSRI is not predictive of the same reaction to another SSRI. Patients showing no improvement after 6 weeks of SSRI treatment at the usual effective dose should switch to another SSRI or to another class of antidepressant (i.e., nefazodone, venlafaxine, bupropion).

On discontinuation, some patients may experience dizziness, lethargy, nausea, irritability, and headaches. These symptoms can be prevented by slowly tapering the medication over several weeks when discontinuing the drug.

Tables 7 and 8 list additional antidepressant medications and their key pharmacological concepts.

TABLE 6   Drug Interactions—SSRI Antidepressants

Interacting drug group	Examples and comments
These Drugs May Increase Serum Levels (and Potential Toxicity) of Various SSRI Antidepressants	
Antidepressants—MAO inhibitors	Serious reactions occurred when various SSRIs used concurrently
Azole antifungal agents	Particularly ketoconazole (also itraconazole) may increase citalopram levels
H_2 antihistamines	Cimetidine may increase paroxetine and sertraline levels
Macrolide antibacterial agents	Erythromycin coadministration may increase citalopram levels
Other drugs	L-Tryptophan (fluoxetine, fluvoxamine, paroxetine), dextromethorphan (fluoxetine) increase drug levels
These Drugs May Decrease Serum Levels of Various SSRI Antidepressants	
Anticonvulsants	Phenytoin and phenobarbital both may decrease paroxetine levels
SSRI Antidepressants May Increase Drug Levels (and Potential Toxicity) of These Drugs	
Anticoagulants	Warfarin activity may be potentiated by all SSRIs
Anticonvulsants	Carbamazepine levels increased by fluoxetine, fluvoxamine, and citalopram
Antidepressants—tricyclic, other	Tricyclic antidepressants (by all SSRIs), buspirone by fluoxetine
Antipsychotic agents	Clozapine and haloperidol levels increased by fluvoxamine and fluoxetine; pimozide levels increased by fluoxetine
Benzodiazepines	Risk probably greatest with alprazolam in combination with SSRIs
Beta-blockers	Most noteworthy is fluvoxamine or citalopram effect on propranolol and metoprolol levels
Bronchodilators	Theophylline clearance may be decreased by up to threefold with fluvoxamine and paroxetine coadministration
Calcium channel blockers	Diltiazem and fluvoxamine concurrent use may induce a bradycardia
Lithium	Both increased and decreased levels reported with various SSRIs
Other drugs	Digoxin, methadone, sumatriptan, tolbutamide
Other Potentially Important Drug Interactions	
Alcohol	No clear-cut interaction proven; however, concurrent use is discouraged
Alternative medical therapies	Concurrent use with St. John's wort may increase sedative-hypnotic effects
Smoking	Smoking significantly increases fluvoxamine metabolism

Source: Ref. 48.

TABLE 7 Pharmacological Profile of Antidepressant Medications

Drug	Brand name	Therapeutic category	Preparations	Dosage
Nefazodone	Serzone	Serotonin antagonist and reuptake inhibitor	Tablet: 50, 100, 150, 200, 250 mg	Begin with 100 mg bid, increase dose after several days to weeks by 50–100 mg/day in partial responders, usual effective dose 150–300 bid, max 600 mg/day
Venlafaxine	Effexor, Effexor XR	Serotonin-norepinephrine reuptake inhibitor	Immediate-release tablet: 25, 37.5, 50, 75, 100 mg; Extended-release capsule: 37.5, 75, 150 mg	Immediate-release: 75 mg/day divided bid-tid, usual effective dose 150–225 mg/day, max 375 mg/day; Extended-release: begin with 37.5–75 mg qd, max 225 mg/day
Bupropion[a]	Wellbutrin, Wellbutrin SR	Norepinephrine-dopamine reuptake inhibitors	Regular release tablet: 75, 100 mg; Sustained-release tablet: 100, 150 mg	Regular Release: begin with 100 mg bid, after 4–7 days can increase to 100 mg tid, usual effective dose 300–450 mg/day, max 150 mg/dose and 450 mg/day; Sustained-release: begin with 100–150 mg qam, after 4–7 days may increase to 150 mg bid, max 400 max/day; allow 8 h between doses, with last dose no later than 5 p.m.

[a]Contraindicated with seizures, bulimia, anorexia. Seizures in 0.4% at 300–450 mg/day.
Source: Adapted from The 2002 Tarascon Pocket Pharmacopoeia.

TABLE 8 Key Pharmacological Concepts—Antidepressant Medications

	Absorption and bioavailability			Elimination		
Drug	Peak levels	Bioavailable	Protein binding	Half-life	Metabolism	Excretion
Doxepin	1–4 hr	13–45%	80–85%	28–52 hr[a]	Hepatic; active metabolite is desmethyldoxepin	Renal
Amitriptyline	1–4 hr	30–60%	90–97%	9–25 hr	Hepatic; active metabolite is nortriptyline	Primarily renal
Bupropion	2 hr	N/A in humans; in animals (rats and dogs) 5–20%	85%	Initial 1.5 hr Second 14 hr	Hepatic; active metabolites are hydroxybupropion, threo-hydrobupropion, erythro-hydrobupropion	Renal 87%
Venlafaxine	Parent 2 hr Metabolite 4 hr	N/A	Parent 25–30% Metabolite 18–42%	Parent 3–5 hr Metabolite 9–11 hr	Hepatic CYP 2D6; active metabolite is O-desmethyl-venlafaxine	Renal 87%
Nefazodone	1 hr	20%	>99%	2–4 hr	Hepatic; active metabolites are hydroxynefazodone, metachlorophenyl-piperazine, and triazoledione	Renal 55%, fecal 20–30%

[a]Half-life of doxepin major metabolite.
Source: Ref. 48.

Nefazodone

Nefazodone (Serzone) has been shown to have the same efficacy as the SSRIs in the treatment of depression. However, it has little to no effect on sexual functioning. Nafazodone is different from the other antidepressants because of its dual actions on the serotonin system. It is a selective serotonin (5-HT2A) receptor antagonist, as well as a serotonin-reuptake inhibitor of moderate potency. In general, it is a well-tolerated medication. The most common side effects are nausea, dry mouth, dizziness, sedation, agitation, constipation, weight loss, and headaches.

Venlafaxine

It has been recognized for many years that most antidepressants are potent reuptake-blocking agents for noradrenergic or serotonergic receptors. Previously in clinical practice, when a particular case of depression proved unresponsive to a norepinephrine-reuptake inhibitor, the patient was tried on medication that preferentially blocks the reuptake of neurotransmitters in the serotonergic system and vice versa. Venlafaxine (Effexor) is a novel antidepressant that is believed to act by selectively inhibiting both norepinephrine and serotonin reuptake with little effect on other neuro-transmitter systems (4). Its efficacy appears to be comparable to that of the SSRIs.

Venlafaxine has a relatively benign side effect profile. The most common side effects are insomnia and nervousness. Nausea, sedation, fatigue, sweating, dizziness, headache, loss of appetite, constipation, and dry mouth are also common. Sexual dysfunction occurs in approximately 10% of patients (4). Seizures occur in 0.3% of patients (4). Venlafaxine has been reported to cause hypertension in about 3–13% of patients and appears to be dose related (4). Blood pressure should be monitored during venlafaxine therapy. Venlafaxine can produce dizziness, insomnia, dry mouth, nausea, nervousness, and sweating with abrupt discontinuation. Consequently, it should be slowly tapered over several weeks.

Bupropion

Bupropion (Wellbutrin) has been shown to be as effective as the SSRIs in the treatment of depression. However, it is associated with less sexual dysfunction than the SSRIs. Bupropion is a relatively weak inhibitor of dopamine reuptake, with modest effects on norepinephrine reuptake and no effect on serotonin reuptake (5).

In general, bupropion is a well-tolerated medication. The most common side effects are insomnia, agitation, headache, constipation, dry mouth, nausea, and tremor. A rare but serious side effect of bupropion is seizure induction. The incidence of seizures in patients receiving buproprion at therapeutic doss of 450 mg/day or less range from 0.33 to 0.44% (6). Bupropion should not be used in patients with a history of seizure or with conditions, such as bulimia, that may potentially lower the seizure threshold. This medication should be avoided in drug or alcohol abusers.

Doxepin

The tricyclic antidepressant (TCA) doxepin (Sinequan) is probably the ideal agent for the treatment of depressed patients with neurotic excoriations. In addition to its antidepressant effect, doxepin has a strong antiprurituc effect because it is a very powerful H1 antihistamine. To stop the excoriating behavior, it is important to treat the patient's depression and to put an end to the itch/scratch cycle. Moreover, the majority of depressed patients who present with excoriations appear to be suffering from an agitated depression in which the patient parodoxically becomes more restless, angry, and argumentative when depressed. For these patients, the most common side effect of doxepin, sedation, can actually be therapeutic.

The usual starting dosage of doxepin for depression is 25 mg at bedtime. The dosage can be titrated with 25 mg increments every 5–7 days, as tolerated, up to the usual therapeutic range for depression, which is anywhere from 100 to 300 mg. In general, it takes at least 2 weeks after the therapeutic dosage is reached before the antidepressant effect can be observed. Some patients may require 6–8 weeks of treatment before responding. However, the other therapeutic effects of doxepin, such as the antipruritic effect, analgesic effect, and effects in calming the patient down and improving insomnia, generally occur immediately. If a patient is showing no response despite taking a large dose of doxepin for several weeks, it may be helpful to check a serum doxepin level to see if it is within the therapeutic range for depression. There can be an up to 20-fold difference in serum blood levels among individuals who are taking the same dose of doxepin (7). Table 9 lists drug interactions for tricyclic antidepressants.

The most common side effect of doxepin is sedation. The sedative side effect can usually be avoided by taking it at bedtime. More persistent sedation may require lowering the dose or changing the time of administration of doxepin. For example, if the patient complains of difficulty waking up in the morning, this can usually be overcome by taking doxepin earlier than bedtime or by dividing the dose so that the patient takes some of the dose when he or she gets home and takes the rest at least 1–2 hours before bedtime. This way the patient is less likely to experience excessively high "peak" serum level and the resultant sedation the next morning. The other side effects of doxepin are similar to those of other older TCAs, including cardiac conduction disturbances, weight gain, orthostatic hypotension, and anticholinergic side effects such as dry mouth, blurry vision, constipation, and urinary retention. TCAs may slow cardiac conduction, resulting in intraventricular conduction delay, prolongation of the QT interval, and AV block. Therefore, TCAs are contraindicated in patients with preexisting conduction defects, arrhythmias, or recent myocardial infarction (MI). A pretreatment electrocardiogram (EKG) is recommended to rule out the presence of prolonged QT for older patients or any patient with a history of cardiac conduction disturbance. In addition, an EKG should be repeated to rule out dysrhythmia if doxepin is used in dosages of 100 mg daily or higher. Doxepin should also be used with caution in patients with a history of seizure disorder or manic-depressive disorder because it can lower the seizure threshold and precipitate a manic episode. Because of the possibility of suicide with an overdose of TCA, it is good practice for clinicians to see these types of patients frequently, such as on a

TABLE 9 Drug Interactions—Tricyclic Antidepressants

Interacting drug group	Examples and comments
These Drugs May Increase Serum Levels (and Potential Toxicity) of Tricyclic Antidepressants	
Anticonvulsants	Valproic acid
Antidepressants—other	Bupropion (various tricyclics), venlafaxine (desipramine)
Antipsychotic agents	Haloperidol may increase levels of tricyclic antidepressants
H_2 antihistamines	Cimetidine may significantly increase levels; no interaction with other H_2 blockers
MAO inhibitors	Concurrent therapy may induce a hyperpyretic crisis with CNS and cardiovascular complications as well
SSRI antidepressants	Various SSRIs, especially fluvoxamine (Luvox)
These Drugs May Decrease Serum Levels of Tricyclic Antidepressants—CYP Inducers	
Anticonvulsants	Carbamazepine, phenobarbital both may decrease tricyclic levels and efficacy
Charcoal[a]	Administration may reduce tricyclic toxicity in an overdose
Rifamycins	Rifampin and rifabutin with similar effect due to enzyme induction
Tricyclic Antidepressants May Increase Drug Levels (and Potential Toxicity) of These Drugs	
Antiadrenergic agents	Clonidine
Anticholinergic agents	Various
Anticoagulants	Dicumarol
Anticonvulsants	Carbamazepine
Fluoroquinolones	Grepafloxacin, sparfloxacin (torsades de pointes—life threatening)
Tricyclic Antidepressants Decrease Drug Levels of These Drugs	
Antiparkinson therapy	Levodopa absorption delayed and bioavailability decreased; may result in hypertensive crisis
Sympathomimetic agents	Various

[a]Charcoal reduces tricyclic levels but is not a CYP inducer.
Source: Ref 48.

weekly basis, so that one can not only closely monitor the patient and titrate the dosage but also avoid giving the patient a large supply of doxepin at one time.

Abrupt discontinuation of TCA may lead to transient dizziness, nausea, headache, diaphoresis, insomnia, and malaise. Consequently, they should be tapered gradually over several weeks after prolonged treatment with TCA. Slow taper also decreases the likelihood of relapse of depressive symptoms.

PHARMACOLOGICAL MANAGEMENT OF PSYCHOTIC DISORDERS IN DERMATOLOGY

The type of psychotic patients most often seen by a dermatologist are those with monosymptomatic hypochondriacal psychosis (MHP). Patients with MHP are psychologically "normal" in every way except for the presence of an "encapsulated" delusional ideation that revolves around one particular hypochondriac concern and, possibly, hallucinatory experiences that are compatible with the delusion (8–10). For example, many patients with delusions of parasitosis also experience formication, which is manifested as cutaneous sensations of crawling, biting, and stinging. MHP is very different from schizophrenia, in which in addition to the delusional ideation, patients have other psychological disturbances.

Tables 10 and 11 list antipsychotic medications and their key pharmacological concepts.

Pimozide

The most common type of MHP seen by dermatologists is delusions of parasitosis. The treatment of choice for delusions of parasitosis is the antipsychotic medication pimozide (Orap) (11–13). Pimozide is marketed in the United States for the treatment of Tourette's disorder, but it is widely used in some European countries in the treatment of schizophrenia.

Careful titration of pimozide dosage is the key to safe use of this medication. Because of the possibility of extrapyramidal side effects, such as stiffness and restlessness, patients should start at a low initial dose of 1 mg daily. The dosage of pimozide can be increased gradually by 1 mg increments every 4–7 days until the optimal clinical response is attained. Most patients experience significant improvement in delusional preoccupation, agitation, and formication by the time the dosage of 4–6 mg/day is reached. Trying to push the dosage of pimozide beyond the 4–6 mg/day range may increase the risk of side effects.

TABLE 10   Pharmacological Profile of Antipsychotics

Drug	Brand name	Preparations	Recommended dosage
Pimozide	Orap	Tablet: 2 mg (scored)	Begin with 1 mg qd, increase by 1 mg every 4–7 days to usual effective dose 1–6 mg/day
Risperidone	Risperdal	Tablet: 0.25, 0.5, 1, 2, 3, 4 mg Solution: 1 mg/mL	Begin with 1 mg bid (0.5 mg/dose in the elderly), slowly increase every 5–7 days to usual effective dose of 4–8 mg/day divided qd-bid, max 16 mg/day
Olanzapine	Zyprexa	Tablet: 2.5, 5, 7.5, 10, 15 mg	Begin with 5–10 mg qd, usual effective dose 10–15 mg/day, max dose 20 mg/day
Quetiapine[a]	Seroquel	Tablet: 25, 100, 200 mg	Begin with 25 mg bid, increase by 25–50 mg every 2–3 days to usual effective dose 150–750 mg/day, max 800 mg/day

[a]Eye exam for cataracts needed every 6 months.
Source: Adapted from The 2002 Tarascon Pocket Pharmacopoeia.

Once the patient shows improvement in his or her clinical state and becomes nondelusional or "quietly delusional," where the delusion or formication no longer significantly interferes with the capacity to work or enjoy life, this clinically effective dosage is maintained for at least 1 month. If the patient persists in his or her improvement, then the dosage of pimozide can be gradually decreased by 1 mg decrements every 1–2 weeks until either the minimum effective dosage is determined or the patient is successfully tapered off pimozide altogether. If the clinical state deteriorates in the future with a new episode of increased mental preoccupation with parasites and formication, the patient can be restarted on pimozide and treated in a time-limited fashion to control that particular episode. Long-term use of pimozide is best avoided to minimize the risk of tardive dyskinesia developing in these patients. Tardive dyskinesia, which consists of abnormal involuntary choreoathetoid movements of muscles of the head, trunk, and extremities, is the most worrisome adverse effect of pimozide, as it may be irreversible. Lindskov (14) reported a patient who had a "slight twitching of her lips" that "has been present since treatment." He never explicitly labeled this as tardive dyskinesia, and there was no follow-up.

TABLE 11 Key Pharmacological Concepts—Antipsychotic Medications

Drug	Absorption and bioavailability			Elimination		
	Peak levels	Bioavailable	Protein binding	Half-life	Metabolism	Excretion
Pimozide	6–8 hr	N/A	N/A	55 hr	Hepatic CYP3A	Primarily renal
Risperidone	1 hr	70%	90%	20 hr	Hepatic CYP2D6 active metabolite is 9-hydroxy resperidone	N/A
Olanzapine	6 hr	N/A	93%	21–54 hr	Hepatic	Renal 57%, fecal 30%
Quetiapine	1.5 hr	100%	83%	6 hr	Hepatic	Renal 73%, fecal 20%

Source: Ref. 48.

Driscoll et al. (15) later cited the case by Lindskov as "tardive dyskinesia," even though Lindskov himself never called it that. Although pimozide can cause tardive dyskinesia, we know of no reported case despite decades of use.

The most common side effects of pimozide are extrapyramidal symptoms such as stiffness and, less frequently, a subjective feeling of restlessness called akathisia. Even though only a minority of patients treated with pimozide experience any extrapyramidal side effects, it is advisable for the clinician to explain the possibility of developing such adverse effects and to write a prescription for either benztropine (Cogentin) 1–2 mg up to 4 times daily or diphenhydramine (Benadryl) 25 mg up to 3 times daily before starting pimozide. The advantage of benztropine over diphenhydramine is that the former agent is not sedating. As long as the extrapyramidal side effects can be controlled with one of the two medications as described, it is fine to continue with treatment with pimozide and even increase the dose until the optimal dosage is reached.

In Canada there have been undocumented reports of sudden unexpected deaths, presumably cardiac related, in schizophrenic patients receiving pimozide in dosages above 10 mg/day (16). Published European studies on the antipsychotic efficacy of pimozide have used dosages substantially higher than 10 mg/day and do not report any adverse cardiac effects (16). If you do not use dosages above 10 mg/day, EKG appears to be optional. As stated previously in this chapter, most patients with delusions of parasitosis experience significant improvement by the time the dose of 4–6 mg/day is reached. We generally do not recommend going beyond the 4–6 mg/day range since the risk of side effects may increase.

The most challenging aspect of managing patients with delusions of parasitosis or any other cases of MHP is to convince delusional patients to take pimozide. Truly delusional patients have little or no insight regarding the psychogenic nature of their condition and therefore are vehemently opposed to even the slightest suggestion that their condition may be psychological. Moreover, if MHP patients previously had negative experiences in their encounters with other physicians, they may be defensive and hostile. Because the question "How do you get someone with delusions of parasitosis to take pimozide?" is one of the most frequently asked questions in psychodermatology, one particular approach is presented here, providing a reference point to be utilized by other clinicians.

The first step in trying to manage patients with delusions of parasitosis successfully is to establish rapport with the patient. In trying to achieve this, it is important to recognize that the patient with delusions of parasitosis is expecting the clinician to treat him or her as having a bona fide skin disease, not as a psychiatric case. Therefore, the most effective approach may be not to spend a long time talking to the patient about psychological issues, but instead to take his or her chief complaint seriously. A careful and complete skin examination is critical not only in ruling out the presence of a true dermatological diagnosis but also to demonstrate to the patient that his or her concerns are being taken seriously. If the patient brings in various specimens as proof of "infestation," it is important to at least look at them, once again to demonstrate to the patient that his or her concerns are being taken seriously. At the same time, it is important to avoid any statement that may inadvertently reinforce the patient's delusional ideation, such as a comment that some type of organism responsible for his or her condition was found. Delusional patients are much more difficult to deal with if they believe that a clinician agrees with them about the delusion.

The process of establishing therapeutic rapport may take several visits. Once the clinician senses that a reasonable working relationship has developed between them, a therapeutic trial of pimozide can be gently introduced. There are many different ways to introduce pimozide. Even when these patients develop some trust in the dermatologist, if the dermatologist presents pimozide bluntly and tactlessly as an antipsychotic medication, they will most likely refuse the medication. In addition, the dermatologist might have irrevocably damaged the therapeutic rapport in that setting. A more pragmatic approach would be to present pimozide as a medication that can help the patient by decreasing the crawling, biting, and stinging sensations, agitation, and mental preoccupation. Once patients start taking pimozide, they usually experience significant symptomatic relief, and this improvement can work as a further incentive for them to continue with the medication.

Atypical Antipsychotic Agents

The use of pimozide and other traditional antipsychotic medications has been limited by serious side effects, most notably extrapyramidal side effects (EPS) and tardive dyskinesia (TD). A new generation of antipsychotic agents referred to as "atypical" antipsychotics has entered clinical practice; they are as effective as conventional agents, such as pimozide, yet better tolerated with a significantly lower incidence of EPS and TD as well as less sedation and less weight gain (17,18). Three atypical antipsychotic medications are now the most prescribed agents for the treatment of psychosis: risperidone (Risperdal), olanzapine (Zyprexa), and quetiapine (Seroquel). These atypical antipsychotics are both dopamine (D_2) and serotonin ($5HT_2$) receptor antagonists. Atypical antipsychotics have greatly reduced the risk for side effects such as EPS and TD because they are much more selective in binding to these receptors, which are thought to be related to antipsychotic effects but not to other receptors related to side effects (18–22). None of these newer agents have been compared to one another in head-to-head clinical trials. In addition, studies comparing pimozide with the newer atypical antipsychotics in the treatment of delusions of parasitosis and other MHP have not yet been done. More research is needed to place these new drugs into clinical perspective.

Differing side effect profiles may guide use of a particular agent for an individual patient. The *Physicians' Desk Reference* (23) and package inserts suggest that atypical antipsychotics should be used with caution in patients with a history of seizures or with conditions such as Alzheimer's disease that potentially lower the seizure threshold. During premarketing testing, seizures occurred in 9 (0.3%) of 2607 risperidone-treated patients, 22 (0.9%) of 2500 olanzapine-treated patients, and 18 (0.8%) of 2387 quetiapine-treated patients (23).

Risperidone

Risperidone (Risperdal) has been administered to over 1 million patients during its postmarketing period, and it appears to be generally well tolerated at therapeutic doses. The most common side effects are anxiety, dizziness, and rhinitis. Dose-related side effects include sedation, fatigue, and accommodation disturbance. Risperidone is known to prolong the QT interval and should be used with caution in patients with abnormal baseline QT intervals or those taking other medications that can prolong the QT interval (e.g., antiarrhythmics such as quinidine or procainamide). At a dose of 6 mg/day or less, risperidone-induced EPS are often negligible, but their incidence rises with higher doses (24,25). As the only currently available atypical antipsychotic with minimal anticholinergic effects (e.g., dry mouth, blurry vision, urinary hesitation, and constipation), risperidone may be considered the agent of choice for the elderly (26,27).

Olanzapine

Olanzapine (Zyprexa) is generally well tolerated with a very low incidence of EPS. The most common side effects are sedation, anticholinergic effects, and weight gain.

Quetiapine

Quetiapine (Seroquel) is a novel antipsychotic drug belonging to a unique chemical class, the dibenzothiazepines. Like the other atypical antipsychotic drugs, it binds to both D_2 and $5HT_2$ receptors in the brain, with a higher affinity for the $5HT_2$ site. Quetiapine also blocks histamine H_1 and α_1-adrenergic receptors. Some patients who fail to respond to other atypical antipsychotics respond to quetiapine. The most common side effects are mild somnolence and mild anticholinergic effects. Quetiapine is associated more often with orthostatic hypotension than the other newer atypical antipsychotics but is usually manageable with careful dose adjustment, and patients frequently become partially or fully tolerant to it (28). Quetiapine does not seem to cause EPS (29–31).

Due to the concern over the development of cataracts in patients treated with quetiapine, the manufacturer recommends slit-lamp eye examinations at the initiation of therapy, shortly thereafter, and then every 6 months. This recommendation was made based on preclinical studies that showed an association between cataracts and the administration of quetiapine to dogs at four times the dose recommended for humans. However, the proportion of patients developing cataracts in Phase II and III trials was not significantly different from those treated with haloperidol (32).

MANAGEMENT OF OBSESSIVE-COMPULSIVE DISORDER IN DERMATOLOGY

There are many different manifestations of obsessive-compulsive disorder (OCD) or tendencies in dermatological practice. These include trichotillomania, onychotillomania, onychophagia, acne excoriée, and some cases of factitial dermatitis and neurodermatitis.

SSRI Antidepressants

In a dermatological setting, a pharmacological approach may be most feasible for patients who refuse to be referred to a psychiatrist. Currently, five SSRIs—fluoxetine (Prozac), paroxetine (Paxil), sertraline (Zoloft), fluvoxamine (Luvox), and citalopram (Celexa)—are the first-line treatment for OCD.

The choice of a particular SSRI depends primarily on the individual side effect profiles, although they are more alike than different (see previous section on SSRIs). Many clinicians find that patients with OCD often require higher doses of SSRIs and take longer to respond than when treating depression. In OCD, initial response to SSRIs can take 4–8 weeks, and maximal response may take as long as 20 weeks. After 6 weeks of therapy, the response should be assessed and the dose increased for patients with partial response. Complete remission is unusual. A 10- to 12-week trial with an SSRI at therapeutic dosage is the minimum necessary to confirm failure to respond. A failure to respond to one SSRI does not predict failure to respond to another (33). For nonresponders, a 10-week trial of a SSRI followed by a switch to another SSRI is the most recommended current practice if a psychiatric referral is not feasible. Therapy should be continued for at least 6 months to 1 year once a therapeutic response is achieved (34). Medications should be tapered slowly during discontinuation and should be restarted if symptoms worsen.

No matter which medication one chooses to use, it is important to tell the patient that these medications are not "magic bullets." They can be very helpful in overcoming one's obsessive thoughts or compulsive behaviors, but these medications are no substitute for the patient's own motivation to stop the destructive behavior. Therefore, patients should be encouraged to keep up their own efforts and vigilance in controlling their compulsive behavior while they undergo treatment with anti–obsessive-compulsive medications.

PSYCHOPHARMACOLOGICAL MEDICATIONS FOR TREATING PURELY DERMATOLOGICAL CONDITIONS

Certain psychopharmacological agents are known to be useful in treating purely dermatological conditions. The class of medications with the most well-documented analgesic effect is the older tertiary TCAs such as doxepin (Sinequan) and amitriptyline (Elavil) (35–40). If pruritus is the primary problem, doxepin is the preferred agent. On the other hand, if various manifestations of pain, such as burning, stinging, biting, or chafing, are the primary sensations, amitriptyline is the preferred agent.

Doxepin is frequently used to treat pruritus when more conventional antipruritic agents, such as diphenhydramine (Benadryl) or hydroxyzine (Atarax), prove inadequate. There are several advantages of using doxepin for the control of pruritus compared with the conventional antipruritic agents. First, doxepin has a much higher affinity for histamine receptors than do the traditional antihistamines and may therefore exert a much more powerful antipruritic effect. The affinity of doxepin for histamine (H_1) receptor in vitro is approximately 56 times that of hydroxyzine and 775 times that of diphenhydramine (41). Second, the therapeutic effect of doxepin is much longer-lasting than either of these H_1-antihistamine medications. Because of its long half-life, doxepin taken once per day, usually at bedtime, is adequate to provide therapeutic benefit for up to 24 hours. Therefore, patients with severely pruritic conditions, such as atopic dermatitis, who complain of waking up in the middle of the night even if they respond to hydroxyzine or diphenhydramine taken at bedtime usually find that when they switch to doxepin, they can sleep through the night. Third, doxepin normalizes sleep curves. When the patient spends more time in a deeper state of sleep, the amount of nighttime excoriation often dramatically diminishes (42). Doxepin can also be helpful in treating patients with chronic urticaria or other disorders mediated by histamines who have failed treatment with traditional antihistamines (43,44). There are no good data regarding the optimal therapeutic blood level of doxepin for treatment of conditions such as pruritus or urticaria. A wide dosage range may be adequate depending on the individual patient. For example, the dosage of doxepin adequate for control of pruritus may range from as little as 10 mg nightly to as much as 300 mg nightly, which is the maximum recommended dose according to package insert. If a patient is not showing an initial desirable therapeutic response, the clinician should gradually titrate the doxepin dose upward as tolerated until the desired therapeutic response is seen.

Amitriptyline is one of the treatments of choice for postherpetic neuralgia. When TCAs are used as analgesics, the dosage required tends to be much less than the dosage required for its antidepressant effect. Therefore, when amitriptyline is used to treat postherpetic neuralgia, the effective dosage range is from 25 to 75 mg at bedtime, which is much less than the usual antidepressant dosage of 100 mg at bedtime or higher (35–37).

Even though the efficacy of TCAs as analgesics is most well established with the older TCAs such as doxepin or amitriptyline, these medications are also the most difficult TCAs to tolerate because they have the most problems with sedative, cardiac, anticholinergic, and α-adrenergic side effects, including orthostatic hypotension, which can be particularly problematic in elderly patients. These side effects can be minimized by the use of the lowest possible effective dose. If the patient cannot tolerate these agents, other TCAs, such as imipramine (Tofranil) or desipramine (Norpramin), may be used (45). The dosage range for these medications is very similar to that of amitryptyline in that the patient can be started at 25 mg at bedtime and titrated to the maximally effective dose. For use as an analgesic, a dosage of 100 mg/day or less should suffice. If the patient still cannot tolerate the newer TCAs, then an SSRI antidepressant, such as fluoxetine (Prozac), can be tried. There are some reports of SSRI antidepressant usefulness as analgesic agents (46,47).

CONCLUSION

In this chapter, relatively detailed explanations regarding the use of selected psychopharmacological agents were given along with their psychodermatological indications. For a more complete description regarding the use of these medications, the reader is advised to consult standard textbooks on psychopharmacology and the *Physicians' Desk Reference*. It should be emphasized that psychiatric consultation should be obtained whenever feasible. Yet for a significant proportion of patients who refuse psychiatric referral, the judicious use of these medications may still provide the much-needed assistance in the recovery from various psychodermatological disorders.

REFERENCES

1. Rocca P, Fonzo V, Scotta M, Zanalda E, Ravizza L. Paroxetine efficacy in the treatment of generalized anxiety disorder. Acta Psychiatr Scand 1997; 95:444–450.
2. Aguiar LM, Haskins T, Rudolph RL, et al. Double-blind placebo-controlled study of once-daily venlafaxine extended release in outpatients with GAD. In New Research Program and Abstracts of the Annual Meeting of the American Psychiatric Association; June 3, 1998; Toronto, Canada. NR643:241.
3. Entsuah R, Derivan AT, Haskins T, et al. Double-blind placebo-controlled study of once daily venlafaxine extended release and buspirone. In: New Research Program and Abstracts of the Annual Meeting of the American Psychiatric Association; June 3, 1998; Toronto, Canada, NR644:241.
4. Montgomery SA. Venlafaxine: a new dimension in antidepressant pharmacotherapy. J Clin Psychiatry 1993; 54:119–126.
5. Richelson E. Biological basis of depression and therapeutic relevance. J Clin Psychiatry 1991; 52(suppl):4–10.

6. Davidson J. Seizures and bupropion: a review. J Clin Psychiatry 1989; 50:256–261.

7. Friedel RO, Raskind MA. Relationship of blood levels of Sinequan to clinical effects in the treatment of depression in aged patients. In: Mendels J, ed. A Monograph of Recent Clinical Studies. Lawrenceville, NJ: Excerpta Medica, 1975.

8. Munro A. Monosymptomatic hypochondriacal psychosis. Br J Psychiatry 1988; 153(suppl):37–40.

9. Munro A, Chmars J. Monosymptomatic hypochondriacal psychosis: a diagnostic checklist based on 50 cases of the disorder. Can J Psychol 1982; 27:374–376.

10. Bishop ER Jr. Monosymptomatic hypochondriacal syndromes in dermatology. J Am Acad Dermatol 1983; 9:152–158.

11. Damiani JT, Flowers FP, Pierce DK. Pimozide in delusions of parasitosis. J Am Acad Dermatol 1990; 22(pt 1):312–313.

12. Hamann K, Avnstorp L. Delusions of infestation treated by pimozide: a double-blind crossover clinical study. Acta Derm Venereol (Stockh) 1982; 62:55–58.

13. Holmes VF. Treatment of monosymptomatic hypochondriacal psychosis with pimozide in an AIDS patient (lett). Am J Psychiatry 1989; 146(4):554–555.

14. Lindskov R. Delusions of infestations treated with pimozide. Acta Derm Venereol 1985; 65:267–270.

15. Driscoll MS, Rothe MJ, Grant-Kels JM, et al. Delusional parasitosis: a dermatologic, psychiatric and pharmacologic approach. JAAD 1993; 29:1023–1033.

16. Schatzberg AF, Cole JO, DeBattista C. Manual of Clinical Psychopharmacology. 3rd ed. Washington, DC: APA Press 1997, 154–155.

17. Stahl SM. Selecting an atypical antipsychotic by combining clinical experience with guidelines from clinical trials. J Clin Psychiatry 1999; 60(suppl 10):31–41.

18. Brown CS, Markowitz JS, Moore TR, Parker NG. Atypical antipsychotics: part II adverse effects, drug interactions and costs. Ann Pharmacother 1999; 33:210–217.

19. Meltzer HY. New drugs for the treatment of schizophrenia. Psychiatr Clin North Am 1993; 16:365–385.

20. Deutch AY, Moghaddam B, Innis RB, et al. Mechanisms of action of atypical antipsychotic drugs: implications for novel therapeutic strategies for schizophrenia. Schizophr Res 1991, 4:121–156.

21. Gerlach J. New antipsychotics: classifications, efficacy and adverse effects. Schizophr Bull 1991; 17:289–309.

22. Davis KL, Kahn RS, Ko G, et al. Dopamine in schizophrenia: a review and reconceptualization. Am J Psychiatry 1991; 148:1474–1486.

23. Physicians' Desk Reference. Montvale, NJ: Medical Economics, 1998.

24. Schotte A, Janssen PFM, Gommeren W, et al. Risperidone compared with new and reference antipsychotic drugs: in vitro and in vivo receptor binding. Psychopharmacology 1996; 124:57–73.

25. Borison RL. Clinical efficacy of serotonin-dopamine antagonists relative to classic neuroleptics. J Clin Psychopharmacol 1995; 15:24S–29S.
26. Casey DE. Side effect profiles of new antipsychotic agents. J Clin Psychiatry 1996; 57(suppl 11):40S–45S.
27. Prescribing information. Risperdal (risperidone). Titusville, NJ: Janssen Pharmaceuticals, 1996.
28. Hansen TE, Casey DE, Hoffman WF. Neuroleptic intolerance. Schizophr Bull 1997; 23:567–582.
29. Arvanitis LA, Miller BG. ICI 204, 636, an atypical antipsychotic: results from a multiple fixed-dose, placebo-controlled trial (abstr). Psychopharmacol Bull 1996; 32(3):391.
30. Hong WW, Arvanitis LA, Miller BG, et al. The atypical profile of ICI 204, 636 is supported by its lack of induction of extrapyramidal symptoms (abstr). Psychopharmacol Bull 1996; 32(3):458.
31. Arvanitis LA, Miller BG, and the Seroquel Trial 13 Study Group. Multiple fixed doses of "Seroquel" (quetiapine) in patients with acute exacerbation of schizophrenia: a comparison with haloperidol and placebo. Biol Psychiatry 1997; 42:233–246.
32. Prescribing information. Seroquel (quetiapine). Wilmington, DE: Zeneca Pharmaceuticals, 1998.
33. Leonard HL. New developments in the treatment of obsessive-compulsive disorder. J Clin Psychiatry 1997; 58(suppl 14):39–45.
34. Rasmussen SA, Eisen JL. Treatment strategies for chronic and refractory obsessive-compulsive disorder. J Clin Psychiatry 1997; 58(suppl 13):9–13.
35. Watson CP, Evans RJ, Reed K, et al. Amitriptyline versus placebo in postherpetic neuralgia. Neurology 1982; 32:671–673.
36. Max MB, Schafer SC, Culnane M, et al. Amitriptyline, but not lorazepam, relieves postherpetic neuralgia. Neurology 1988; 38:1427–1432.
37. Watson CPN, Chipman M, Reed K, et al. Amitriptyline versus maprotiline in postherpetic neuralgia: a randomized, double-blind crossover trial. Pain 1992; 48:29–36.
38. Feinmann C, Harris M, Cawley R. Psychogenic facial pain: presentation and treatment. Br Med J 1984; 288:436–438.
39. Urban BJ, France FD, Maltbie AA, et al. Long-term use of narcotic/antidepressant medication in the management of phantom limb pain. Pain 1986; 24:191–196.
40. Eberhard G, von Knorring L, Nilsson HL, et al. A double-blind randomized study of clomipramine versus maprotiline in patients with idiopathic pain syndromes. Neuropsychobiology 1988; 19:25–34.
41. Bernstein JE, Whitney DH, Soltani K. Inhibition of histamine-induced pruritus by topical tricyclic antidepressants. J Am Acad Dermatol 1981; 5:582–585.
42. Savin JA, Paterson WD, Adam K, et al. Effects of trimeprazine and trimipramine on nocturnal scratching in patients with atopic eczema. Arch Dermatol 1979; 115:313–315.

43. Figueiredo A, Ribeiro CA, Goncalo M, et al. Mechanism of action of doxepin in the treatment of chronic urticaria. Fundam Clin Pharmacol 1990; 4(2):147–158.

44. Lawlor F, Greaves MW. The development of recent strategies in the treatment of urticaria as a result of clinically oriented research. Zeitschr Hautkrankh 1990; 65(1):17–27.

45. Kishore-Kumar R, Max MB, Schafer SC, et al. Desipramine relieves postherpetic neuralgia. Clin Pharmacol Ther 1990; 47:305–312.

46. Boyer WI. Potential indications for the selective serotonin reuptake inhibitors. Int J Clin Psychopharmacol 1992; 6(suppl 5):5–12.

47. Bernstein JE, Whitney DH, Soltani K. Inhibition of histamine-induced pruritus by topical tricyclic antidepressants. J Am Acad Dermatol 1981; 5:582–585.

48. Wolverton SE. Comprehensive Dermatologic Drug Therapy. Philadelphia: WB Saunders 2001:402–425.

Index

About the Editors

JOHN Y. M. KOO is Professor and Vice Chairman, Department of Dermatology and Director of the Psoriasis Treatment Center and Phototherapy Unit, University of California, San Francisco. He is Board Certified in Psychiatry and Dermatology. The author or coauthor of more than 200 professional publications, he serves on the editorial board of the *Journal of the American Academy of Dermatology* and *Dermatology and Psychosomatics* and is coeditor of the journal *Psoriasis Forum*. Dr. Koo is a member of the American Psychiatric Association and the American Academy of Dermatology and an advisory board member for the National Psoriasis Foundation, as well as first and founding chairman for the American Academy of Dermatology task force on psychodermatology. A founding member of the Association for Psychocutaneous Disorders of North America, Dr. Koo graduated as the Harvard National Scholar from Harvard University, Cambridge, Massachusetts.

CHAI-SUE LEE serves at Henry Ford Hospital, Detroit, Michigan, and has published several articles and chapters on psychodermatology with Dr. Koo. Dr. Lee received the M.D. degree from the University of California, San Francisco, and completed a fellowship at the Psoriasis and Skin Treatment Center, University of California, San Francisco.